Contents

Preface / vii
Acknowledgments / ix

1. An Introduction to Health Communication 1

Definitions of Communication / 1
Basic Assumptions about Human Communication / 4
Selected Models of Communication / 8
Selected Health-Related Models / 11
A Model of Health Communication / 17
Summary / 20

2. Communication Variables in Health Care / 23

Empathy / 23
Control / 30
Trust / 41
Self-Disclosure / 49
Confirmation / 60
Summary / 71

3. Communication in Health Care Relationships 79

Professional–Patient Relationships / 79
Professional–Professional Relationships / 93
Professional–Family Relationships / 103
Patient–Family Relationships / 111
Summary / 120

4. Nonverbal Communication in Health Care Settings..................... 127

The Importance of Nonverbal Communication in Health Care / 127
The Nature of Nonverbal Communication / 129
Dimensions of Nonverbal Communication / 135
Summary / 157

5. Interviewing in the Health Care Context 163

Interviewing Defined / 163
Types of Interviews in Health Care Settings / 165
Phases in the Interview Process / 170
Communication Techniques in Interviews / 180
Summary / 192

6. Small Group Communication in Health Care 195

Definition of Small Group Communication / 196
Types of Health Care Groups / 196
Components of Small Groups / 198
Phases of Small Groups / 215
Summary / 222

7. Conflict and Communication in Health Care Settings 225

Conflict Defined / 226
Kinds of Conflict / 228
Theoretical Approaches to Conflict / 235
Styles of Approaching Conflict / 243
Communication Approaches for Conflict Resolution / 249
Summary / 255

8. Ethics and Health Communication................................... 259

Dimensions of Biomedical Ethics / 259
Informed Consent: A Communication Issue / 266
Honesty and Truth Telling: A Communication Responsibility / 271
Ethics Committees: The Process of Ethical Decision Making / 274
Summary / 280

9. Intercultural Communication and Health Care......................... 285

Intercultural Communication Defined / 286
Related Concepts / 286
Two Major Characteristics of Culture / 289
Elements in Intercultural Communication / 293
Ways to Promote Effective Intercultural Communication / 300
Summary / 306

Author Index / 311
Subject Index / 316

Preface

Since the publication of the first and second editions of this book, a great deal has changed in health care. In the mid-1980s when the book first came out, there was much talk in health care about diagnostic related groups (DRGs) and efforts to contain health care costs. By the early 1990s, DRGs were accepted as standard and talk shifted to finding other ways to put the brakes on spiraling costs. After a failed effort by the government to package health care delivery in a new way, talk shifted to the role of managed care and its advantages and disadvantages.

Although change in health care has been dramatic, one thing has remained constant: effective communication is central to every aspect of the health care delivery process. We have written this book to explain the communication process that occurs in health care settings and to give health professionals theory-based strategies they can use to improve communication with patients, families, and with other health care professionals.

The approach we have taken to describe communication is a systems perspective, emphasizing that communication is a transactional process that significantly affects health care outcomes. Furthermore, we provide a dual perspective on health communication since one author's work is in the communication field and the other author's work is in the field of nursing.

Although the format and structure of this edition is consistent with the earlier editions, the third edition presents a new and substantially expanded discussion of communication issues in health care. The changes are largely the result of changes in the field as well as changes suggested by colleagues, students, and reviewers.

Major changes in this edition include a new chapter on "Intercultural Communication and Health Care," which provides discussions of ethnocentrism, prejudice, individualism–collectivism, and contexts. In addition, we discuss how culture affects perception of health care problems and how it influences verbal and nonverbal communication. The chapter provides specific strategies for effective intercultural communication in health care.

The third edition also includes: over 100 new citations with the latest research-based information on communication issues in health care settings;

many new examples and case studies, particularly related to acquired immunodeficiency syndrome (AIDs) and community-based health care; and
new figures and tables to clarify and summarize material in the text.

In updating the various chapters, we have added the following:

(1) an expanded discussion of the health belief model as it applies to
    clinical practice issues;
(2) new material to clarify the concepts of empathy, control, trust, self-
    disclosure, and confirmation;
(3) an expanded discussion of patients' preferences for control and in-
    volvement in their care with health professionals;
(4) a new section on how providers and patients come to find shared
    meanings in their interactions with each other;
(5) a new section on ways to foster better communication between
    providers in acute care and community-based settings;
(6) an expanded and clarified discussion of the nature of conflict and
    how it is defined; and
(7) new information on the role of core values in communication re-
    lated to informed consent.

Overall, we believe that this edition will provide readers with a comprehensive understanding of the communication that occurs in our complex, ever-changing health care arena as it readies itself for the 21st century.

Acknowledgments

We would like to express our appreciation to many individuals who played a role in the development of the third edition. First, we would like to thank the editors and staff at Appleton & Lange for their professional guidance and support on this project. Lauren Keller, Eileen Pendagast, and Elisabeth Church facilitated getting the third edition into production. We are especially grateful to Joan Kmenta, who has given us feedback and editorial assistance on all three editions.

For comprehensive reviews of the manuscript, we would like to thank Jan Taylor Fox, University of Texas at Austin; Duane Pennebaker, University of Washington–Bothel; and Wendy Skiba-King, Rutgers University–New Brunswick. Critiques by these reviewers helped to focus our thinking as we developed the third edition.

A special acknowledgment goes to Terry Hammink, St. Paul-Ramsey Medical Center, Minneapolis, for his insights and suggestions in the development of the new chapter on intercultural communication.

For their continued encouragement and interest in this project, we would also like to thank our colleagues at Wayne State University and Western Michigan University.

Peter G. Northouse
Laurel L. Northouse
Ann Arbor, Michigan

An Introduction to 1
Health Communication

This is a book about communication between people in health care organizations. It is an attempt to answer such questions as, How can better communication be created in health care settings? Is it possible to eliminate the problems that lead to communication breakdowns? What changes are needed to make interpersonal communication more effective in professional–client and professional–professional relationships? To address these questions and the issues related to them, we will present selected concepts and theories of human communication and apply them to the communication that occurs in health care settings.

Communication is a complex and multifaceted process. Although the word *communication* is often used in a general way to describe a variety of events, it is actually a term that refers to an identifiable process that has specific characteristics. Explaining the process of communication and how communication functions among individuals in health care organizations is the focus of this book.

In this chapter, we define different kinds of communication and then describe basic assumptions about human communication. In addition, we present several models that have been developed to explain communication and health-related processes. These models provide the background for the model of health communication that appears in the final section of this chapter.

▶ DEFINITIONS OF COMMUNICATION

In some ways, the word *communication* is similar to universal words such as *freedom*, *love*, or *democracy*. Although each of us intuitively knows what he or she means by such words, they can have different meanings for different people. Because communication has multiple meanings, it is important to identify a specific meaning and also to distinguish among different kinds of communication. Proceeding from general to specific, we now turn to definitions of communication, human communication, and health communication.

Communication

Since the late 1940s, many definitions have been used by researchers to capture the precise meaning of the phenomenon called communication. Common to many of these definitions is the idea that communication involves a transfer of information between a source and a receiver. In addition, many definitions suggest that communication requires that meanings be shared between the source and the receiver based on a common set of rules. For example, a social worker and a nurse who collaborate to assure the quality of life for a person with end-stage kidney disease need to have a similar understanding of the meaning of quality of life. They also need to use a language system, or set of rules, that is common to both of them. Incorporating these definitions, we will be using the following definition of communication in this text: *Communication is the process of sharing information using a set of common rules.*

In later chapters, we will discuss how various factors influence the communication process as we define it here. For example, situational pressures can interfere with the transfer of information; differences between the client's perspective and the professional's perspective can get in the way of shared meanings; and certain inappropriate responses can change the rules of the communication process.

Human Communication

Human communication is a special case, or subset, of communication (Fig. 1–1). It refers to the interactions between people. Human communication differs from some forms of communication, such as animal communication, because it involves the use of symbols and language. The ability to use symbols or other representational language is unique to the communication behavior of human beings. The use of symbolic language also accounts for much of the complexity in human interaction.

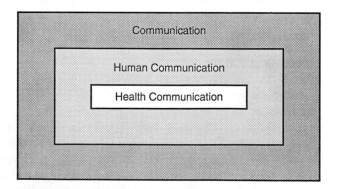

Figure 1–1. Relationship among three kinds of communication.

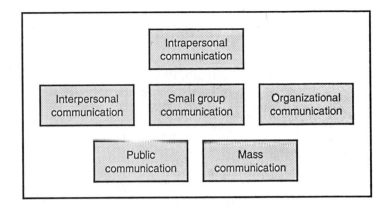

Figure 1–2. Basic human communication contexts.

Human communication has to do with how individuals interact with each other through the use of symbolic behavior—through language. The process is transactional and affective in nature. In other words, it is ongoing, not static, and it involves human feelings and attitudes as well as information.

Before proceeding to define health communication, we would like to identify several contexts (situations) in which communication typically occurs (Fig. 1–2). These categories are presented to give you a frame of reference for the areas into which human communication is usually subdivided. Although we will address issues related to all the contexts represented in Figure 1–2, our discussions will focus primarily on the interpersonal and small group contexts of communication.

Health Communication

Health communication is narrower in scope than human communication (see Fig. 1–1). Health communication is a subset of human communication that is concerned with how individuals deal with health-related issues. It refers to "any type of human communication whose content is concerned with health" (Rogers, 1996, p. 15). In health communication, the focus is on specific health-related transactions and factors that influence these transactions (Pettegrew, 1982). Transactions can be verbal or nonverbal, oral or written, personal or impersonal, and issue oriented or relationship oriented, to name a few of their characteristics. In general, health communication is concerned with the application of communication concepts and theories to transactions that occur among individuals on health-related issues.

Health communication occurs in all of the contexts illustrated in Figure 1–2. At the level of mass communication, health communication refers to areas such as national and world health programs, health promotion campaigns, and public health planning. Finnegan and Viswanath (1990) suggest that health communication at this level "is the dissemination and interpretation of health-related messages" (p. 4). It is closely aligned with social marketing and it is grounded in the larger theory of diffusion of innovations (Clift & Freimuth, 1995).

In the area of public communication, health communication refers to presentations, speeches, and public addresses made by individuals on health-related topics. For example, when the Surgeon General gives a speech on the detrimental effects of smoking he or she is engaged in public communication.

In organizational contexts, health communication may be involved with areas such as hospital administration, staff relations, and organizational communication climates. Within small group contexts, health communication refers to areas such as treatment planning meetings, staff reports, and quality circles. Health communication in interpersonal contexts includes those variables in the human communication process that directly affect professional–professional and professional–client interaction. Finally, health communication in the intrapersonal context would refer to our inner thoughts, beliefs, and feelings, and our "self-talk" about issues that influence our health-directed behaviors. Communication in these contexts has a common health-related focus; however, the specific aims of the communication as well as the number of people involved in the process may vary considerably.

The field of health communication, since its inception 25 years ago as a specialty in communication study, has accomplished a great deal and continues to exhibit rapid growth (Rogers, 1996). The discipline of health communication parallels several other newer fields of study including health psychology, medical sociology, biomedical communication, behavioral medicine, behavioral health, and medical communications. These newer fields are building on the groundwork laid by professional disciplines such as nursing, social work, psychology, sociology, medicine, and public health. Health communication overlaps with these other fields, but maintains a focus primarily on communication issues in health care settings. In an extended discussion of the status and scope of the field of health communication, Ratzan, Payne, and Bishop (1996) suggest that the field is continuing to evolve, and that pragmatic steps need to be taken to continue to define and refine it.

► BASIC ASSUMPTIONS ABOUT HUMAN COMMUNICATION

In studying how people communicate with each other, researchers have found that human communication has several identifiable properties. These properties represent the fundamental assumptions or axioms upon which theories of human communication are built.

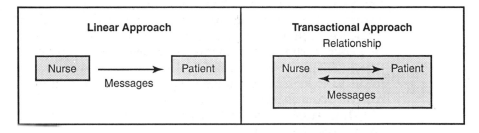

Figure 1–3. Comparison of linear versus transactional approaches.

Human Communication Is a Process

To many persons, the word *communication* triggers an image of an individual talking to someone else on the telephone. This image of one person sending a message along a channel to another person is based on a linear approach to communication (Fig. 1–3), which might be compared to a "hypodermic needle" model of human communication. In this approach, person A instills his or her message into person B. Communication occurs in one direction, with one person directly influencing a second person through the use of specific messages. However, the linear approach has been criticized for being too restrictive. Human communication is more than a one-way event.

In fact, human communication is an ongoing, continuous, dynamic, and ever-changing process. "It does not have a beginning, an end, a fixed sequence of events. It is not static, at rest. It is moving" (Berlo, 1960, p. 24). This implies that communication between person A and person B should be viewed as continuous and involving many variables, all of which continually change during a communication event. Stated another way, communication as a process means that when person A communicates with person B, the physical, emotional, and social states of A and B change during their communication; these changes in turn induce further changes in their interaction.

In health care, the assumption that communication is a process directs our attention to professional–professional and professional–client communication as ongoing dynamic processes rather than one-way, fixed sequences of events. The process assumption directs us not only to look at factors that affect the client but also to analyze factors that affect the nurse, social worker, or physical therapist, and to examine how the ongoing interchange between all of these people will vary depending on the nature of the situation.

Human Communication Is Transactional

A second assumption about human communication, which is an extension of the first assumption, is that human communication is transactional (see

Fig. 1–3). By this we mean that both individuals in an interaction affect and are affected by each other. Transactional communication involves reciprocal influence. Each individual is both a source and a receiver at the same time. As person A constructs a message for person B, A is receiving cues from B that influence how A formulates the message. A transactional approach forces us to look at the simultaneous interplay between the sender and the receiver of a message.

If we accept a transactional perspective, we shift our focus away from an analysis of the ways in which one person affects another; instead we focus on the relationships between individuals that are developed and maintained through their mutual influence on one another. To study communication as a transactional process involves emphasizing the communication behavior of individuals *in relationships*. The transactional viewpoint focuses on the combined properties of the participants in an interaction, not on their individual characteristics (Millar & Rogers, 1976, p. 90). When describing human communication from a transactional perspective, it is important that we think of individuals together in a relationship rather than separately.

To illustrate this point, consider what occurs in a health care situation when a health professional is having a conversation with a client. Each individual perceives the other in the context of what occurs in the interaction. If the nurse, for example, chooses to be dominant with a client, it may be because the nurse desires to be dominant, or it may be because the nurse picks up cues from the client that seem to indicate the client would prefer to be submissive. In other words, the nature of the interaction could be influenced by the desires of the nurse or client, by their perceptions of the other person's desires, or by both of these factors working together simultaneously.

We are saying that in relationships, communication outcomes are mutually determined. Human communication in relationships is a *two-person process*. Health professionals do not make clients submissive and they do not make themselves dominant. Clients and health professionals engage in human interaction, and by doing so they establish how they are related and how they want to communicate.

Human Communication Is Multidimensional

A third assumption is that human communication is multidimensional. When human communication takes place, it occurs on two levels. One level can be characterized as the *content dimension* and the other as the *relationship dimension* (Watzlawick, Beavin, & Jackson, 1967, p. 54). In human communication, these two dimensions are inextricably bound together. The content dimension of communication refers to the words, language, and information in a message; the relationship dimension refers to the aspect of a message that defines how participants in an interaction are connected to each other.

To illustrate the two dimensions, consider the following hypothetical statement made by a nurse to a patient: "Please take this medication." The content dimension of this message refers to taking medication. The relationship dimension of this message refers to how the nurse and the patient are affiliated—to the nurse's authority in relation to the patient, the nurse's attitude toward the patient, the patient's attitude toward the nurse, and their feelings about one another. It is the relationship dimension that implicitly suggests how the content dimension should be interpreted, since the content alone can be interpreted in many ways. The exact meaning of the message emerges for the nurse and patient as a result of their interaction. If a caring relationship exists between the nurse and the patient, then the content "please take this medication" will probably be interpreted by the patient as helpful suggestion from a nurse who is concerned about the patient's well-being. However, if the relationship between the nurse and the patient is distant or strained, the patient may interpret the content of the message as a rigid directive, delivered by a nurse who enjoys giving orders. These two interpretations illustrate how the meanings of messages are not in words alone but in individuals' interpretations of the messages in light of their relationships.

The content and relationship dimensions of messages are illustrated further in the following example of professional–professional communication. A physician says to a nurse, "Why didn't Mr. Jones get the sleeping pill I prescribed last night?" The content dimension of the physician's question could be interpreted in different ways depending on the nature of the nurse–physician relationship. If the physician and nurse have an effective, collegial relationship, the nurse could interpret the content of the question as a request for factual information about the patient. If, however, a competitive relationship marked by repeated power struggles exists between the physician and the nurse, then the content of the same question could be interpreted by the nurse as an attempt by the physician to challenge the nurse's judgment or as an attempt to exert control over the nurse. Although the content dimension of a message is often easier to identify than the relationship dimension, it is often the relationship dimension that is critical to the ultimate interpretation of the message.

Watzlawick, Beavin, and Jackson (1967) believe that in healthy relationships, the relationship dimension of communication recedes into the background and the content dimension of messages becomes more important to the participants. In troubled relationships, the opposite occurs: there is a continuous struggle on the relationship dimension, while the content dimension recedes into the background (p. 52).

It is important that health professionals recognize that the relationships they develop with clients and with other health professionals significantly influence the effectiveness of their interpersonal communication. The *meaning* in health transactions emerges from the interplay between the content and relationship dimensions of messages. Developing relationships is important because it influences how content will be interpreted. Given the multidimensional assumption of human communication, effective communication is more likely to be achieved when health professionals are equally attentive to both the content and the relationship dimensions of messages.

► SELECTED MODELS OF COMMUNICATION

Researchers have constructed many models in attempts to reduce the complexity of the human communication process. These models, which are primarily word–picture diagrams, try to impose some pattern on a process that is intricate and complex.

However, models are never perfect. Because of their very nature, models cannot include *all* the elements of the process they are supposed to represent. Selecting certain attributes to be a part of a model unavoidably results in excluding other attributes. In addition, because models are attempts to represent complex events in a simplified way, there is a tendency for models to oversimplify the process or the event being described.

Recognizing the advantages and the limitations of models, we have chosen to present and discuss three models: (1) the Shannon–Weaver model, (2) the SMCR model, and (3) the Leary model.

Shannon–Weaver Model

One of the first models of communication, and in many ways one of the most influential, was a linear model developed by Shannon and Weaver in 1949. In the Shannon–Weaver model (Fig. 1–4), communication is represented as a system in which a *source* selects information that is formulated (encoded) into a message. This message is then *transmitted* by a signal through a *channel* to a *receiver*. The receiver interprets (decodes) the message and sends it to some *destination*. A unique feature in this model is the concept of *noise*. Noise refers to those factors that influence or disturb messages while they are being transferred along the channel from the source to the destination. In a human communication model, noise could refer to any disturbance, such as audible sound, perceptual distortions, or psychological misinterpretations, that changes the meaning of a message as it is sent from one person to another.

One strength of this early model is the uniform manner in which it attempts to describe the pathway of a communication message from source to receiver. A limitation of this model, however, is that it does not show the transactional relationship between the source and the receiver. Because the model is linear, it implies that communication is a one-way event. As later communication theorists have noted, and as we discussed earlier in this chapter, communication in human relationships is an interactional process.

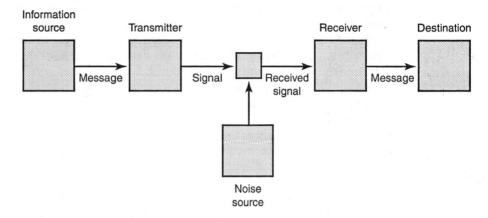

Figure 1–4. Shannon–Weaver communication model. *(Reprinted with permission from Shannon, C. E., & Weaver, W. [1949]. The mathematical theory of communication (p. 98). Champaign, IL: University of Illinois Press.)*

SMCR Model

In his book *The Process of Communication* (1960), Berlo presented what is now a classic model of communication—one that emphasizes, as the title of the book suggests, that communication is a process. Berlo's model is called the SMCR model, standing for the first letter in the words source, message, channel, and receiver (Fig. 1–5). Berlo views these four components as being intertwined.

The SMCR model represents a communication process that occurs as a *source* formulates messages based on his or her communication skills, attitudes, knowledge, and sociocultural system. These *messages,* which have unique elements, structure, content, treatment, and codes, are transmitted along *channels,* which can include seeing, hearing, touching, smelling, and tasting. A *receiver* interprets messages based on her or his own communication skills, attitudes, knowledge, and sociocultural system.

The strength of this model is the manner in which it represents the complexity of communication and treats communication as a process rather

Source	Message	Channel	Receiver
Communication skills	Elements	Seeing	Communication skills
Attitudes	Structure	Hearing	Attitudes
Knowledge	Content	Touching	Knowledge
Social system	Treatment	Smelling	Social system
Culture	Code	Tasting	Culture

Figure 1–5. SMCR model. *(Adapted from The process of communication: An introduction to theory and practice (p. 72) by David K. Berlo, copyright © 1960 by Holt, Rinehart and Winston, Inc. and renewed 1988 by David K. Berlo.) Reproduced by permission of the publisher.*

than a static event. The model is limited by omitting the feedback component of communication, and by not vividly illustrating the process function. If this model were applied to health care settings, it would enable us to see the many factors that influence a client's communication, such as his or her attitudes and sociocultural background Similarly, this model helps to explain how experience and education affect professional-to-professional communication (e.g., the communication between a new baccalaureate nurse and an experienced practical nurse) but is less helpful in highlighting how feedback influences ongoing professional–professional dialogue.

Leary Model

The reflexive model of human interaction developed by Leary is quite different from the previous models we have discussed. Leary's model, which first appeared in the mid-1950s, has received considerable attention in recent years. It is truly a transactional and multidimensional model, stressing relationships and the interactional aspects of interpersonal communication. It states, in effect, that human communication is a two-person process in which both individuals influence and are influenced by each other.

Leary developed this model as a result of his experience as a therapist with patients in psychotherapy. He observed that his own behavior was different in his sessions with different patients—that is, he found that patients influenced the way he behaved toward them. Leary concluded that individuals actually train others to respond to them in particular ways—ways that are pleasing for the individual's own preferred interpersonal behavior. For example, if we like to be submissive, we condition others to behave in dominant ways toward us; conversely, if we like to be dominant, we condition others to behave submissively.

Leary's model is designed to classify certain aspects of interpersonal behavior used in communication. Figure 1–6 gives a simplified version of the Leary model. (See Leary's article "The Theory and Measurement Methodology of Interpersonal Communication" [1955] for an extended description of the theory.)

From the perspective of the Leary model, every communication message can be viewed as occurring along two dimensions: dominance–submission and hate–love. Two rules govern how these dimensions function in human interaction. *Rule 1:* Dominant or submissive communicative behavior usually stimulates the *opposite* behavior in others. Stated in another way, acting autocratically (dominantly) usually stimulates others to act submissively, and acting powerlessly usually stimulates others to act dominantly. *Rule 2:* Hateful or loving behavior usually stimulates the *same* behavior from others. This means that being kind usually encourages kindness from others, while being hostile usually stimulates aggressiveness from others. Leary states that these rules operate reflexively—our responses toward each other are involuntary and immediate. Our own communication behaviors

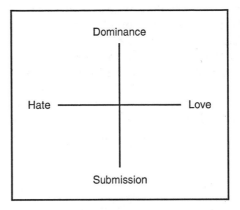

Figure 1–6. Leary's reflexive model. *(Adapted from Leary, T. [1955]. The theory and measurement methodology of interpersonal communication.* Psychiatry, 18, *152. Copyright © 1955 by the William Alanson White Psychiatric Foundation.) Used by permission.*

automatically stimulate dominant or submissive and love or hate reactions in others.

The Leary model can be directly applied to communication in health care settings. For many years, patients in acute care settings often assumed or were placed in the submissive role, while health professionals often assumed a dominant role. Current trends in consumerism are causing a shift in the balance of power between professionals and patients. As patients have become more assertive in health care matters, providers have had to relinquish some of their control and authority. The strength of the Leary model is the transactional way in which he describes these power and affiliation issues in human interactions. If we are really going to understand our communication with others, we need to look at the qualities that both persons bring to the interaction.

▶ SELECTED HEALTH-RELATED MODELS

Up to this point we have been primarily concerned with models of human communication. However, we believe that it is important to look specifically at health-related fields and see how these fields have portrayed communication in their models. Obviously, the focus of these models will not be solely on the common elements of communication, but on the broader goal of maximizing health outcomes.

For our discussion we have selected three models developed by researchers to explain human behavior as it pertains to health and illness. The three are (1) the therapeutic model, (2) the health belief model, and (3) the King interaction model. We recognize that there are many other health-related models that could have been selected. For example, in nursing alone, theories developed by Orem, Rogers, and Roy have all added to our understanding of human behavior in health care situations. The three models we selected were chosen because each provides a different focus or emphasis in health care and each has a direct relationship to human communication.

Therapeutic Model

The therapeutic model emphasizes the important role that *relationships* play in assisting clients and patients to adjust to their circumstances and to move in the direction of health and away from illness. When used by health professionals, *therapeutic communication* can be defined as a skill that helps people cope with stress, confront psychological obstacles, and learn how to relate effectively to others. Although therapeutic communication appears to be a term that describes communication in traditional psychotherapeutic settings, it also describes communication between health professionals and clients in other health care contexts.

Although many models have been developed to describe the various kinds of psychotherapeutic theories, not all of these therapeutic models are pertinent to health-related interaction. One model that is pertinent and has proved useful in explaining the interactions that occur in health care settings is the Rogerian model. Carl Rogers (1951) believes that if a therapist communicates honest, caring understanding to the client, it will help the client adjust in a healthy way to his or her circumstances. This Rogerian model is labeled *client centered* because the focus of the interaction is on the client. In this model, the helper is encouraged to communicate with empathy, positive regard, and congruence. These three behaviors, together, comprise the necessary conditions to help the client successfully. We have depicted these components in Figure 1–7.

For Rogers, *empathy* is the process of communicating to clients the feeling of being understood; it is standing in the shoes of the client. *Positive regard* is the process of communicating support to the client in a caring and nonjudgmental way. It is communication that is genuine, nonthreatening, and unconditional. Communicating *congruence* involves the honest expres-

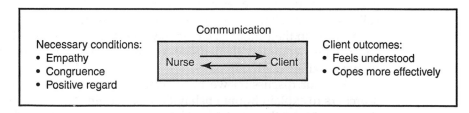

Figure 1–7. A therapeutic model.

sion of the helper's own thoughts and feelings. Congruence requires that the helping professional will respond honestly to the client and attempt to be real in his or her relationship with the client.

In health care settings, the therapeutic model can be directly applied to professional–client communication. The Rogerian model describes how health professionals should communicate if they choose to be client centered. According to the Rogerian model, when health professionals communicate empathy, positive regard, and congruence, clients feel understood and are better able to cope with their illnesses.

Health Belief Model

The health belief model, formulated by Rosenstock and his colleagues (1966, 1974), is broader, more complex, and has a very different focus than the therapeutic model. The frequent use of this model in health care settings and its heavy emphasis on the client's perceptions are two reasons that it is being examined here. This model was designed to explain the nature of individuals' preventive health actions. Since the model appeared in the late 1950s, it has been the focus of a great deal of research; it has come to be recognized as one of the most influential social–psychological theories formulated to explain how healthy individuals seek to avoid illness.

As Figure 1–8 illustrates, the health belief model consists of three major elements: (1) an individual's perception of susceptibility to and severity of the disease, (2) an individual's perception of the benefits and barriers to taking a preventive health action to prevent disease, and (3) the cues available to an individual that would stimulate him or her to engage in preventive health activity (Becker & Maiman, 1975). At the top of the diagram a fourth element of the model appears, containing demographic and social-psychological variables. These variables, called modifying factors, indirectly influence individuals' perceptions and beliefs. In essence, the health belief model is designed to predict the likelihood of an individual's adopting a particular health behavior as a function of perceived threat and perceived benefit.

The following example may help clarify how the health belief model is used in health communication research. Hypothesize for a moment that we are interested in studying the safe sex habits of college students. We are particularly interested in knowing whether college students use condoms during sexual intercourse; a recommended preventive health action.

The model in Figure 1–8 gives us a conceptual framework for addressing this question. The likelihood that college students will engage in this behavior is influenced by the degree to which they see acquired immunodeficiency syndrome (AIDS) as a threat. AIDS is seen as threatening to students when they perceive themselves to be susceptible to it and when they see it as life threatening. Whether students see AIDS as a threat is also influenced by their age, sex, and ethnicity, as well as by social and psychological vari-

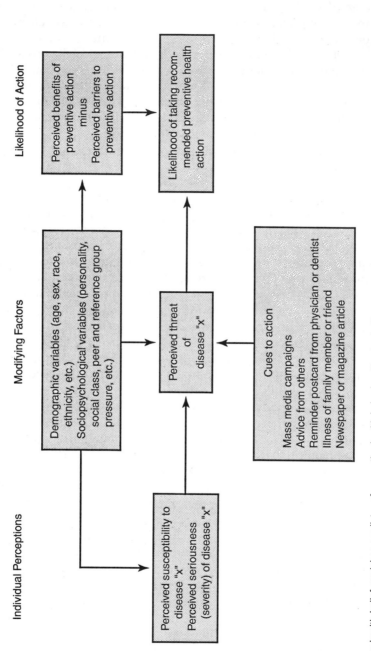

Figure 1–8. The health belief model as predictor of preventive health behavior. *(Reprinted with permission from Becker, M. H., & Maiman, L. A. [1975]. Sociobehavioral determinants of compliance with health and medical care recommendations. Medical Care, 13 (1), 12.)*

ables. Students are also influenced by other factors such as mass media campaigns, magazine articles, or knowing someone with AIDS. The likelihood of students engaging in safe sex is further influenced by whether they see the benefits for using condoms as greater than the barriers. In this example, you can see how the health belief model provides a structured way to analyze different factors that contribute to the likelihood of individuals engaging in selected preventive health behaviors.

Although many aspects of the health belief model involve communication, two aspects are distinctively communication centered. First, the Cues to Action element of the model includes mass media campaigns, advice from others, newspaper articles, and similar message-related variables, all of which are types of communication. Communication is essential if individuals are to receive cues that have potential for motivating them to take health action. For example, newspaper articles on the importance of fastening seat belts may persuade people to buckle up while driving their cars. In the same way, messages on the radio about the links between cancer and cigarette smoking may influence persons to quit smoking. A second element of the model that is particularly relevant to health communication pertains to Modifying Factors, which include social–psychological variables. Many of these variables are important elements in the communication process. Becker and Maiman (1975) refer to a series of studies showing that compliance behavior in patients is associated with the communication in health professional–client relationships. For example, patients' failure to comply has been found to be related to communication patterns in which the health professional is described as formal, rejecting, or controlling; the professional strongly disagrees with the patient; the professional interviews the patient at length without allowing for feedback, or engages in nonreciprocal interaction. Clearly, communication has an impact on the health behavior of clients.

The health belief model has certain merits and also certain limitations. On the positive side, the model illustrates the importance of broader modes of communication, such as the impact of mass media, on health behavior. The health belief model also focuses on the perceptions and beliefs of clients that can be altered to enhance certain health behaviors. On the negative side, the health belief model has been criticized for placing too much emphasis on abstract, conceptual beliefs. Overall, this model highlights the clients' perceptions of preventive health care measures rather than the transactional nature of the client–professional interaction in promoting health care.

King Interaction Model

King's work (1971, 1981) on the development of a conceptual framework for nursing provides the basis for a third health-related model, which can be described as an interaction model. King's model places strong emphasis on the communication process between nurses and clients and, therefore, was selected as an important model for understanding health communication. King uses a systems perspective to describe how health professionals (nurses) assist clients to maintain health. She provides a conceptual framework that discusses the interrelationships among personal, interpersonal, and social systems. Although King describes the nature of each of these three systems, she gives particular emphasis to interpersonal systems in health care.

The paradigm King employs to discuss the role of interpersonal systems in health care is represented in Figure 1–9. Essentially the model suggests that in nurse–patient interactions both the nurse and the patient simultaneously make *judgments* about their circumstances and about each other, based on their *perceptions* of the situation. Judgments, in turn, lead to verbal or nonverbal *actions* that stimulate reactions in the nurse and the patient. At this point, new perceptions are established and the process repeats itself. *Interaction* is the dynamic process that includes the reciprocal interplay between the nurse's and the clients' perceptions, judgments, and actions. *Transactions* are the result of the reciprocal relationships established by nurses and clients as they participate together in determining mutual health-related goals.

King's model is particularly valuable for explaining communication between a health professional and client. It represents the nurse–patient interaction process in a manner similar to the models formulated by the communication theorists. This model encompasses the important dimensions of relationship, process, and transaction that have been identified as crucial elements in the communication process. The feedback loop in the model also indicates the importance of shared meaning between the nurse and client. Although King does not show in this diagram how interpersonal relations

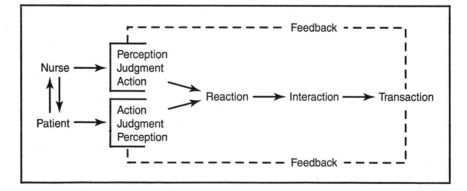

Figure 1–9. An interaction model. An approach to the nurse–client communication process. *(Reprinted with permission from King, I. M. [1971]. Toward a theory of nursing: General concepts of human behavior (p. 92). New York: Wiley.)*

are affected by situational factors, nor how interpersonal relations are related to the patient's health behavior, she does explain these issues in *A Theory For Nursing* (1981).

▶ A MODEL OF HEALTH COMMUNICATION

The communication and health-related models we have described in the previous sections provide the foundation for constructing a model of health communication. The model in Figure 1–10 illustrates health communication as we presently conceptualize it. Health communication refers specifically to transactions between participants in health care about health-related issues. Our primary focus is on the health communication that occurs within various kinds of relationships in health care settings. In contrast to previously described models, this model of health communication takes a broader systems view of communication, and it emphasizes the way in which a series of factors can impact on the interactions in health care settings. The health communication model in Figure 1–10 illustrates the three major factors of the health communication process: relationships, transactions, and contexts. Included within each major factor are several subelements that describe the composition of each factor more fully.

Relationships

From a systems perspective, the health communication model illustrates four major types of relationships that exist in health care settings: professional–professional, professional–client, professional–significant other, and client–significant other. As a rule, when an individual is engaged in health communication, he or she is involved in one of these four types of relation-

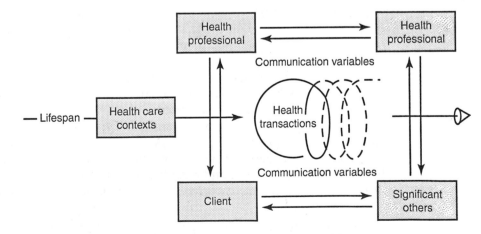

Figure 1–10. Health communication model.

ships. The model also indicates that these interpersonal relationships can influence other types of relationships in the health care setting. For example, how health professionals communicate with each other can affect how health professionals and clients interact. Similarly, how a client reacts with members of his or her social network can influence later interactions between the client and health professionals.

In our model, the term *health professional* is used to identify any individual who has the education, training, and experience to provide health services to others. *Health professional* includes a wide range of individuals— nurses, health administrators, social workers, physicians, health educators, occupational and physical therapists, pharmacists, chaplains, public health personnel, health psychologists, technicians, and other specialists. Each health professional brings unique characteristics, beliefs, values, and perceptions to health care settings, which will affect how he or she interacts with clients and with members of the health care team. For example, the age, sociocultural background, and past experiences of the health professional will affect the way in which he or she responds to clients and coworkers.

Clients are individuals toward whom health services are directed. In acute care settings the client is usually, but not always, referred to as the *patient*. In other health care settings, the individuals who are receiving services are simply referred to as *clients*. In the health communication model, the term *client* is used to designate the individuals who are the focus of the health care services that are being provided. The term encompasses the specific characteristics, values, and beliefs that these individuals bring to the health care setting. Just as the personal characteristics of health professionals influence *their interactions,* the unique characteristics of clients influence the interactions clients have with others.

The social network of the client includes a third set of individuals who are participants in health communication. *Clients' significant others* have been found to be most essential in supporting clients as they seek to maintain health. These social networks include family members (spouses, sisters, brothers, and other relatives), roommates, friends, co-workers, and other individuals connected in a significant way to the person using health services. In short, clients' social networks are composed of all those individuals who are significant in their lives, but who are not health professionals.

Too often in the past health professionals have overlooked the important role played by family members and other significant individuals in enhancing the health of the ill person. We have included the client's significant others in our model of health communication because we believe that these persons are frequent and essential participants in the health communication process. In fact, if current trends continue, significant others will assume an even more central role as patients are discharged sooner and with a greater number of acute care needs into the care of their family members or others.

Transactions

Transactions are a second major element in the health communication model. *Transactions* refer to the health-related interactions that occur between participants in the health communication process. Health transactions involve any interactions between individuals about health-related information. Health transactions include both verbal and nonverbal communication behavior. Both types of communication are equally important, and health transactions are most effective when verbal and nonverbal aspects of messages are compatible with each other.

Health transactions also include both the content and relationship dimensions of messages. Health transactions deal with health-related content—how a client seeks to attain and maintain health over a life span. The relationship dimension of health transactions is established within the various relationships represented by the model and this dimension influences how the content of the messages should be interpreted.

In the center of the health communication model, health transactions are represented by a circle from which an unending spiral emerges. This illustrates the ongoing, transactional nature of health communication. Health communication is not a static event but an interactive process that occurs at various points in time during the course of a person's life. It includes continual feedback, which allows participants to adjust and readjust their communication. Health transactions are constantly moving forward and turning back to make changes and alterations in the message.

At the top and bottom of the health communication model, there are many communication variables that influence the participants and their messages. In Chapter 2, we will discuss selected communication variables that have a significant impact on health communication.

Contexts

A third major element of the health communication process is health care *contexts*—the settings in which health communication takes place and the systemic properties of these settings. Health care contexts actually have a great influence on the communication among health professionals, clients, family members, and others involved in the process.

At one level, health care contexts refer to health care settings, such as hospitals, nursing homes, and outpatient clinics. Health communication may be affected by the specific setting in which it occurs, such as a hospice, a hospital room, a physician's office, a clinic, or a waiting room, to name a few possibilities. For example, an intensive care unit, with its accelerated pace and lack of privacy, will affect patterns of communication in a different way from an ambulatory care unit where private office space is available and the pace may be less hectic. Each particular health care setting affects the dynamics of health transactions that take place within it.

At another level, health care contexts can refer to the number of participants within a particular health care setting. Health communication may take place in a one-to-one situation, in triads, in small groups, and among larger collections of individuals. The number of persons present within a given context also influences interactions in the context.

Together, the components of our health communication model include relationships, transactions, and contexts; they provide a systems perspective on communication in health care. It is our belief that as the complexity of health care continues to increase, health communication can be better understood from this broader systems perspective. This is not to negate the importance of messages, channels, or characteristics of the source and receiver of the message, but rather to propose that these factors be studied while keeping in mind the many contextual factors and relationships that affect the health transaction.

► SUMMARY

For purposes of our discussion, communication is the process of sharing information according to a common set of rules. When information is shared between individuals using a common system of symbols and language, the process is called human communication. Health communication refers to health-related transactions between individuals who are attempting to maintain health and avoid illness.

Three basic assumptions can be made concerning human communication. First, human communication is a process, which means it is ongoing, dynamic, and always changing. Second, human communication is transactional, which means each participant in an interaction is simultaneously affected by every other participant. Third, human communication is multidimensional, which means it has both a content and relationship dimension. Both dimensions (content and relationship) are inextricably bound together in human interaction.

Selected models of communication provide ways of illustrating different aspects of the process. Shannon and Weaver's model depicts communication as a one-way, linear event. Berlo's SMCR model indicates elements that affect the source, message, channel, and receiver in the communication process. Leary's reflexive model illustrates how dominance–submission and hate–love are central in each human communication interaction.

Although they are widely different in form and structure, the selected health-related models we presented are useful in describing issues of communication as they pertain to health. Rogers's therapeutic model sets forth ways of communicating that are effective for health professionals who choose to be client centered. A paradigm that is useful in explaining why individuals do or do not engage in certain health-related behaviors is found in Rosenstock's health belief model. King's interaction model depicts what occurs in nurse–patient interactions and emphasizes the transactional and feedback features of health professional–client communication.

Together, the selected communication and health-related models provide the basis for the health communication model, which has three major elements: relationships, health transactions, and contexts. Considered together, these elements illustrate that health communication is a transactional multidimensional process by which individuals (both health professionals and clients) interact with each other on health-related issues in a mutual effort to maintain the client's health.

▶ REFERENCES

Becker, M. H., & Maiman, L. A. (1975). Sociobehavioral determinants of compliance with health and medical care recommendations. *Medical Care, 13*(1), 10–24.

Berlo, D. K. (1960). *The process of communication: An introduction to theory and practice.* New York: Holt, Rinehart & Winston.

Clift, E., & Freimuth, V. (1995). Health communication: What is it and what can it do for you? *Journal of Health Education, 26*(2), 68–75.

Finnegan, J. L., & Viswanath, K. (1990). Health and communication: Medical and public health influences on the research agenda. In E. B. Ray & L. Donohew (Eds.), *Communication and health: Systems and applications* (pp. 9–26). Hillsdale, NJ: Erlbaum.

King, I. M. (1971). *Toward a theory for nursing: General concepts of human behavior.* New York: Wiley.

King, I. M. (1981). *A theory for nursing: Systems, concepts, process.* New York: Wiley.

Leary, T. (1955). The theory and measurement methodology of interpersonal communication. *Psychiatry, 18,* 147–161.

Millar, F. E., & Rogers, L. E. (1976). A relational approach to interpersonal communication. In G. R. Miller (Ed.), *Explorations in interpersonal communications* (pp. 87–103). Beverly Hills, CA: Sage.

Pettegrew, L. S. (1982). Some boundaries and assumptions in health communication. In L. S. Pettegrew, P. Arntson, D. Bush, & K. Zoppi (Eds.), *Explorations in provider and patient interaction.* Louisville, KY: Humana.

Ratzan, S. C., Payne, J. G., & Bishop, C. (1996). The status and scope of health communication. *Journal of Health Communication, 1*(1), 25–41.

Rogers, C. R. (1951). *Client-centered therapy.* Boston: Houghton Mifflin.

Rogers, E. M. (1996). The field of health communication today: An up-to-date report. *Journal of Health Communication, 1*(1), 15–23.

Rosenstock, I. M. (1966). Why people use health services. *Milbank Memorial Fund Quarterly, 44*(3), 94–124.

Rosenstock, I. M. (1974). Historical origins of the Health Belief Model. *Health Education Monographs, 2*(4), 354–386.

Shannon, C. E., & Weaver, W. (1949). *The mathematical theory of communication.* Champaign, IL: University of Illinois Press.

Watzlawick, P., Beavin, J., & Jackson, D. D. (1967). *Pragmatics of human communication.* New York: Norton.

Communication Variables 2
in Health Care

The communication process includes numerous variables, each of them important to an understanding of the overall process of communication. As illustrated in the health communication model discussed in Chapter 1, these variables affect the health transactions that occur in various health care relationships. Because it is not possible to discuss all of the variables, we have chosen to consider five which we think are central to effective health communication. We are aware that we have selected only a few out of many possible variables, and that our readers might have chosen different variables. However, the variables we discuss can be studied in light of communication research and can be directly applied to health care settings.

We have chosen to examine the following variables; (1) empathy, (2) control, (3) trust, (4) self-disclosure, and (5) confirmation. In our discussion, we will describe each variable, present a conceptual framework for it, and then apply the variable to health care settings. In keeping with our belief that communication is a transactional process, the application section will consider each variable from the client's and the health professional's perspective.

▶ EMPATHY

Of all the variables that comprise health communication, empathy is regarded as one of the most essential and at the same time one of the most complex variables operating in the communication process (Forsyth, 1980; Kalisch, 1973; LaMonica, 1981; Morse et al., 1992; Wheeler, 1988). Empathy is believed to affect communication outcomes in all types of relationships— from our everyday social relationships to intense therapeutic encounters. It is well established that empathy plays an important role in effective, interpersonal communication. Without empathy, the communication between people lacks the essential quality of understanding.

The term *empathy* is credited to Theodor Lipps (1909), who defined *Einfuhlung* as the process of "feeling into." However, much of the recent interest in empathy is a result of Carl Rogers' pioneering work (1951, 1959) on client-centered therapy. In his description of empathy, Rogers defines empathy as a process that involves

---

entering the private perceptual world of the other and becoming thoroughly at home in it. . . . It includes communicating your sensings of his world as you look with fresh and unfrightened eyes at elements of which the individual is fearful. It means frequently checking with him as to the accuracy of your sensings, and being guided by the responses you receive. . . .

To be with another in this way means that for the time being you lay aside the views and values you hold for yourself in order to enter another's world without prejudice. . . . (Rogers, 1975, p. 4)

This extensive definition indicates the complexity of the empathic process.

Other researchers have defined empathy in ways that differ from Rogers; some of the definitions focus on empathy as emotional sensitivity (Mehrabian & Epstein, 1972), accuracy of understanding (Hobart & Fahlberg, 1965), a fantasy process (Stotland et al, 1978), or a personality trait (Hogan, 1969), to name a few. Although different definitions emphasize different aspects of the empathic process, all of the definitions include the element of *understanding*.

It is important to clarify that empathy is *not* sympathy. These two words are frequently used interchangeably although their meanings are very different. Sympathy is the concern, sorrow, or pity shown by an individual for another individual. It is the expression of one's *own* feelings about another person's predicament and the urge to alleviate his or her suffering. Empathy is an attempt to feel *with* another person, to understand the other person's point of view. It involves taking the role of another and attempting to feel the way that other person feels. In empathy, the focus is on the client with the problem, whereas with sympathy, the focus shifts away from the client to the listener. (See Wispe [1986] for an in-depth discussion of this distinction.) In short, empathy is observing the world from another person's point of view.

Conceptual Frameworks of Empathy

To further understand empathy, we will examine how researchers and theoreticians have conceptualized it. What are the major components of empathy and how can its influence be explained? Research suggests two primary ways of explaining empathy: (1) as a unitary trait, and (2) as a multidimensional process (Table 2–1).

Personality theorists view empathy as a unitary trait, as one personality trait among many other traits, such as dogmatism, introversion–extroversion, or aggressiveness, that people possess in varying degrees. Because of their personality makeup, some people may possess a high degree of un-

TABLE 2–1. CONCEPTUALIZATIONS OF EMPATHY

Conceptual Frameworks of Empathy
Unitary personality trait
Multidimensional process
• Cognitive
• Affective
• Communicative

derstanding of other peoples' problems and predicaments, whereas other people may have little ability to empathize with others. According to personality theorists, this difference in empathic ability is due to the amount of the empathy trait that each person possesses.

A second way of looking at empathy is as a multidimensional process. This approach is grounded in the pioneering work of Rogers who contends that empathy is one of the core conditions of successful psychotherapy (1957) and one of the major elements in establishing a helping relationship (1958, 1961). For Rogers, empathy involves cognitive, affective, and communication components. The *cognitive* perceptual process involves observing a client's behavior and processing the obtained information. The *affective* process involves being sensitive to a client's feelings. The *communication* component, which has been of special interest to researchers and clinicians in the helping professions, focuses on the language and responses of the listener. By focusing on the communication dimension of empathy, researchers have been able to design specific strategies and techniques to assist professionals in developing and enhancing their empathic skill. Many of the common therapeutic techniques (reflection, restatement, and paraphrasing) are actually communication skills.

Similar to Rogers, the works of Barrett-Lennard (1981), Gladstein (1983), and Davis (1983) all support a multidimensional view of empathy. Collectively, the research of these scholars lends support to Rogers' position that empathy involves trying to feel what others feel (affective component), trying to adopt their point of view (cognitive component), and communicating this understanding to others (communicative component). To measure empathy as a multidimensional process, Davis (1983) has developed a 28-item self-report instrument called the Interpersonal Reactivity Index.

Several attempts have been made to measure the amount of empathy that nurses demonstrate toward clients. One approach is to ask a panel of experts to judge tape-recorded interactions between nurses and clients and to determine the degree to which the nurse is responding to the client in an empathic manner (Williams, 1979). Another approach is to ask nurses to read several case studies of counseling situations and to choose, from a list of several responses, the response that would be the most empathic

(Forsyth, 1979). Another way of measuring empathy and one of the more widely used approaches is to ask clients to rate the amount of empathy that they perceive from nurses. Most investigators using this approach use the Barrett-Lennard Relationship Inventory, a 16-item questionnaire that asks one person (e.g., client) to rate another person (e.g., the nurse) on such items as "She/He tries to see things through my eyes" and "She/He understands me" (Barrett-Lennard, 1962).

Empathy is indeed complex and may occur at several points within the communication process. Because of this, many qualities—observational skill, communication skill, perceptual skill, emotional sensitivity, and caring, to mention just a few—are needed by those who are asked to exhibit empathy.

Applications of Empathy in Health Care

Given the complexity of the empathic process, how can theoretical information about empathy best be applied in health care settings? We believe that it is important to address empathy both from the client's perspective and from the professional's perspective. The common premise to both perspectives is that understanding is achieved through empathy. In fact, it is an essential factor in effective interpersonal communication. For clients, empathy is important because illness is confusing and frightening, and being understood helps clients cope with these emotions. For professionals, empathy is essential because it helps professionals to understand clients and their problems, as well as to understand other professionals and themselves.

Empathy: The Client's Perspective

Clients in health care settings have many needs that range from physiological to psychosocial. One of their strongest psychosocial needs is the need to be understood. Yet the impersonal nature of health care organizations makes this need the hardest to fulfill. Many things (e.g., availability of time, advanced technology, staff shortages, demands for efficiency) may hinder and prevent health professionals from attending fully to clients. Nonetheless, clients' negative reactions to the strange and highly technological health care system are reduced significantly when health professionals are sensitive to clients' points of view. Expressing empathy helps clients satisfy their need for understanding.

Researchers have established that showing empathy produces positive therapeutic outcomes for clients (Olson, 1995; Williams, 1979). First, showing empathy reduces clients' feelings of alienation (Rogers, 1975) and of being "all alone" with their predicament. When clients feel understood, they feel connected to others and a part of life. Empathy breaks down the sense of being an isolated island that people with illness often experience, and it also provides clients with a sense of confirmation. When health professionals empathize with clients, clients feel understood; they know that they exist and that their point of view has value (Kalisch, 1973).

In a recent study, Olson (1995) examined the relationship between nurse-expressed empathy and two outcomes: patient-perceived empathy and patient distress in an acute care setting. The results indicated that as nurses expressed more empathy, patients felt more understood and reported less anxiety, depression, and anger. Olson's research highlights the important role that empathic communication plays in patients' response to illness and also lends support for continued efforts to teach empathy skills to nurses.

Similar to the Olson study, Raudonis (1993) found empathic relationships had a positive impact on patients in a hospice setting. Using in-depth interviews of 14 terminally ill adults, Raudonis determined that empathic relationships were important to patients because they acknowledged their personhood and value. She found that the mere initiation of a relationship with a terminally ill person was validating and highly valuable. In addition, the findings showed that empathic relationships also resulted in the improvement and maintenance of patients' overall physical and emotional well-being.

At times, however, health professionals may become too caught up in their own feelings and expectations and fail to see the values and expectations of the client. The following example illustrates this problem.

John is a 25-year-old man who was hospitalized for numerous diagnostic tests to rule out the possibility of Hodgkin's disease. John and his new wife of 2 months anxiously awaited the results of a biopsy of a neck node. They expressed much relief and hope when the pathology report returned and showed that the results were negative.

The thoracic surgeon who did the biopsy, however, was convinced that John's symptomatology was still characteristic of Hodgkin's disease and suggested that another biopsy from a different location be done. When the pathology report from this second biopsy was completed, the surgeon accompanied by two residents and a nurse rushed into John's room and loudly announced, with a wide smile on his face, "I found the specific cell that confirms my diagnosis. I was right—it is Hodgkin's disease." Possibly noting the look on John's face, the physician said, "You should be glad it's Hodgkin's disease; it could have been a lot worse! You've got a good 10 years ahead of you." John and his wife thanked the physician for being so thorough and persistent that an accurate diagnosis could be made.

However, moments after the health team left the room, John and his wife burst into tears. Later, when he recalled the incident, John said "I was mystified by the situation. I felt such shock, fear, horror—yet it seemed inappropriate to have these feelings—it would have spoiled the surgeon's celebration of having found what he was searching for. Thank God that the nurse in the background had tears in her eyes, although she never said anything. It was the only thing that let me know that my inner feelings weren't crazy."

This surgeon became preoccupied with the diagnostic process and failed to be sensitive to the meaning of the diagnosis to the patient and his family. In this case, the surgeon was oblivious to the patient's anxiety and fear about the results of the pathology report on the second biopsy. On the other hand, the nurse in the example was sensitive to the patient's feelings, and she did communicate her understanding of the patient's feelings by her actions. As the patient said, it was the empathic response of the nurse that validated his own emotions.

The following example captures many of the important aspects of how individuals should exhibit empathy toward others. It describes what one of our students wrote when asked how she would like others to listen to her problems.

"I was diagnosed with diabetes over 12 years ago. Although I live a relatively normal life, my disease has also brought on some complications with my health, and at times I wonder if I can deal with it all. Every little bit of stress can elevate my blood sugar. Last December I landed myself in the hospital due to complications with my diabetes and I almost died because of it. Inside my right eye I have a blood vessel hemorrhaging and soon I will have to have surgery on it so I don't go blind. I must watch every aspect of my health, because if I don't, it could ruin my life.

I usually don't let my diabetes bother me; it is basically a way of life for me now. At times though, when I can't get my blood sugar under control for no apparent reason, or when I find out some other problem has arisen, I get really frustrated.

At these times, I need someone to listen to me rant and rave about how much I resent having to go through these small problems. I don't want pity, I just want someone to listen. I don't want advice, I get enough of that from my doctors. I just want someone to tell me that it's okay to get angry and that I don't have to put a strong face on every time. I need someone to listen to what I'm saying without putting judgement on me, without them telling me they know how I feel, when really they don't.

I think these are the best ways for someone to show me empathy. By just letting me talk, without really saying anything. By standing behind me through the tough days, and letting me go through all the emotions that I have to go through to get by. But most of all, by showing me and letting me know that I have a shoulder to lean on if I need it.

This example clearly illustrates how important it is for all of us to be sensitive to the subtle and complex struggles others are facing on a daily basis.

For the most part, empathy helps clients feel that others care about them, which leads to greater self-acceptance (Rogers, 1975). Empathy enhances clients' feelings of being understood and facilitates their adjustment to very stressful situations. Being understood in a nonjudgmental way assists clients in feeling positive about their own value and worth. Finally, empathy gives clients a sense of control. If professionals have listened to them without making judgments, clients gain a sense of control by expressing their own thoughts without opposition or evaluation. They become less dependent on others and feel more in charge of the way they want to respond to life events (Kalisch, 1973).

Despite the importance of therapeutic empathy for patients in general, it has been suggested by Morse and associates (1992) that empathy may be difficult to express in some health care settings. For example, in acute care settings, clinicians are often involved in many complex procedures, which leaves little time for relationship development. Similarly, the transient nature of some settings, such as outpatient clinics, works against the development of rapport, a necessary prerequisite for effective therapeutic empathy. In spite of these difficulties, research suggests that empathy is an important goal for provider–patient relationships.

Empathy: The Professional's Perspective

Empathy also has an impact on health professionals, who, like clients, have a need to be understood. Health professionals desire understanding not because they are confronting an illness but rather because they desire to be more effective helpers to clients and also to have better interpersonal relationships with co-workers. Empathy, then, enables health professionals to improve the accuracy of their communication with clients and to reduce communication problems with other health professionals.

When a professional is able to empathize with another, he or she adopts a new frame of reference for the other. This new frame of reference in turn increases the probability that the professional will be able to interpret the other person's communication more accurately because the professional has been sensitized to the uniqueness and nuances of the other person's point of view. Empathy assists professionals to see the problems of clients and other professionals more clearly.

In addition, empathy helps professionals to build effective interpersonal relationships with each other—an almost universally desired goal. Many examples can be cited to illustrate how professionals have a need for empathic communication. In hospitals, pharmacists wish nurses understood the pressures pharmacists face when asked to fill a certain prescription immediately while at the same time they must fill thousands of daily hospital prescriptions. Nurses wish patients and families understood why it takes time to respond to call lights when there are staff shortages. Nurses wish physicians would acknowledge the nurses' unique areas of expertise. Physicians wish nurses understood the responsibility they feel for patient care. Staff in radiology departments would like personnel on the floors to understand the importance of preparing patients properly for complex X-ray procedures. In nursing homes, administrators wish families understood staffing difficulties and why there are sometimes delays in having patients ready for visitation hours. Staff members wish administrators would understand their desire for fair scheduling. Public health nurses would like clients to understand the importance of programs to prevent communicable diseases.

These examples illustrate only a few of the many situations in which health professionals desire understanding. In each situation, the wish being expressed by the professionals is for others to accurately perceive them and what they are doing in the health care setting. Health professionals are justified in wanting to be fully understood by other health professionals, because the misunderstandings between professionals often lead to communication breakdowns, interpersonal conflict, personal stress, and, in the end, to ineffective patient care.

Health professionals at all levels within the health care system need to share in the responsibility for giving empathic understanding to others. Several techniques can be employed in showing empathy. The techniques themselves will not automatically result in empathic communication, but they will assist professionals to improve their empathic skills. Empathic behavior is complex, but it can be learned. In Chapter 5, we will present specific communication approaches that can increase a person's ability to empathize with clients and others.

► CONTROL

The second major communication variable is control—a subtle but powerful factor in health communication. Control is an integral part of every communication event and an intrinsic component of human interaction. Whenever an individual is influenced by or influences another person or event, aspects of control are present. Previous work on control in health care has analyzed control primarily from the perspective of the individual. Does the client have a sense of control over life events? Do clients want more control in managed health care decision-making? How can clients' health-related behaviors be controlled? In this section we will take a new approach to looking at control: We will consider not only the individual perspective, which we have called *personal control*, but also the interpersonal or transactional perspective, which we have called *relational control*. This approach will allow us to discuss more fully the issues involving control in health care.

Personal control is the perception people have that they can influence the way in which circumstance affect their lives or the way in which they respond internally to external events. Personal control, in effect, increases people's feelings of potency about their actions and minimizes their feelings of powerlessness. Control is crucial to an individual's psychological as well as physical well-being (Langer, 1983). Control is important to patients because it gives them a feeling of competence in a context filled with events that create feelings of incompetence. Control does not need to be exercised, or even be real, to have an effect on the individual; it only needs to be *perceived* (Thompson, 1981). Although both clients and professionals express a need for personal control, most of the research on personal control has been done from the perspective of the client.

Relational control refers to the perception individuals have about how they are connected to others, and it includes the degree to which they feel able to influence the nature and development of relationships. This type of control resides within interpersonal relationships, rather than as a characteristic of individuals. Through communication, individuals in professional–professional and professional–client relationships establish who is in control, that is, who is most able to influence the relationship in a given situation (Thompson, 1986). If individuals within a relationship share similar definitions of relational control, more effective interpersonal communication will result.

In the following section, we provide a discussion of the conceptual frameworks for personal and relational control (Table 2–2).

Personal Control

Two areas of research which are particularly useful in conceptualizing personal control are: (1) the Thompson typology of control, and (2) the locus of control perspective.

First, Thompson (1981) has devised a typology of control that categorizes personal control into four separate areas: (1) *behavioral control*, (2) *cognitive control*, (3) *informational control*, and (4) *retrospective control. Behavioral control* is the belief that one can behave in such a way as to alter the proba-

---

TABLE 2–2. CONCEPTUALIZATIONS OF CONTROL

Conceptual Frameworks of Control
Personal control
• Thompson typology
• Locus of control
Relational control
• Complementary
• Symmetrical
• Parallel

bility, intensity, or duration of a threatening event. An example of behavioral control might be a patient who has had abdominal surgery who faithfully walks back and forth to the nurses' station because the nurses have told her it will help in the recovery process. *Cognitive control* is the belief that one can develop mental strategies that will influence the circumstances that affect one's life. Cognitive control could be demonstrated by a patient who is anxious about an upcoming procedure but can practice distraction (such as thinking about a pleasant event) to reduce some of the anxiety. Naber and colleagues (1995) found that children undergoing painful procedures experienced less stress during cancer diagnosis and treatment when parents were close to them and assisted them in practicing distraction techniques. Langer (1983) found that surgical patients who engaged in cognitive control through cognitive reappraisal, calming self-talk, and selective attention reported less postoperative stress and needed fewer pain relievers after surgery. *Informational control* is the belief that an individual can acquire knowledge about external events that affect that person's situation. Teaching preoperative patients about forthcoming procedures and sensations would be one means of assisting them to increase their informational control. *Retrospective control* is the belief that a person can accept responsibility for events in the past, thus mastering the situation after it has happened. Accident victims who have a need to understand what caused their accident and to determine if it could have been prevented may be exercising retrospective control. Elderly patients who engage in reminiscence therapy are another example of individuals who are engaging in retrospective control. Many researchers believe that the way individuals exhibit these four different types of control is related to the way they handle life stress and illness (Seligman, 1975; Thompson, 1981; Wortman & Brehm, 1975).

A second field of research on personal control is the *locus of control* perspective. Research on locus of control originated with Rotter (1954) and social learning theory. According to this theory, individuals develop certain expectations about the influence or impact of their own behaviors through a learning process. For individuals who believe that their own behavior determines what happens to them, the locus of control is said to be *internal*. For individuals who believe that outside forces or factors primarily determine what occurs in their lives, the locus of control is called *external*. For example, the person who believes that engaging in exercise routines and diet alterations will limit the occurrence of heart problems is operating from an internal control perspective. Conversely, the person who assumes that heart problems are due to heredity and nothing can be done to prevent them is operating from an external perspective. Locus of control, then, is a personality variable that discriminates between internally oriented and externally oriented individuals.

Locus of control in general has been measured by Rotter's Internal–External (I–E) scale (1966). More specifically, the locus of control of an individual's health beliefs has been measured by the Health Locus of

Control (HLC) scale (Wallston, Wallston, Kaplan, & Maides, 1976) and by a more refined version of this scale, the Multidimensional Health Locus of Control (MHLC) scale (Wallston, Wallston, & DeVellis, 1978). The items on the MHLC instrument directly assess individuals' beliefs about whether responsibility for health-related matters lies within themselves, with others, or in external events.

Research on locus of control has been of interest to health professionals because it is believed that locus of control may contribute to an understanding of individuals' health-related behavior. For example, research has shown that locus of control is associated with a multitude of health behaviors and health outcomes including engaging in health-promoting actions (Strickland, 1978), quitting smoking (Mlott & Mlott, 1975), showing less dependence on physicians (Seeman & Seeman, 1983), learning health information (Seeman & Evans, 1962), influencing health care professionals' decisions (Johnson & Levanthal, 1974), gaining knowledge about disease (Wallston, Maides, & Wallston, 1976), using medications effectively (MacDonald, 1970), and getting inoculations (Dabbs & Kirscht, 1971).

Research on locus of control has its limitations, however (Lewis, 1982a; Lowery, 1981). First, internal–external locus of control is regarded as a personality variable, and it is therefore questionable whether or not individuals can learn to change their locus of control even if they would benefit from doing so. Second, there is a tendency for researchers to imply that it is good to be "internal" and bad to be "external" (Rotter, 1975). Yet there may be situations in which it is not always healthy to maintain a high internal perspective (Lowery, 1981) or in which it may be more realistic to relinquish some personal control in health matters (Lewis, 1982b). For example, to assume that a client could have prevented certain progressive diseases or natural disasters could be unrealistic and could generate a great deal of guilt or self-blame in the client. Wortman and Brehm (1975) have suggested that overemphasizing a person's sense of control in these types of situations may be maladaptive, and they recommend that an accurate assessment of a person's potential for control in a specific situation is more useful for individuals. A final criticism is that measures of locus of control have not been reliable predictors of health-related behaviors (Lowery, 1981; Rock, Meyerowitz, Maisto, & Wallston, 1987).

Relational Control

Relational control differs from personal control in that it focuses on relationship or interpersonal characteristics, whereas personal control focuses on characteristics of individuals. Relational control is regarded as a transactional process—an interaction that occurs between individuals in a relationship—and is therefore part of the relationship dimension of messages.

As we discussed in Chapter 1, every message has two dimensions: a content dimension and a relationship dimension, inextricably bound together. In interpersonal communication, participants determine where they

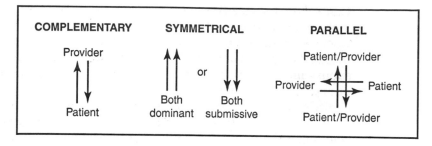

Figure 2–1. Kinds of relationships established through relational control.

stand with each other on the *relationship* dimension through the sharing of information on the *content* dimension. For example, when individuals talk about seemingly unimportant matters, such as school, weather, sports, or general news, they are in essence finding out how they feel about their relationship. The point is that individuals decide how they are related to each other and decide who is in control in a relationship through interaction. Healthy relationships are based on a mutual agreement, either spoken or unspoken, regarding the issues of control between the participants (Morton, Alexander, & Altman, 1976). Good relationships are free of constant conflict regarding who is dominant or who is in charge in the relationship.

The kinds of relationships that individuals establish through relational control can be complementary, symmetrical, or parallel (Watzlawick, Beavin, & Jackson, 1967). (Fig. 2–1).

In *complementary relationships,* the control is unequally distributed: One person exhibits more control and the other exhibits less control. In the classic medical model, health providers are typically the individuals with the control and patients are encouraged to be submissive and without control. In other health care models, clients are taking more responsibility for health-related decisions; it is no longer the norm for the provider to be in the dominant position in complementary provider–client relationships. There are several advantages to complementary relationships. They are stable, efficient, and predictable because individuals in these kinds of relationships know where they stand and need not spend time negotiating who is in charge in every particular situation. On the negative side, complementary relationships are repressive because they inhibit the independence and creativity of the subordinate member in the relationship.

In *symmetrical relationships,* control is shared equally by participants, and the power differences between individuals are minimized. Symmetrical relationships are sometimes characterized by competition for control or submission. It is not always clearly established who is in control in symmetrical relationships; the relationship may constantly be redefined. In health care settings, professional–professional relationships are frequently symmetrical. While this kind of relationship appears ideal initially, power struggles can occur as participants compete for control or compete to give up control. For example, in a symmetrical nurse–physician relationship, if both assume equally dominant positions toward one another, conflict can occur as they try to determine who will have final say in a treatment decision. The advantage of symmetrical relationships is that they promote mutual sharing of thoughts and feelings; both interactants are free to express their own values. However, symmetrical relationships may be inefficient and may promote needless competition. When making decisions, it can be time consuming to debate and discuss the implications of each person's position on every issue or decision.

A third kind of relationship is a *parallel relationship* in which control is transferred back and forth between participants. This kind of relationship may shift between being complementary and being symmetrical. Individuals distribute control to one another in some areas and share control equally in other areas. For example, in a parallel nurse–physician relationship, the nurse may assume greater control than the physician in patient education areas whereas the physician may assume greater control in diagnostic decisions. Parallel relationships result in communication patterns that are more flexible and less likely to result in dysfunctional interaction (Wilmot, 1979). Health professionals who take turns at holding and giving up control, depending on the situation, rather than competing for control would be an example of a parallel relationship.

Applications of Control in Health Care

Issues involving personal and relational control constantly confront both the client and the professional in health care settings. Control is important to clients primarily because they are experiencing the loss of it. For professionals, control is important because it is through the negotiation of control that they are able to work effectively with clients and with other health professionals. In the previous section we discussed personal and relational control. Now we would like to answer the obvious next question: How can health professionals use these concepts regarding control to improve their communication with clients and other professionals?

Control: The Client's Perspective

Loss of personal control is a major obstacle that confronts every client, whether the individual has a serious illness, such as cancer or kidney disease, or a less serious ailment. In a study of cardiac patients, Johnson and Morse (1990) found that regaining control was the key factor in the process of adjustment following a myocardial infarction. Similarly, Moser and Dracup (1995) found that when cardiac patients had perceptions of higher control they had lower levels of stress and anxiety, and better overall psychosocial adjustment.

However, illness makes clients confront the reality that they do not always have mastery of their destinies. Illness introduces uncertainty into the lives of clients—and with uncertainty comes the loss of control, which in turn leads to feelings of fright, anger, helplessness, and incompetence. Losing control takes from clients a primary means of ascribing meaning to their lives. Unless individuals feel potent and able to influence events in their lives, they will feel victimized by outside forces, see life as senseless, and view their own lives as insignificant (Cantor, 1978).

Although clients may experience loss of control in many health care settings, it is even more pronounced in a hospital setting. S. E. Taylor (1979) has suggested that "the hospital is one of the few places where an individual forfeits control over virtually every task he or she customarily performs" (p. 157). In her research on hospital patient behavior, Taylor found that loss of control results in depersonalization in patients and that patients typically respond to depersonalization by acting helpless (a "good patient" role) or by acting angry (a "bad patient" role).

The following example illustrates the loss of control experienced by a nursing home resident and his daughter, who had reluctantly placed him in the nursing home 2 days before the visit she describes below.

I found a man slumped in a chair, tears in his eyes, looking very alone. I was devastated. As his story began to unfold, I became overcome with many emotions—anger, dismay, disbelief. He said the nurse aide removed all of his private belongings from his bedside table. First, she took a laundry pen and put large black marks on each item of clothing, not caring whether the mark would be apparent when worn. (My father had dressed each day of his life in a crisp white shirt, tie, and trousers, with matching colored socks.) She told him to ask his family to provide him with wash pants and white socks, so in case his clothes got "mixed up" or lost, he could wear what came back from the laundry. (I cannot remember my father ever wearing wash pants.)

The nurse aide removed his Alka-Seltzer and denture cleaner from his drawer, explaining that none of the residents can have chemicals in their room—a protection against overdose or inappropriate use. She then removed his fingernail clippers; again citing safety as a reason. He was assured these items would be at the nurse's station and would be available upon request.

My father requested a second blanket, stating he was cold, but was told, "One per resident is enough. We keep the heat turned up high." He became tearful as he talked.

I went to the administrator who recited state statues and policy ad nauseam, and who was certain these practices were well within reasonable guidelines. I was assured my father would adjust and was reminded I should give him 2 weeks to get acclimated.

I knew I had to take my father back home and somehow we would all make it work. We did.

....

As health professionals, it is crucial that we be sensitive to the effect that loss of control has on clients in health care settings. To help clients cope with this, health professionals need to address not only the causes for feelings of loss of control but also ways to restore clients' sense of control. In treatment settings it may be useful to assess clients' preferences for control. For example, a nurse could ask a patient if he or she normally likes to "take charge" of events (internally oriented) or if he or she prefers to take a "wait and see" attitude and let events run their own course (externally oriented). Degner and Russell (1988) studied cancer patients' preferences for control and found that most patients wanted to maintain some control or active participation in the decisions made about their treatments.

In some situations, however, the control desires of patients are not easily ascertained. For example, Montbriand (1995) conducted a qualitative study of how cancer patients utilized alternative therapies as control behaviors. She found that taking control in the form of searching for cures was not necessarily an adaptive coping behavior. Only 7 of 252 patients indicated that they wanted full control of their illness. Many patients were inclined to give their control away even though they indicated they wanted control. Patients expressed that it was uncomfortable for them to feel responsible and in control of their cancer. Montriand's study underscores the need for professionals to be sensitive to the nuances that surround patients' control needs.

It is also useful to assess the patient's environment, the patient's relationships, and other factors that may affect the amount of control that is realistically available to the patient. For example, some patients may wish to control the layout of the furniture in their hospital room, the time and scheduling of various treatments, or simply the degree of privacy in their room. Other patients may wish to control how they talk about their illness. These patients may gain a stronger sense of control if they are allowed to set the pace in their conversations with others. Giving patients free control in areas they can manage alone and a participant role with a health professional in areas they cannot manage alone would be the outcome of this assessment process.

Based on observations drawn from taped interviews of 15 terminally ill patients with acquired immunodeficiency syndrome (AIDS) and cancer, Pepler and Lynch (1991) suggest that it is important for nurses to offer patients control over "small things" when they find themselves unable to control "big things." Consistent with the work of Antonovsky (1988), Pepler and Lynch postulate that patients do not necessarily need control themselves, but they need to feel as if their situation is being controlled—that their illness is being managed and that their circumstances are not chaotic. This is similar to Antonovsky (1988), who has suggested that manageability of life circumstances is integrally related to building a sense of coherence, control, and therefore health.

Another unique perspective on patients' need for control is suggested by Bowker's (1996) metaphor analysis of her own experience with Hodgkin's Disease. Bowker writes about her illness using metaphors, such as insanity, chaos, natural disaster, battle, and splitting apart. All of these metaphors underscore how deeply she experienced the loss of control when she was sick. This study underscores the need for providers to be sensitive to the overwelming feelings of irrationality, uncertainty, and disintegration that some patients feel. It is essential that providers find ways to assist patients to regain a sense of control about their circumstances.

An important way of providing control for patients is to assist them in becoming competent about their own health decision making. Based on an analysis of over 250 provider–patient conversations in Great Britain, Makoul, Arntson, and Schofield (1995) found that physicians neither give nor elicit the full information that patients need to make optimal health care decisions. In addition, they found that patients seldom initiate discussions with providers about these concerns. Their study suggests that the key to helping patients achieve appropriate control is to enhance the information exchange process between providers and patients. By sharing more information, providers can enable patients to make better decisions about their health.

An interesting approach to relational control has been reported by Lazure and Baun (1995) who tried to determine if patient control over visitor entry could alleviate stress in cornary care patients. Randomly assigned patients who received a visitor control device communicated their wishes to visitors by lighting a hallway light; red lights restricted visitors and green lights allowed visits. Patients who used the device perceived greater control over visiting and experienced lower blood pressure than patients who did not use the device. This study was unique because it illustrates that when patients have control over the initiation of their conversations with others they experience positive benefits.

By using behavioral, cognitive, informational, and retrospective dimensions of personal control, professionals may encourage clients to become more involved in their own care, and to learn new behaviors or skills that will enable them to be less dependent on health professionals. Other clients may gain a sense of cognitive control by learning to control their attitudes to their circumstances, although they may not be able to control specific health outcomes. Providing clients with information about treatments and procedures will help them by increasing their sense of predictability. Finally, being with clients and encouraging them to express their thoughts and feelings as they struggle with the meaning of illness in their lives may enable them to gain a degree of retrospective control.

The fundamental advantage of giving patients a chance to exercise legitimate control is that it allows patients to feel more independent, to feel less helpless, and thereby to feel more worthwhile. Secondly, patient participation appears to improve the physical and psychological adjustments of patients (Langer, 1983; Thompson et al., 1993). For example, research on patient-controlled analgesia (PCA) indicates that when surgical patients are taught to regulate the amount of intravenous pain medication they receive, patients reported better relief of pain and higher levels of physical activity after surgery (Attwell et al., 1984). Similarly, Kaplan, Greenfield, and Ware (1989) found that specific aspects of patient–physician communication were related to patients' health outcomes. The researchers found that control, when expressed through questions and answers during office visits, was associated with improvements in patients' blood sugar and blood pressure levels. Finally, it can be argued that there may be a decrease in malpractice litigation and a decrease in health care costs when patients are encouraged to be active participants in their care.

Control: The Professional's Perspective

The issues of control that professionals confront are different from those confronting clients. For professionals, *loss* of control is not as crucial a problem as finding effective ways to *share* control with other professionals and clients. Thus relational control becomes the predominant issue for health professionals.

Learning to share control in professional–professional relationships is not an easy process. Over the years, health care organizations have functioned with hierarchical lines of authority clearly established. Sharing control was not common. It was usually clear who had control, how much control they had, as well as who did not have control. More recently, this has changed, and health care professionals now confront the issue of how to share control. Many factors (patient rights, changing roles of health professionals, self-help groups, holistic orientations) have put pressure on the authoritarian structures of health care systems to become more democratic and allow greater participation. In addition, the increased emphasis on managed health care programs has added to the struggles for control between providers and administrators and providers and patients. Not only has this resulted in a breakdown of traditional roles, but it also has created an increased need for negotiations and communication to clarify issues of control in relationships (Beisecker, 1990; Katon & Kleinman, 1981).

The difficulties that health professionals experience in learning to share control are compounded by the nature of the environment in which they are required to practice. Much of what occurs in health settings has a life and death dimension. Health professionals who function under these critical conditions "believe they require total control in order that the environment in which they attempt to save lives be maximally efficient and predictable" (Friedman & DiMatteo, 1979, p. 8). Yet health professionals also practice in organizations in which professionals must depend on one another if they are to function with the most effectiveness. It seems then that the task for health professionals is to learn how to share control, because through *sharing* control interdependence can be achieved without any individuals *losing* control.

Agreement regarding who is in control is the key to effective professional–professional and professional–client relationships, and arriving at this agreement takes place through interaction. Sometimes the content of interactions may be an important issue, such as the need for a computerized axial tomographic (CAT) scan, or it can be a less important issue, such as parking problems. Whatever the issue, in interactions with each other, professionals have a need to feel that their ideas and opinions are of value and that they are competent. Through sharing information, professionals are able to define where they stand with each other. If they can do this in mutually acceptable ways, more productive interpersonal communication is likely to result.

How control is shared depends on the nature of the relationships, that is, whether they are complementary, symmetrical, or parallel. In the following example, examine the responses to determine what the nature of the relationships may be.

Physician to Nurse: I want the most recent lab reports on Mr. Johnson. Could you find them for me?

Nurse to Physician:

    Response A: No, I'm doing meds. You'll have to find them yourself.

    Response B: Yes, I'll look them up for you right now.

    Response C: No . . . But perhaps you could find them over there *(nods head)* on the latest printout from the lab.

Obviously there are numerous responses that could be made to the physician's request in this example. We have chosen these three hypothetical responses to illustrate how the control dimensions of a message are negotiated depending on the nature of the relationship. Response A represents a straightforward rejection of the physician's assertion of control. Although the physician would like to be in control in this situation, the nurse exerts his or her own control. This characterizes a symmetrical relationship. This symmetrical relationship (in which both people seek dominance) can lead to interpersonal conflict, however, as they compete for control. In response B, on the other hand, the nurse accepts the physician's request for control. The nurse in this case essentially accepts the physician's definition of the relationship, which places the physician in the dominant controlling position and the nurse in the submissive controlled position. This represents the complementary relationship. Who has control in this case is clearly established and also agreed upon mutually. Although this response may preserve harmony in their relationship, it can also negate the importance of the nurse's role or place it secondary to the physician's role. Response C represents an attempt on the part of the nurse to share control with the physician. The nurse rejects the physician's request for dominance but offers the alternative of assisting the physician, which does acknowledge the physician and his or her request. In essence, the nurse is saying that the physician can have control, but not at the overall expense of the nurse, who retains control in this exchange. This may characterize a parallel relationship.

Relational control is often manifested in the degree of collaboration that occurs among health professionals. Collaboration is the ongoing interaction between professionals in which each person contributes to the problem-solving effort that results in a new assessment, definition of the problem, or plan (Lamb & Napodano, 1984). Collaboration implies a distribution of control or a give-and-take of control rather than a fixed dominance of one professional over another. More and more professionals are realizing that in order to solve the complex health care problems confronting clients, there is a need for expertise and input from a variety of health professionals.

Sharing control in health care relationships is a complex and difficult process. While there are no simple prescriptions for how it is best done, being aware of professionals' and clients' needs for control is a first step in the process. This awareness, coupled with flexibility and willingness to adapt one's own needs for control to the needs of others, will result in better interpersonal communication and more productive professional-professional and professional-client relationships.

▶ TRUST

Trust is another central variable in the human communication process. Trust involves accepting others without evaluating or judging them. It plays an essential part in establishing effective counseling relationships. Pearce (1974) points out in his review of the literature that trust exists when a person feels that another individual will behave in ways that are beneficial to the relationship, without attempting to control or direct it. For our discussion, *trust* is defined as an individual's expectation that he or she can rely on the communication behaviors of others. Trust creates the belief that events are predictable and that people are basically sincere, competent, and accepting. Trust gives relationships a special, unique, positive quality that sets them apart from other relationships.

In health care settings, trust is particularly important to clients because clients often feel helpless, extremely vulnerable, and in need of support. The act of trusting health professionals gives clients a bridge to building relationships that lessen their feelings of depersonalization or vulnerability. Clients will also feel that they can depend on professionals to behave in predictable ways, and that they can rely on professionals' knowledge and integrity. For these reasons, trust appears to be an important variable to study in health care.

Conceptual Frameworks of Trust

Researchers have approached trust from three different orientations: game theory (Deutsch, 1958; Vinacke, 1969), source credibility (Giffin, 1967), and interpersonal trust (Pearce, 1974; Wheeless, 1978) (Table 2–3). In the game theory literature, trust has been studied most often by having individuals play what is called the Prisoner's Dilemma game (Luce & Raiffa, 1957)[1] and observing participants' behaviors during the game. Prisoner's Dilemma is a two-person game in which individuals are asked to choose between two alternatives, both of which produce gains or losses for the individual and for the individual's partner. The key psychological element of the game is that mutual trust must exist between the players in order to solve the game, since independent individual behavior does not result in a reasonable solution to the game (Deutsch, 1960, p. 138). The theorists measure trust in the game setting through the choices participants make that let them maximize the potential gains for one another. In the game, trust is the reliance that one individual places on another in a risky situation in which the individual has a lot to lose.

Game theory is useful because it provides researchers with an easy method for establishing a variety of conditions under which trusting behavior can be observed. However, the overall value of this approach is limited because it is difficult to interpret and apply the outcomes of these games to trust in ongoing personal relationships.

A second way of conceptualizing trust emerges from the research that has been conducted on what is called *source credibility*. Source credibility actually originated with Aristotle, who argued that audiences would believe and trust speakers who exhibit intelligence, character, and good will. From this perspective, trust is seen as the degree to which one individual per-

---

[1] Luce and Raiffa (1957) describe the Prisoner's Dilemma game as follows: "Two suspects are taken into custody and separated. The district attorney is certain they are guilty of a specific crime, but he does not have adequate evidence to convict them at a trial. He points out to each prisoner that each has two alternatives: to confess to the crime the police are sure they have done or not to confess. If they both do not confess then the district attorney states that he will book them on some very minor trumped-up charge. . . . ; if they both confess, they will be prosecuted, but he will recommend less than the most severe sentence; but if one confesses and the other does not, then the confessor will receive lenient treatment for turning state's evidence whereas the latter will get the book slapped at him" (p. 95).

TABLE 2–3. CONCEPTUALIZATIONS OF TRUST

Conceptual Frameworks of Trust
Game theory
Source credibility
Interpersonal trust
• General
• Specific

ceives another to have certain positive characteristics. For example, if certain colleagues are perceived as sincere in their interactions with clients or conscientious about professional responsibilities, then they would be described to others as colleagues who are credible and trustworthy. Put another way, we learn to trust certain individuals because we have seen them act in positive, consistent, and reliable ways.

Research into trust has also been approached from an interpersonal perspective. This line of research, taken by Wheeless and Grotz (1975, 1977) and Northouse (1979), indicates that interpersonal trust occurs and can be measured at two levels: *general trust* (the trust an individual has of other people in a global sense), and *specific trust* (the trust an individual has of a particular person in a relationship). For example, you may consider yourself to be basically trusting because you openly accept people you meet (high general trust), while at the same time you may have a particular supervisor or colleague whom you distrust at times (low specific trust). Similarly, some paranoid clients may have a general mistrust of other persons, yet they are able to develop a specific trust in a particular mental health nurse or psychiatric social worker.

To measure *general trust,* researchers have employed the widely used Rotter Interpersonal Trust Scale (Rotter, 1967). To measure *specific trust* in the context of interpersonal communication, researchers have used a variety of word-choice scales. Using both types of measures, researchers are able to compare and contrast individuals with regard to the general trust and specific trust they exhibit in interpersonal situations. Unlike the other research frameworks that view trust more as a quality that a person either does or does not have, the interpersonal trust perspective approaches trust as a variable that may change when an individual is involved in specific relationships and specific situations.

Applications of Trust in Health Care

Two positive outcomes emerge when trust is present in interpersonal relationships. First, trust helps individuals to experience a sense of security and connectedness, to feel that they are not alone and that others care about them. Second, trust creates a supportive climate in relationships, which reduces defensive communication: It makes individuals more open and honest about their attitudes, feelings, and values. In health care settings, the first outcome—security—is especially important to clients; the second outcome—a supportive climate—is important to both health professionals and clients.

Trust: The Client's Perspective

The nature of various health care situations can increase clients' needs to establish trusting relationships with professionals. Undergoing brain surgery, selecting a treatment regimen, receiving an intravenous medication, or having their chest X-rays read are just a few of a multitude of complex and disturbing situations in which clients need to depend on and trust health professionals. Cantor (1978), describes how important it is for cancer patients to establish a relationship with a skilled and competent oncologist: "Being able to trust those upon whom we must depend is essential. . . . We seek out the best in others and attach our hopes to their abilities" (p. 75). Clients are simply unable to do many of the things that health professionals do, and in many ways they are forced to depend on the competent skills of the professionals. Being able to trust the professionals reduces some of the fear and uncertainty that is inherent in this forced dependence. Furthermore, clients have a need to be able to see professionals as competent, sincere, and caring individuals (Tagliacozzo & Mauksch, 1979). Being able to trust professionals produces in clients the sense of being connected to others and the feeling of not being alone.

Trust: The Professional's Perspective

Knowing that trust reduces uncertainty in clients and helps them to feel secure is important for professionals to understand. But in addition, professionals will want to be aware of ways in which they can help clients to develop that trust.

As we described in the preceding section on conceptual frameworks, clients trust professionals if they believe professionals are worthy (source credibility) and if they develop caring relationships with health professionals (interpersonal trust). Health professionals who want to establish trust with clients will try to build both their professional credibility as well as trusting interpersonal relationships. Too often these two kinds of trust are fostered separately from one another or not fostered at all. For example, the health professional may go to great lengths to convince the client of his or her expertise or credibility in technical matters, while totally disregarding the elements of a caring relationship that are necessary to develop interpersonal trust. The following example illustrates a situation in which neither credibility nor a caring atmosphere was present.

A young brain surgeon hurriedly walked into the room of a 75-year-old woman, and introduced himself as the neurosurgeon who had been asked by another physician to assess her neurological condition. The woman and her family had never heard of this neurosurgeon and were immediately skeptical about his competence because he was quite young. After quickly assessing the woman's physical status and giving her the results of the CAT scan and laboratory reports, the surgeon recommended that the woman be scheduled for surgery at 8:00 a.m. the next morning. The woman and her family were startled at this sudden suggestion for surgery, since another physician had previously diagnosed the woman as having had a stroke and had prescribed outpatient physical rehabilitation for the past 3 months. The woman and her family expressed their concern to the physician, stating that events were moving too fast and that they needed time to think and talk about the situation. The surgeon appeared dismayed at the woman's hesitation and the request for more time. He told her that he had two accident victims with severe head injuries waiting for him in the emergency room and he had no more time to talk with her. . . . The woman refused the surgery.

In the next few days, the family members called different health professionals they knew to gather more information on the neurosurgeon. They learned that he was noted for his surgical skills but not for his interpersonal skills. Also, over the next few days, the neurosurgeon altered his approach to the woman and her family, spent a little more time discussing the pros and cons of surgery and building rapport. After learning about the surgeon's expertise and after building a limited rapport with the surgeon, the woman consented to surgery.

This example vividly illustrates the importance of trust in professional–client communication. The patient and her family find themselves in a situation in which they must depend on a health professional to perform a difficult operation. They do not understand the details behind the two different diagnoses they have received, and they are frightened. Naturally, they want to trust the surgeon and they know they need to trust him; yet his attitude and approach reduce his credibility in the minds of the patient and her family.

By the initial refusal of surgery, the message is sent to the surgeon "We don't trust you. . . . Show us that we can trust you." The surgeon responds to the patient and family by demonstrating an increased degree of concern.

The additional time he spends helps the patient and family feel more a part of the treatment process and more secure with the surgeon. Also, as the family hears other health professionals' opinions of the surgeon's competence, his source credibility increases. In the end, the surgeon is trusted for both his competence and his supportive behavior, and the patient and her family agree to the surgery.

Building trust with clients is not an easy task for health professionals, especially because of the many demands on their time. Nonetheless, health professionals need to realize that their behavior toward others does influence, either positively or negatively, the development of trust. For example, health professionals who actively try to be knowledgeable, sincere, honest, predictable, and caring can enhance their source credibility with others. In a similar way, health professionals who try to nurture supportive relationships can encourage others' trust.

Up to this point, we have been discussing the importance of developing trust in relationships. Now we would like to assess which communication factors in professional–client and professional–professional relationships will foster trust. Our primary source for this discussion will be a classic article by Gibb (1961), which divides different types of communication behaviors into only two categories: those communication behaviors that produce a *supportive climate* and those that produce a *defensive climate* (Table 2–4).

Trust is enhanced in health care relationships when professionals use supportive communication behaviors (e.g., description, problem orientation, spontaneity) and trust is hindered when they use defensive communication (e.g., evaluation, control, strategy). In the next section, each trust-producing behavior is described and contrasted with its opposite distrust-producing behavior.

EVALUATION VERSUS DESCRIPTION. Professionals whose communication is evaluative in tone or content will increase defensiveness in others. "If by expression, manner of speech, tone of voice, or verbal content the sender seems to be

TABLE 2–4. CATEGORIES FOR COMMMUNICATION BEHAVIORS THAT PRODUCE TRUST AND DISTRUST

Defensive Climates	Supportive Climates
1. Evaluation	1. Description
2. Control	2. Problem orientation
3. Strategy	3. Spontaneity
4. Neutrality	4. Empathy
5. Superiority	5. Equality
6. Certainty	6. Provisionalism

Reprinted from Gibb, J. R. (1961). Defensive communication. Journal of Communication, 11(3), 143. Reprinted with permission of the International Communication Association.

evaluating or judging the listener, then the receiver goes on guard" (Gibb, 1961, p. 143). Descriptive communication, on the other hand, reduces defensiveness in the receiver and increases trust. The message communicated is free of moral or value judgments; it does not prescribe what the listener ought to do differently. For example:

Evaluation: You haven't positioned this patient properly. You have to do it this way. *(Demonstrates.)*

Description: I have found that patients experience less pain when they are turned on their unaffected sides with two pillows placed between their legs like this *(demonstrates)* and another pillow behind their back.

CONTROL VERSUS PROBLEM ORIENTATION. Professionals whose communication attempts to control the receiver will create a reaction of distrust. When the listener senses that the professional is trying to change his or her attitudes, values, or behaviors through the communication, it implies that the listener is inadequate, less informed, immature, or unable to make independent decisions—and the listener will set up resistance. The opposite of this is problem-oriented communication, which reduces resistance and builds trust because it involves the listener in defining the problem and finding solutions. For example:

Control: John, you know that desserts are not a part of your diabetic diet. You must cut them out of your diet completely or your diabetes will not stabilize at a manageable level.

Problem Orientation: John, I gather that you are very fond of desserts. Have you thought of any alternate ways to manage your craving for desserts that would fit into your diabetic diet?

STRATEGY VERSUS SPONTANEITY. Listeners distrust communicators who appear to have hidden intentions or specific plans in their messages. Listeners prefer to have professionals communicate with them in uncomplicated ways that are marked by openness, honesty, and directness. Although spontaneity is not always common among health professionals, it is effective in reducing the defensive barriers put up by clients and by other health professionals. For example:

Strategy: Jean, you have such great skill in writing nursing care plans, would you mind writing up care plans on Mr. F. and Mr. M. in addition to those other patients?

Spontaneity: Jean, I really feel frustrated and pressed for time about writing those two care plans. Would you be willing to help me out and show me how to develop the nursing diagnoses?

NEUTRALITY VERSUS EMPATHY. When the tone and content of communication express neutrality, the listener tends to resist it. In essence, neutrality makes others feel as if they are not valued as unique persons. Clients resent the clinical, detached patient-as-object approach. On the other hand, empathic communication increases trust because it indicates that others value the listener enough to set their own thoughts and values aside and attempt to place themselves into the listener's personal world. For example:

Neutrality: For patients like your husband who have had a stroke, we typically expect eight out of ten to survive the initial phase and about 30 to 60 percent of the patients to return to a productive work life. It is also likely that your husband will regain only 65 percent of the movement of his right arm.

Empathy: Mrs. B., even though this has been a difficult period for you and the family, Mr. B.'s condition seems to be improving now. I am hoping that with some intensive physical rehabilitation, he will be able to regain much of his arm movement, and be able to return to his office on a limited basis.

SUPERIORITY VERSUS EQUALITY. People whose communication gives the impression that they feel superior to the listener in some way will be met with a defensive response. Communicating superiority indicates an unwillingness to participate and share in a mutual problem-solving relationship. On the other hand, communicating equality suggests that the speaker is interested in others' perspectives and is willing to participate in planning that will involve mutual trust and respect. As we discussed before, the nature of health care settings actually works against equality between communicators. Nevertheless, attempts to reduce superiority will usually increase trust and have a positive impact on the development of relationships. For example:

Superiority: I know you have worked with the family a long time Mrs. L., but my work toward a specialist degree gives me a broader perspective. Here are my ideas about how the family dynamics can be altered.

Equality: Your experience with the family is extremely important in helping me to understand the family relationships. Perhaps we could work together to find some ways to deal with their problems.

CERTAINTY VERSUS PROVISIONALISM. When individuals communicate in a way that indicates absolute, unquestionable certainty, they often evoke distrust in the listener. If professionals imply that their way is always correct and their approach to a problem is the only approach, this belittles the clients' ideas. On the other hand, communication that sounds more provisional will create more trust in the client, because it implies willingness on the professionals' part to share control in analyzing a problem. The client then has a chance to participate in the outcome of the interaction. For example:

Certainty: I give *my* mastectomy patients all the information that they need to know about their rehabilitation from breast surgery. Mrs. K. doesn't need this "touchy-feely" support group you are suggesting!

Provisionalism: You mentioned a support group for mastectomy patients for Mrs. K. Although I don't think she needs it, tell me what you think these groups offer to patients.

All the different types of communication behaviors that health professionals use will have a major impact on the development—or the lack of development—of trust between client and health professional, as well as on trust between professionals. Health professionals cannot automatically assume that others will immediately trust them and grant them credibility just because they occupy a particular position. By attending to others' needs and communicating in ways that will create positive reactions, health professionals can foster trust and credibility.

▶ SELF-DISCLOSURE

The fourth communication variable we have chosen to discuss in this chapter is self-disclosure. Self-disclosure is included because of its critical importance in facilitating open communication, which is essential in the development of healthy interpersonal relationships. The recognition of self-disclosure as a communication variable can be traced to Sidney M. Jourard's book, *The Transparent Self*, first published in 1964. A central tenet of Jourard's work is that people can attain health only insofar as they gain the courage to be themselves with others, that is, to self-disclose.

The variable, self-disclosure, can be characterized as any message about the self that one person communicates to another (Cozby, 1973). For our discussion, self-disclosure will be defined as a process whereby an individual communicates personal information, thoughts, and feelings to others.

Conceptual Frameworks of Self-Disclosure

The research that has been conducted on self-disclosure provides a relatively clear picture of what self-disclosure is and how it affects communication. Researchers have studied self-disclosure from two viewpoints: (1) a relational perspective, and (2) a message perspective (Table 2–5).

Jourard's studies of self-disclosure (1964, 1968, 1971) represent a relational perspective, which emphasizes that disclosure to others benefits individuals because it enables them to find meaning and direction for their lives. Through the process of sharing, individuals discover their true selves in relation to others. Jourard believes that individuals remain healthy as long as they are able to develop human relationships in which self-disclosure is possible. People become less healthy when they are estranged from other human beings and when the opportunities for self-disclosure are no longer possible: In effect, self-disclosure is directly linked to the healthy personality. Although he has reported some evidence that suggests self-disclosure is curvilinearly related to mental health (i.e., that the benefits taper off at high and low levels) (Jourard, 1971, p. 234), Jourard's *theoretical* position emphasizes the positive relationship between self-disclosure and personality adjustment as illustrated in Figure 2–2 (D. A. Taylor, 1979).

In contrast to the position taken by Jourard and others, who assert that increased amounts of self-disclosure are related to increased levels of mental health, other researchers have stressed that self-disclosure is curvilinear (Fig. 2–3) with extremely high or low levels of self-disclosure being related to adjustment problems in individuals (Chaikin & Derlega, 1974a, 1974b; Cozby, 1973). Chaikin and Derlega (1974a) contend that certain factors, such as the nature of interpersonal relationships themselves and different types of situational contexts, mediate or influence the relationship between self-disclosure and mental health. Although there has not been a great deal of research on the general rules governing appropriate self-disclosure, there are some indications that disclosing personal information at an inappropriate time or to the wrong persons may in fact reflect some kind of maladjust-

TABLE 2–5. CONCEPTUALIZATIONS OF SELF-DISCLOSURE

Conceptual Frameworks of Self-Disclosure
Relational perspective
Message perspective
• Intention
• Amount
• Valence
• Honesty
• Depth

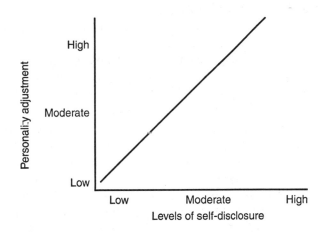

Figure 2–2. A positive relationship between self-disclosure and personality adjustment.

ment (Chaikin & Derlega, 1974a; Wortman, Adesman, Herman, & Greenberg, 1976).

The relational approach to self-disclosure taken by Wenburg and Wilmot (1973) also acknowledges both the benefits and risks of self-disclosure. They maintain (1) that situational constraints cannot be ignored, and (2) that self-disclosure should be reasoned. "In reasoned self-disclosure, one is concerned with the other person as well as himself/herself" (Wenburg & Wilmot, 1973, p. 227). In this perspective, the individual is encouraged to disclose only the amount and kind of information that he or she feels is appropriate to others and to the situation. Wenburg and Wilmot believe that it is legitimate for individuals to keep some things to themselves. Reasoned

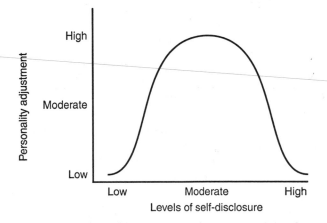

Figure 2–3. A curvilinear relationship between self-disclosure and personality adjustment.

self-disclosure means the individual can be honest about his or her true feelings without being expected to disclose everything.

In addition to studies from the relational perspective, other studies have examined the nature of self-disclosing *messages* (Cozby, 1973; Wheeless & Grotz, 1976). These studies revealed that self-disclosure is composed of at least five separate dimensions or aspects: (1) intention, (2) amount, (3) valence, (4) honesty, and (5) depth.

1. The *intention* aspect of self-disclosure refers to a person's demonstrated willingness to disclose to others. Sometimes individuals disclose information that they had not really planned to share with someone else, such as an unintentional slip of the tongue. However, when individuals consciously choose to reveal their personal thoughts and feelings, they are engaged in intentional self-disclosure.
2. The *amount* aspect refers to the quantity of information a person communicates to others. Individuals who share a lot of information about themselves when talking with others are demonstrating greater amounts of self-disclosure. A client who tells you little about his or her feelings would exemplify a low degree of self-disclosure.
3. The *valence* aspect refers to the positive or negative content of the self-disclosure. If individuals tend to disclose good aspects about themselves, the valence would be labeled positively (+), whereas it would be labeled negatively (−) if the information provided about themselves was primarily unfavorable.
4. The *honesty* dimension refers to the accuracy of the disclosures that an individual makes to others. Self-disclosure may vary in the degree to which what is said accurately matches what an individual really thinks or feels. For example, some individuals find it difficult to reveal their true experiences to others and may cloak some of their feelings, while other individuals are comfortable "telling it like it is."
5. The *depth* dimension refers to the intimacy level of the content of disclosures. Information of a very personal nature is described as being of greater depth than less personal information.

To assess self-disclosure, researchers have most frequently used Jourard's Self-Disclosure Questionnaire (Jourard & Lasakow, 1958), consisting of 60 items that measure the extent to which individuals share specific kinds of information with significant others. It should be pointed out, however, that this instrument and subsequent shorter versions of it have been criticized by researchers who have found little evidence that the test is valid—that it actually measures what it claims it does (Cozby, 1973). Wheeless and Grotz (1976) have developed a more reliable measuring instrument, consisting of 16 statements that measure the intention, amount, valence, honesty, and depth of self-disclosure. For specific use in a health care interview, Dawson, Schirner, and Beck (1984) have developed a 21-item patient self-disclosure instrument, which assesses the degree of difficulty that patients have disclosing personal problems and feelings to health care providers.

Applications of Self-Disclosure in Health Care

In the preceding section, we discussed ways of thinking about or conceptualizing self-disclosure. Now we will look more closely at how self-disclosure applies to interpersonal relationships in health care settings. Those health care organizations that support open communication among professionals and clients will foster the positive outcomes that can result from self-disclosure. In health care, clients and professionals often approach the self-disclosure process from distinct perspectives, which we will discuss in the next two sections.

Self-Disclosure: The Client's Perspective

Self-disclosure is important for clients for a number of reasons. First, it allows catharsis, the draining of emotional tension and anxiety that often accompanies illness. Second, it allows clients to receive feedback from others that their reactions to their illness are normal. Third, it promotes problem solving and enables clients to examine their situation from a more objective perspective.

Although disclosing feelings helps clients adjust to their illness, often they feel inhibited (Spiegel, *et al.* 1989). For example, in a study of 256 patients with cancer, only 52 percent of the patients told their friends and neighbors about the diagnosis; 32 percent told only their closest friends; and 16 percent did not reveal the diagnosis to friends (Cassileth, Zupkis, Sutton-Smith, & March, 1980). In a study of patients having radiation therapy, the majority of the patients reported that they wished they could discuss their situation more openly with someone (Mitchell & Glicksman, 1977).

Given the many positive outcomes of self-disclosure, what makes the process of self-disclosure so difficult? Part of the answer lies in the feelings of vulnerability and uncertainty experienced by clients who may wish to share feelings with other clients or health team members. For example, clients often wonder if their reactions to illness and stress are normal (Northouse & Northouse, 1987). They worry that if they disclose their feelings about their illness, others will evaluate them and find them to be responding in weak, excessive, or strange ways.

Clients may also fear that their self-disclosure could disrupt relationships they have already established with health professionals (Tagliacozzo & Mauksch, 1979). For example, a client who is concerned about some aspects of the health services being provided may fear that a complaint or negative reaction could disrupt the relationship that he or she has with the health team member and could also have a negative impact on the kind of care he or she receives. The point is that clients, because they feel vulnerable, are careful about what they say to health professionals; therefore, they may refrain from self-disclosure because they fear negative repercussions in their care.

Clients' concerns about how others will respond to their self-disclosures are not totally unfounded. In a study of people's reactions to victims, Coates, Wortman, and Abbey (1979) noted that when victims disclose their misery and their need for support, others often evaluate them as less well adjusted and less attractive than victims who do not disclose. Similarly, Wortman and Dunkel-Schetter (1979) noted that cancer patients often receive mixed messages or confusing feedback from others in response to the personal concerns that they voice. Breast cancer patients in one study reported that other people often tried to cheer them up; this forced cheerfulness frequently made the patients feel less normal and hindered them from revealing their true feelings (Peters-Golden, 1982). Perhaps it is not surprising, then, that disclosing feelings can be a difficult process for some patients. Clients may want to self-disclose and yet fear to do so because of the risks that make it so difficult. Despite the problems surrounding disclosure, there is some indication that the more patients are able to discuss their illness with others, especially family members, the better their psychosocial adjustment to illness (Gotcher, 1992).

Given their concerns about how others will respond, it appears that patients attempt to "test the water" by disclosing in small amounts over an extended period of time. In a qualitative study of 29 individuals with either AIDS, herpes, or a history of family violence, Limandri (1989) found that there seemed to be an "unlayering" process to disclosure. In other words, these individuals would conceal for a while, then disclose, retract back, and then disclose further, depending on the situation or on the response of others. Individuals disclosed more easily when they felt compassion, acceptance, and knowledge in their listeners. Also, it was sometimes helpful when respondents asked these individuals to tell more about themselves.

To assist clients in dealing with disclosure, it is important to assess the context of the situation and the nature of the relationship. It is unrealistic for professionals to expect clients to freely disclose information about their health or personal matters to anyone at anytime. Based on interviews with 24 physically disabled individuals, Braithwaite (1988) contends that individuals with disabilities should not be advised to freely disclose but rather to actively choose what and how they want to disclose to others about their circumstances. By regulating self-disclosure, individuals can maintain better control of the boundaries of their selves and their self-identities (Derlega & Chaikin, 1977).

Furthermore, it is important for clients to identify trustworthy people who may give them personal support in settings where there is enough privacy for self-disclosing communication. Clients need to be encouraged to participate actively in the process of choosing people and places for self-disclosure, so that the experience is comfortable and positive for them, rather than threatening and nonproductive.

Consider the following example in which a woman is encouraged by an acquaintance to self-disclose in a very public setting. As you read the example, assess the difficulties faced by the woman who is being asked to talk about a personal health-related matter.

Joanne was a 30-year-old woman who miscarried in her eighth month of pregnancy. One month after the loss of her baby, Joanne was asked to serve punch at a reception in a hospital dining room.

A former colleague and acquaintance of Joanne's came to the reception. Upon arriving at the reception, she went to the punchbowl where Joanne was serving and expressed her sympathy to Joanne. She told Joanne that she was sorry about the loss of her baby and then proceeded to ask questions such as, "What do the doctors feel the problem was that caused you to lose the baby?" and "This won't affect your ability to have children in the future, will it?" Joanne gave brief responses to the questions and excused herself from the punchbowl saying she had to use the bathroom. In the bathroom Joanne tried to gain back the composure that she had lost while choking back the sad feelings these questions rekindled.

Later, when discussing this incident, Joanne said that she wished the woman had waited until she was not in the middle of serving punch, or she wished the woman had visited her in her office, instead. She felt very uncomfortable sharing such private information in such a public setting. Joanne also noted that she and this woman had never really talked about personal things before, even when they had worked together, and that it seemed quite unnatural to discuss those kinds of things now.

This case illustrates a situation in which neither a trusting relationship nor privacy was available, and the person found self-disclosure almost impossible. Health care settings are notorious for the lack of privacy available to clients and their families. Large four-bed wards and semiprivate rooms make disclosure of personal information very difficult. Giving families information in front of other families in waiting rooms, or asking them to step into hallways to hear results of surgical procedures obviously inhibits self-disclosure. The clinic waiting room is another example of a public setting that could hinder not only clients' disclosures to professionals, but also professionals' disclosures to clients. If health professionals accept the importance of self-disclosure for clients, it is important for professionals to work toward creating contexts in health care settings in which self-disclosure can be fostered, and then to nurture trusting relationships in which client disclosure can be facilitated.

Another aspect to take into consideration is that clients vary in their preference for self-disclosure (Bradac, Tardy, & Hosman, 1980). You may know some people who are comfortable sharing personal information with many people without any hesitation. You may also know people who are comfortable disclosing information to only one or two close family members and, even then, do so with great difficulty and restraint. Because of this variability among individuals, health professionals need to assess clients' readiness and preferences for self-disclosure. Expecting immediate self-disclosure from clients who seldom self-disclose to anyone or who have not yet developed a comfortable rapport with us may be an unrealistic expectation (Klotkowski, 1980). Only as we take into consideration the preferences of the other person, the nature of our relationships, and the settings of the interactions will we be able to assist clients in showing reasoned self-disclosure.

Self-Disclosure: The Professional's Perspective

Most health professionals see self-disclosure as important for clients. As professionals they are faced with the problem of creating contexts in which clients feel free to self-disclose, building relationships that foster self-disclosure in these situations, and doing both without failing to meet their other professional obligations. At the same time, however, professionals need to find ways to self-disclose and ventilate their own feelings. Even though there is not a long tradition to support professional self-disclosure in the health care fields, there is evidence that it is important for professionals (Jourard, 1964). A closer examination of the professional's perspective may provide some insight into why self-disclosure is a difficult aspect of the communication process for professionals in health care.

In a study of self-disclosure at a large public urban hospital, Johnson (1980) noted three explanations that were commonly given by staff nurses who were asked whether they self-disclosed to patients or whether they encouraged patients to self-disclose to staff. First, nurses in this study indicated that they did not have sufficient time to listen to clients once the clients started to talk about personal matters and feelings. Second, nurses indicated that other nursing care activities were given higher priority than self-disclosure. Last, nurses pointed out that they did not have the skills to handle self-disclosure from clients and they could do little to change clients' personal problems. Health professionals' discomfort with patients' disclosures is illustrated in the following example. An oncologist describes his interactions with cancer patients and the approach that he takes toward their self-disclosure.

I know that patients who have cancer have much going on inside themselves about the meaning of life, death, and their cancer experience. I value these feelings. . . . But I don't feel prepared to respond to them, so I don't encourage patients to talk about their feelings. Allowing patients to talk about the existential anxiety they feel is important, but I don't really deal with this aspect.

The physician acknowledges patients' needs to air their feelings, yet he expresses personal concern about how he should handle patients' self-disclosures. This illustration is not an isolated case, but may represent the response of many health professionals to patients' self-disclosure. Health professionals can recognize the importance of self-disclosure for clients and yet find it hard to feel comfortable with it or know how to react.

Some professionals are concerned about their own ability to remain objective or to remain composed in response to client self-disclosure. Other professionals fear that being in touch with clients' feelings can be an obstacle to good treatment. Yet, as the following example from a cancer patient's unpublished journal so clearly suggests, patients do want health professionals to help them in the self-disclosure process.

The emotional support I received during my experience with cancer was limited. I wanted to talk to someone who could put the medical facts in the proper perspective for me. My need for support was most overwhelming when I started receiving radiation treatments. Yet this is when I had the least support.

I felt hostile, desperate, frightened, and totally alone. I needed answers to my questions about the "machines." The technicians later told me they did not talk much to me because they were not supposed to talk with patients and they thought leaving me alone was the best thing! I think they were as frightened of me as I was of them.

I don't know why people were afraid to talk with me about my cancer. I'm the one who had the disease, not them; I'm the one who had to walk away from the clinic and live with it.

It seemed like there was no place for me to release my daily anxieties. At 29 years old, I felt that I did not belong in the waiting room with the "old" people with "cancer." Even if I wanted to talk to them I couldn't because it was blatantly discouraged by the sign on the wall which read: *Please do not talk about your problems with other patients.* What help we might have been to each other! It would have outweighed any harm. Certainly a cancer patient did not make that sign and hang it on the wall.

In essence, this patient is expressing her desire to be heard by health professionals. Her remarks suggest that clients do not want health professionals to be insulated; they want professionals to help them in the self-disclosure process and to communicate with them about personal and health-related subjects.

Up to this point in our discussion we have been focusing on possible explanations for why health professionals find it difficult to promote client self-disclosure. Another aspect that deserves consideration is the approach health professionals themselves take toward self-disclosing to clients and to other professionals. Several questions are commonly raised in this regard: For example, should health professionals engage in self-disclosure at all? Is it appropriate for them to self-disclose to clients? What is the role of self-disclosing communication in professional–professional relationships?

Based on our preceding discussion of conceptual frameworks for self-disclosure, these questions would be answered affirmatively. It is helpful when health professionals share their personal feelings with other professionals and to some extent with clients. All the positive outcomes of self-disclosure, so strongly espoused by Jourard and others, are available to professionals just as they are to clients. So, too, the rules for appropriate self-disclosure apply to professionals as they do to clients. Too much or too little self-disclosure is maladaptive for professionals just as it is for any individual.

In communication between professionals and clients, the focus of the interaction needs to remain on the client. Fostering patient disclosure does not require that professional disclosure be inhibited—in fact, to be fully effective, self-disclosure needs some element of reciprocity. However, reciprocal disclosure does require that professional self-disclosure be appropriately expressed. It does *not* mean that the professional "tells all" to the client or switches the focus of the interaction onto the needs of the professional— only that the professional uses self-disclosure to facilitate empathic understanding. Therefore, reciprocity of disclosure calls for sharing honest feelings and observations with clients, as in the following statements:

- "The situation you're telling me about sounds really frightening. I probably would have felt the same way you did."
- "I'm glad that you told me about that. It gives me a better understanding of what you are going through. I really sense you have deep inner strength that was untapped before this crisis."
- "I know you're angry about the missing laboratory report. I'm also very mad and frustrated at the way this thing has worked out."
- "I can understand your hesitancy to see a marriage counselor. A few years ago I was in a similar crisis and found my talks with a mental health professional very helpful. . . . You may want to give the idea a little more thought."

In these situations, the focus of the interaction remains on the client, even though the professional is sharing some of his or her own feelings and perceptions.

Even in the area of treatment decisions, sharing concerns and questions can create a participatory relationship between the professional and the client. According to Thompson and Seibold (1978), self-disclosure increases attraction between participants and reduces tension and uncertainty. The following example illustrates a form of reciprocal self-disclosure.

A 55-year-old man who had had surgery for an obstructed bowel exhibited symptoms including nausea, distended abdomen, and moderately severe pain. Three days after surgery, the following brief conversation took place between the man and the surgeon.

Patient: I'm still feeling bad. My pain isn't going away and I don't feel any better than I did before surgery. What do you think is the matter? *(Puzzled look on his face.)*

Surgeon: I just don't know; I'm concerned too. I know the bowel has been reattached properly, so that couldn't be causing these problems. I can't figure it out. *(Sitting with a frown on his face, arms closed in front of his chest, one hand supporting his chin.)*

Patient: Well, I'm glad to know that you think the bowel attachment is OK. . . . Anything I can do to get rid of some of this bloated feeling? *(Looking at physician.)*

Surgeon: We might increase your exercise a little to help with the peristalsis. I'll check back with you tonight. We'll work this one out. *(Touches patient's shoulder as he leaves.)*

The following day the symptoms subsided and the patient went on to a complete recovery. Later, in recalling his postsurgery complications, the patient graphically described how the surgeon, while pacing at the foot of the patient's bed, had expressed his bewilderment with the complications. He said that although he was concerned that the surgeon didn't know exactly what was wrong, he felt assured by the physician's open, honest approach and willingness to involve him in the problem-solving process.

In disclosing his concerns about the postsurgery problems, the surgeon allowed the patient to perceive him as fallible. This disclosure encouraged the patient to become actively involved in his care and also let him see a very human side of the physician. To honestly express his frustrations and concerns about the patient's progress in this way was appropriate professional–client self-disclosure, and it had a positive impact on their relationship.

In addition to the importance of professionals using disclosure with clients, it is also important for professionals to feel that they can self-disclose to other professionals. When professionals engage in self-disclosure with other professionals, they can express their feelings and talk about things that concern them with others who are likely to understand and be supportive. Although it is more common for professionals to share feelings and concerns with their own colleagues (nurses with nurses, social workers with social workers, and administrators with administrators), it is also important for interdisciplinary sharing to take place. Through interdisciplinary communication and self-disclosure, nurses can increase their sensitivity to social workers, and physicians can increase their sensitivity to nurses, to name only a few possibilities. Through appropriate self-disclosure, health care professionals can begin to exchange some of their true concerns and feelings. The result may well be increased cooperation and understanding among the staff, and higher quality care for their clients.

► CONFIRMATION

Confirmation, the final human communication variable we have selected to discuss, overlaps in some ways with the variables we have already presented (empathy, control, trust, and self-disclosure). Confirmation involves dimensions of showing empathy, sharing control, exhibiting trust, and disclosing personal thoughts and feelings to others. However, confirmation is also a distinct variable that plays a unique role in health communication (Thompson, 1986). Confirmation is a way of communicating acknowledgment and acceptance to others. It is a relatively new concept that is starting to receive more emphasis in health care (Garvin & Kennedy, 1988; Heineken, 1982; Loveridge & Heinekin, 1988).

In our discussion, confirmation will refer to specific kinds of verbal and nonverbal responses that one individual makes to another. *Confirming responses* acknowledge and validate the other person's perspective. They are responses that enable someone else to value himself or herself more fully as a human being (Cissna & Sieburg, 1981; Sieburg & Larson, 1971). Engel (1980) has suggested that confirming responses include acceptance of the other individual's self-definition despite the fact that this definition may be very different from one's own definition of the other. On the other hand, *disconfirming responses* express indifference to and denial of the presence and experiences of another. They are responses that cause another person to place less value on himself or herself as a human being (Cissna & Sieburg, 1981; Sieburg & Larson, 1971).

As we discussed in Chapter 1, every communication event occurs on two levels: content and relationship. Confirmation can be thought of as occurring on the *relationship* level. Individuals define who they are through other people's responses to them (Sieburg, 1975). Thus it is satisfying if others respond in ways that affirm the receiver's own experience, and it is

TABLE 2–6. CONCEPTUALIZATIONS OF CONFIRMATION

Conceptual Frameworks of Confirmation
Existential perspective
Confirmation/disconfirmation behavior perspective

painful if others respond in a disconfirming manner that negates the receiver's self-experience.

In the following sections, we will try to make the meaning of confirmation clearer by presenting two frameworks for understanding it: (1) the existential perspective, and (2) the confirmation/disconfirmation behavior perspective (Table 2–6). In addition, we will examine how health professionals can apply theoretical information about confirmation to improve their communication in health care situations.

Conceptual Frameworks of Confirmation

Confirmation has its historical roots in existentialism. The writings of existentialists, such as Martin Buber, Viktor Frankl, and R. D. Laing, provide a conceptual orientation for understanding confirmation. According to Buber (1957), all individuals wish to be confirmed and accepted for what they are and what they can become. Societies in which confirmation flourishes are the most human. In addition, Buber believes that every person in society is able to fulfill this wish *in others* by confirming them as unique human beings (p. 102). Approaching confirmation from a different perspective, Viktor Frankl (1963), in a moving account of how he and others survived Auschwitz and the Nazi concentration camps, describes the importance of being able to ascribe meaning to one's *own* existence, whether it be through doing a deed, through experiencing the love of another human being, or through suffering (p. 176). For Frankl, the essence of life revolves around our ability to find meaning through actively choosing the way in which we respond to life's circumstances. The meaning we establish for our lives—and our actions and responses—all become more meaningful when they are acknowledged and *validated* by others. R. D. Laing, a psychiatrist, was also interested in confirmation. He was particularly interested in the consequences of disconfirming communication on patients. He has focused on finding ways to prevent people from disconfirming others. Laing (1967) describes the opposite of confirmation as being those "attempts to constrain the other's freedom, to force him to act in the way we desire, but with ultimate lack of concern, with indifference to the other's own existence or destiny" (p. 36). From the existential point of view, individuals search for meaning in their lives and this search is often confirmed or disconfirmed by others.

A second way of conceptualizing confirmation is by examining specific communication behaviors that have been described by researchers as either confirming or disconfirming communication. Confirming and disconfirming responses were first identified in studies by Sieburg (1969) and Sieburg and Larson (1971). Sieburg's initial work included a factor analytical study of a list of "ways of responding" and people's preferences for these ways of responding in their interactions with others. Two major factors that described the communication responses emerged from her analysis: The first factor, identified as *confirming responses*, included items labeled direct acknowledgment, agreement about content, supportive responses, clarification, and expression of positive feelings (Table 2–7). The second factor, identified as *disconfirming responses*, included imperviousness, interruption, irrelevance, tangential responses, impersonal responses, incoherence, and incongruous responses (Table 2–8).

Receiving confirming responses can validate an individuals' experience in three ways (Sieburg, 1975, pp. 9–10):

1. Confirming responses decrease a person's fears of depersonalization by acknowledging that person's presence; they confirm the receiver's feeling, "I exist." For example, health professionals who show confirmation to clients are communicating to clients the obvious but extremely important message that the professional is aware of the presence of the client as a unique human being.
2. Confirming responses relieve the individual's fears of being blamed

TABLE 2–7. CONFIRMING RESPONSES

Confirming responses make another person value himself or herself more as an individual. They acknowledge the other's existence as a unique person.

The following responses are characterized as confirming:

1. *Direct acknowledgment.* To respond directly to what the other person communicated. To attend directly to another.
2. *Agreement about content.* To reinforce or support what the other person is talking about. Examples: "Yes, that is an important area." "At least now I can see your side of the issue."
3. *Supportive response.* To express understanding, reassurance, or to try to make the other person feel better. Examples: "I think I know what you mean." "With your attitude, I know you'll do well." "I'm impressed with the progress you are making."
4. *Clarification.* To attempt to make the content of another's message or the other's present or past feelings more understandable. This may include asking for further information or encouraging the other person to express in greater detail how he or she feels. Examples (content): "Tell me more about your reasoning for that point." "I'm not sure I understand; could you explain it further?" Examples (feelings): "Could you describe for me how you feel about that person?" In attempting to clarify the other person's feelings, the emphasis is on description, not on interpreting the feelings.
5. *Expression of positive feelings.* To respond to another person with affirming uncritical feelings. Example: "I'm glad you told me that." "What you said makes me want to look further into this."

Adapted from Sieburg, E. (1969). Dysfunctional communication and interpersonal responsiveness in small groups. (Doctoral dissertation, University of Denver, 1969.) Dissertation Abstracts International, 30, 2622A. University Microfilm No. 69-21, 156.

TABLE 2–8. DISCONFIRMING RESPONSES

Disconfirming responses deny the other person's existence. These responses are inappropriate or irrelevant to what the other person has communicated. They make the other person value herself or himself less as an individual.

Disconfirming responses may be characterized as follows:

1. *Impervious.* To ignore or disregard the other person's attempt to communicate by making no verbal or nonverbal acknowledgment of what they have communicated.

2. *Interruptive.* To cut the speaker off before she or he has a chance to finish a statement or fully elaborate on a point.

3. *Irrelevant.* To respond in an unrelated way to what another person has communicated. This can be done by introducing a new topic or shifting to a previous topic without warning.

4. *Tangential.* To acknowledge what the other has said, but to immediately take the conversation in another direction. Examples: "Yes, I know you're having pains in your stomach, but I'm concerned that you're not getting enough exercise." "Yes, I see the problem, but I'm sure it will go away. Let me tell you how another one of my friends got around this problem."

5. *Impersonal.* To respond in the third person in an intellectualized tone. This type of response often contains many cliches and euphemisms. Examples: "The problem with working double shifts is that one is always tired and prone to make many mistakes." "In debating that particular position, you people need more evidence."

6. *Incoherent.* To respond in incomplete sentences or long, rambling speeches. This response is often difficult to follow because it contains much retracing and rephrasing which adds nothing to the content of the message.

7. *Incongruous.* To act in a way that differs from what you say. It is sending two messages (verbal and nonverbal) that are not consistent. Examples: "No, you're not bothering me" *(stated in a high voice with shaky hands).*

Adapted from Sieburg, E. (1969). Dysfunctional communication and interpersonal responsiveness in small groups. (Doctoral dissertation, University of Denver, 1969.) Dissertation Abstracts International, 30, 2622A. University Microfilm No. 69–21, 156.

or rejected, by validating the individual's own way of experiencing events. Individuals learn to feel that their own perspective is legitimate and that it is all right for them to be who they are.

3. Confirming responses reduce feelings of loneliness, alienation, and abandonment by creating in the receiver the undeniable feeling that he or she is engaged in a human relationship with another person. In essence, the confirming response is saying to the receiver, "I see you, you are OK, and you and I have established a relationship."

Applications of Confirmation in Health Care

Throughout this book it has been stressed that health professionals have a responsibility to be sensitive to the circumstances of clients and to assist clients in finding ways to participate in their own treatment. Of all the variables discussed in this chapter, confirmation is probably the most important in this process.

Confirmation: The Client's Perspective

Only a limited amount of research has been conducted on confirmation in health care settings. Heinekin (1982) studied confirmation in the context of nursing practice by comparing the interpersonal responses of four groups of psychiatric clients with the responses of a group of "normal" individuals. She found that psychiatric clients engaged in significantly more disconfirming communication than did the people in the control group. An important implication of this study was that when psychiatric clients used primarily disconfirming communication, they were likely to receive disconfirming responses from others. Based on her research, Heineken encourages health providers to observe clients' interactions and, where necessary, to teach clients ways to use more confirming communication with others.

Drew (1986) studied confirming and excluding (i.e., disconfirming) responses between hospitalized patients and their caregivers. She found that patients who felt excluded by a caregiver experienced fear and anger and saw themselves as a bother to the caregiver. In addition, disconfirmed patients hesitated to ask the caregiver questions and found their interactions tiring. On the other hand, patients who received confirming responses from caregivers said that the caregivers' warm, nurturing responses gave them feelings of strength and relaxation. Patients who were confirmed also had more confidence in their ability to cope with their situations, and they felt that they had more energy to direct toward their recovery.

When health professionals' communication is confirming, it helps clients in a variety of ways. First, through communicating in confirming ways, health professionals provide recognition of clients as unique persons with real problems. Clients often feel like inanimate objects, as if they were objects rather than people. A vivid illustration of this is provided in the following example of a nurse who was a patient in a rehabilitation hospital.

One day, as I was sitting on the toilet, a volunteer brought a group of visitors through the bathroom. The volunteer threw back the curtain that served as the door of the toilet stall, exposing both me and my wheelchair (the latter of which was slightly more socially acceptable at that moment). Then the volunteer proudly announced to the group of visitors, "This is one of our quadriplegics!" I literally felt as though I was nothing, and as far as meaning anything, I did not. I might just as well have been a resident on Monkey Island at the zoo. In order to reconfirm that I was indeed somebody, I shouted a few phrases that would have made a longshoreman blush. The volunteer and the visitors retreated while uttering comments about what an ungrateful, uncouth wretch I was. Well, at least "ungrateful and uncouth" constitutes an identity of sorts and one which at that moment I preferred to no identity at all.[2]

---

[2] Jean A. Werner-Beland, *Grief Responses to Long-Term Illness and Disability*, 1980, p. 181. Reprinted with permission of Reston Publishing Co., a Prentice-Hall Co., 11480 Sunset Hills Road, Reston, VA 22090.

In the above situation, the nurse loudly voiced a desire to be treated as a person and not as an object to be studied. Clients are vulnerable and, unfortunately, easily viewed only as cases—the "gallbladder in room 518," "the triple bypass in the stepdown unit," or the "C-section in 306"—which negates their humanness. Although these labels are not intended to be harmful in any way, they are examples of the subtle ways in which health professionals disconfirm clients. Health professionals have a responsibility to recognize clients as *people* with unique, innate human needs.

Second, by confirming communication, health professionals assure clients that their responses to illness and their concerns are normal, and that they will not be rejected for the feelings they experience. Clients in health care settings find themselves in a strange environment, and they are often expected to do things they would not normally have to do in their home setting, such as wearing identifying wristbands, urinating in plastic cups, and exposing their bodies to the scrutiny of numerous people. Not only do these new situations and relationships produce stress, but they also can result in clients' developing feelings of being different. It is not unusual for clients to wonder if they are coping adequately with these changes and if their responses are appropriate.

For example, the woman who is experiencing acute grief over the loss of her husband may sometimes hear the voice of her deceased husband and wonder whether she is going crazy. An informed health professional who understands the grieving process can confirm her response as being perfectly normal. In another situation, while clients are waiting for laboratory results, X-ray readings, or pathology reports that sometimes take a long time to return, they may react to the uncertainty of the situation by conjuring up their own reasons for the delays. For example, a client may think, "They must have found something bad that they don't want to tell me about." Or, "It must mean that something really unusual is going on." Clients will interpret the events around them in their own unique way and probably much differently from the way in which we health professionals would interpret the same event. A health professional can give a confirming response to clients' reactions in these uncertain situations. Confirmation does not have to mean that health professionals *agree* with clients—just that it is all right for clients to respond in their own way.

Third, we have observed that confirmation is also important in providing clients in health care settings with a sense of connectedness. In our communities, we confirm those "in need" when we help them maintain a connectedness to their health care system. Jezewski (1995), for example, in a study of how to facilitate health care for homeless persons, suggests that "staying connected" is the *essence* of what nurses and other providers do to help homeless individuals cope with health concerns. In hospitals, clients can feel disconnected, not only from family and work, but even from the health professionals who are caring for them. These feelings are illustrated in the following comments a patient made to one of the authors about her intense feelings of alienation while undergoing a series of exploratory surgeries.

I wish I knew what was happening. No one seems to know what's going on around here. Are they going to have to operate on me again? What did the last biopsy show? Why are they doing more X-rays? Will the same person operate if they choose to do more surgery? Who is coordinating all of this? I feel like no one is in charge of what's happening to me. No one cares a bit. I'm a cabbage sitting here in a field: I'm left out and no one even knows it.

This client was describing deep feelings of fear that things were happening to her and that the health professionals around her did not seem to be concerned. She wanted and needed information and confirmation. Information concerning her X-rays, biopsies, and surgeries would have helped to lessen her fears of being a meaningless object (a cabbage in a field) that no one cared about. Acknowledging her circumstances (the lack of coordination) through confirming responses would have reduced her feelings of alienation and helped her to feel involved with health professionals in her own treatment.

The professional–client conversations provided in Tables 2–9 and 2–10 illustrate the difference between disconfirming and confirming responses. In the first conversation (Table 2–9), the nurse unintentionally disconfirms the client and leaves the client feeling that his concerns are unimportant. In

TABLE 2–9. EXAMPLE OF DISCONFIRMING INTERACTION BETWEEN PROFESSIONAL AND CLIENT

Interactants	Disconfirming Interaction	Kind of Response
Male Patient:	You know, I'm kind of worried about this knee surgery. . . . Seems a little silly, doesn't it, compared to all those other guys who have to have back surgery and heart surgery . . . ?	
Nurse:	There is nothing for you to worry about. . . . The surgery is fairly easy and won't take too long *(straightening up the room).*	Impervious Irrelevant
Male Patient:	I guess you're right. It's kind of crazy of me to worry. I've got to stop overreacting to things, I guess *(nervously laughing).*	
Nurse:	Why don't you try to watch a little TV? Watching TV helps to keep your mind off other things *(walking out of the room).*	Irrelevant Impersonal

TABLE 2–10. EXAMPLE OF CONFIRMING INTERACTION BETWEEN PROFESSIONAL AND CLIENT

Interactants	Confirming Interaction	Kind of Response
Male Patient:	You know, I'm kind of worried about this knee surgery. . . . Seems a little silly, doesn't it, compared to all those other guys who have to have back surgery and heart surgery . . . ?	
Nurse:	No, I can understand that you might be worried. What are you especially concerned about?	Direct acknowledgment Clarification
Male Patient:	Well, I kind of wonder how I'm going to get around at home. My wife hasn't been too well, and she depends on me to do a lot of things for her. Kind of crazy of me to be so worried about this surgery, isn't it?	
Nurse:	No, I think it's very understandable to wonder how the surgery is going to affect your life, especially with your wife depending on you the way she does.	Direct acknowledgment Supportive

the second conversation (Table 2–10), because the nurse is more confirming, the client is able to express his underlying concerns and will probably be able to solve his problems more productively.

Based on a study of patients and their caregivers, Drew (1986) developed a list of caregivers' behaviors that confirm rather than exclude clients. Caregivers who engaged in confirming behaviors used a wide range of affective responses, had a relaxed yet energetic manner, maintained eye contact, used an expressive tone of voice, avoided jargon, and kept a close position to the patient while speaking. Conversely, caregivers who engaged in excluding behaviors lacked warmth, seemed hurried, avoided eye contact, used a flat tone of voice and an abrupt manner of speaking, used jargon as a distancing maneuver, and avoided physical closeness to the patient. Clearly, confirming behaviors will promote more effective interpersonal relationships between clients and health professionals.

Although it is important to show confirmation to others, it is not always easy for providers to do so. Many clients present challenges that make confirmation difficult for providers. For example, Fraser and Gallop (1993) found that psychiatric patients with the diagnosis of borderline personality disorder (BPD) received significantly less confirming responses from nurses than patients with affective disorder or other diagnoses. Interactions with the patients with BPD was difficult for providers because these patients were overly controlling and manipulative. Showing confirmation to patients in contexts such as these takes a great deal of understanding and a high degree of interpersonal competence.

Confirmation: The Professional's Perspective

Confirmation is essential for clients, but it is also important for nurses and other health professionals. Perhaps one of the reasons for this is that health professionals themselves experience so little confirmation from clients and other health professionals. Time pressures, rotating shifts, and staff shortages make it difficult for professionals to share in meaningful communication with others. In this environment, it is not surprising that nurses and other health professionals often feel as if they are just one of many cogs in a wheel.

Just as clients have a need to be treated personally, professionals also have a need to be seen by others as fully human and able to make unique professional contributions to the health care process. Health professionals dislike being treated as insignificant persons. For example, a psychiatric nurse who develops a treatment plan for a depressed client does not like to hear that the psychologist working with the patient has cancelled the treatment plan because it did not originate with him or her. The psychologist's decision to invalidate the treatment plan disconfirms the psychiatric nurse as an independent professional who is competent to make assessments and formulate treatment plans. Similarly, a medical social worker who arranges a discharge planning meeting with an entire staff to discuss procedures for placing patients in nursing homes does not want to learn at the start of the meeting that the attending physician on the unit is not going to be present. In this example, the physician's absence communicates that the social worker's professional actions (to call a planning meeting) are without value and significance. These examples by no means exhaust the impersonal and disconfirming ways in which professionals treat each other.

Furthermore, health professionals, like clients, also have a need to feel accepted and worthwhile. Although they seldom say it out loud, many professionals have a strong desire to be viewed as integral members of the health care team. They want to participate, make contributions, and be involved. Nurses, social workers, health educators, chaplains, physicians, pharmacists, physical therapists, occupational therapists, and others, each have unique contributions that they want to offer the health care team and that they think deserve feedback from others on the team.

Health care settings sometimes demand that professionals work in isolation from each other in order to fulfill professional responsibilities. The tasks to be performed by professionals can become so numerous and so complex that professionals seem to have little or no time for personal interaction. Nonetheless, professionals want and need to be related to others. Being confirmed by other professionals satisfies health professionals' desire to be humanly connected to the helping process.

There is some indication that confirming and disconfirming responses are reciprocal in nature (Garvin & Kennedy, 1986; Sundell, 1972). As a result, a chain reaction can occur, which begins when health professionals who feel disconfirmed lack the emotional energy to become involved with

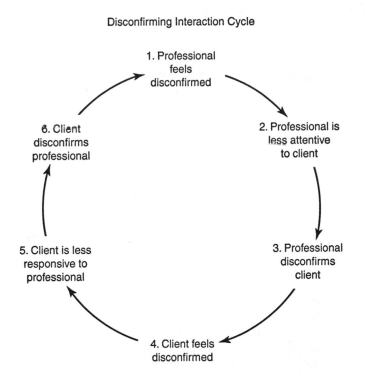

Disconfirming Interaction Cycle

1. Professional feels disconfirmed

2. Professional is less attentive to client

3. Professional disconfirms client

4. Client feels disconfirmed

5. Client is less responsive to professional

6. Client disconfirms professional

Figure 2–4. The cyclical process of disconfirming communication showing the negative effect it has on communication between professionals and clients.

clients, whom they then treat as objects (Fig. 2–4). Clients who are experiencing emotional isolation will increase their own disconfirming responses toward the staff. Health professionals interpret these responses as further evidence that they are misunderstood and not appreciated. This chain of reactions can continue until the client is discharged or until one of the persons in the interaction actively seeks to alter this "vicious cycle."

Interrupting a disconfirming cycle is not easy because system pressures often keep it going. Although changing system pressures is not always possible, learning to alter interpersonal communication patterns is possible. A change toward showing more confirmation of others is not a cure-all for health communication problems, but confirmation can definitely benefit professionals as well as clients. Tables 2–11 and 2–12 illustrate how confirmation can significantly affect professional–professional interaction. In the first conversation (Table 2–11), the night supervisor fails to acknowledge the pressures being experienced by the staff nurse and hence reacts to the nurse with impervious, irrelevant, tangential, and impersonal disconfirming responses. The end result of the conversation is distant communication, more similar to monologue than dialogue. In the second con-

TABLE 2–11. EXAMPLE OF DISCONFIRMING INTERACTION BETWEEN TWO PROFESSIONALS

Interactants	Disconfirming Interaction	Kind of Response
Staff Nurse:	We're really busy here tonight. We're short of staff and E.R. has sent up three new patients to be admitted. I'm feeling hassled and in need of some help.	
Night Supervisor:	You wouldn't believe it but things are that way throughout the hospital. You should have been here last night.	Impervious Irrelevant
Staff Nurse:	It couldn't have been much worse than tonight. It seems like it's impossible to do everything. It's really a problem.	
Night Supervisor:	I know, but it's always going to be this way when the census is up. One just has to stay with it and do what one can do.	Tangential Impersonal

versation (Table 2–12), the night supervisor, using confirming responses, is able to have a more meaningful interaction with the staff nurse, and identifies strong feelings and concerns of the nurse. The scenario in the first interaction perpetuates a disconfirming cycle, while in the second encounter, the night supervisor alters the interaction, and both people feel confirmed.

TABLE 2–12. EXAMPLE OF CONFIRMING INTERACTION BETWEEN TWO PROFESSIONALS

Interactants	Confirming Interaction	Kind of Response
Staff Nurse:	We're really busy here tonight. We're short of staff and E.R. has sent up three new patients to be admitted. I'm feeling hassled and in need of some help.	
Night Supervisor:	I can see you're under pressure here. This place is really busy. As far as additional staff to help out, I don't know what to tell you. All the float-staff have already been assigned.	Direct acknowledgment Agreement about content
Staff Nurse:	On nights like this, trying to fulfill *all* my responsibilities really makes me feel uptight. I want everything to get done but I just can't do it all by myself.	
Night Supervisor:	I understand your situation. You're trying to do *everything* but it's impossible. I'm glad you've made me aware of this. I'll try to get more staff up here to relieve some of this pressure, if I can.	Supportive response Expression of positive feelings

Some research suggests that health professionals are starting to use more confirming communication with one another. Garvin and Kennedy (1986) analyzed videotapes of interactions between nurses and resident physicians in a laboratory setting and found that 87 percent of their communication was confirming rather than disconfirming. Although the investigators point out that the laboratory setting was not the same as a complex clinical practice setting, they believe that the results of their study indicate that nurses and physicians have the potential to interact with one another in mutually respectful ways (Garvin & Kennedy, 1988).

Effective communication in health care depends on health professionals who will continuously assess their interactions with clients and peers. Conscious attempts to use confirming communication responses that are based on the underlying belief in the uniqueness of people and the uniqueness of their responses to situations provide the means for clients and professionals to experience connectedness with others and for them to experience minimal alienation and rejection.

▶ SUMMARY

In this chapter, conceptual frameworks of five selected communication variables were presented and the effects of these variables on the communication of clients and professionals in health care settings were discussed. Our intention has been to demonstrate how the application of these variables—empathy, control, trust, self-disclosure, and confirmation—can enhance health communication.

Empathy is the process of observing the world from another person's point of view. It is a complex variable that involves cognitive, affective, and communicative components. Through empathy, clients are helped to feel that they are understood, accepted, and that they have a sense of control over their circumstances. For professionals, empathy improves the accuracy of communication and reduces misunderstanding.

Control is an intrinsic part of human interaction. There are two kinds of control: personal and relational. When individuals sense that they can influence the circumstances surrounding their lives, they have personal control. In health care, clients have intense needs for personal control. Relational control is the process whereby individuals share influence with other individuals within relationships. Three kinds of relationships can be established through different approaches to relational control: complementary, symmetrical, and parallel. A willingness to adapt one's own needs for control to the needs of others is the key to building productive relationships. Effective professional–professional and professional–client relationships are usually based on shared control.

Trust is present in relationships when individuals feel that they can rely on others. Being able to trust health professionals as competent and caring helps clients face the fears and uncertainties of illness. In professional–professional and professional–client relationships, building trust requires that individuals' communication be descriptive rather than evaluative, problem oriented rather than control oriented, spontaneous rather than strategic, empathic rather than neutral, equal rather than superior, and provisional rather than certain.

Self-disclosure is a process in which an individual communicates personal information, thoughts, and feelings to others. If exhibited appropriately, self-disclosure has many benefits for clients and professionals. If there is too much or too little disclosure, or if it is given in inappropriate circumstances, it can be maladaptive. In health care settings, many factors make it difficult for both clients and professionals to self-disclose. Nevertheless, it is important for health care organizations to foster reasoned self-disclosure in client–professional and professional–professional relationships.

Confirmation refers to the communication that enables others to value themselves more fully as unique human beings. By communicating in confirming ways, health professionals help clients to cope with feelings of depersonalization, rejection, and alienation. Confirming responses show to others direct acknowledgment, agreement about content, supportiveness, clarification, and expression of positive feelings. Disconfirming responses are impervious, interruptive, irrelevant, tangential, impersonal, incoherent, and incongruous. Professionals need confirmation from other professionals just as much as clients need confirmation from professionals.

Each of these five variables describes a different component in the highly complex process of health communication. By observing these variables from both the client's perspective and the professional's point of view, the communication that takes place in health care settings can be enhanced.

► REFERENCES

Antonovsky, A. (1988). *Unravelling the mystery of health.* San Francisco: Jossey-Bass.

Attwell, J. R., Flanigan, R. C., Bennett, R. L., Allen, D. C., Lucas, B. A., & McRoberts, J. W. (1984). The efficacy of patient-controlled analgesia in patients recovering from flank incisions. *Journal of Urology, 132,* 701–703.

Barrett-Lennard, G. T. (1962). Dimensions of therapist response as causal factors in therapeutic change. *Psychological Monographs, 76*(43), 1-36.

Barrett-Lennard, G. T. (1981). The empathy cycle: Refinement of a nuclear concept. *Journal of Counseling Psychology, 28*(2), 91–100.

Beisecker, A. E. (1990). Patient power in doctor–patient communication: What do we know? *Health Communication, 2*(2), 105–122.

Bowker, J. (1996). Cancer, individual process, and control: A case study in metaphor analysis. *Health Communication, 8*(1), 91-104.

Bradac, J. J., Tardy, C. H., & Hosman, L. A. (1980). Disclosure styles and a hint at their genesis. *Human Communication Research, 6*(3), 228–238.

Braithwaite, D. O. (1988). *Just How Much Did That Wheelchair Cost? Management of Privacy Boundaries and Demands for Self-Disclosure by Persons with Disabilities.* Paper presented at the annual meeting of the Speech Communication Association, New Orleans, LA.

Buber, M. (1957). Distance and relation. *Psychiatry, 20*, 97–104.

Cantor, R. C. (1978). *And a time to live: Toward emotional well-being during the crisis of cancer.* New York: Harper & Row.

Cassileth, B. R., Zupkis, R. Y., Sutton-Smith, K., & March, Y. (1980). Information and participation preferences among cancer patients. *Annals of Internal Medicine, 92,* 832-836.

Chaikin, A. L., & Derlega, V. J. (1974a). Liking for the norm-breaker in self-disclosure. *Journal of Personality; 42,* 117–129.

Chaikin, A. L. & Derlega, V. J. (1974b). Variables affecting the appropriateness of self-disclosure. *Journal of Consulting and Clinical Psychology, 42,* 588–593.

Cissna, K. N., & Sieburg, E. (1981). Patterns of interactional confirmation and disconfirmation. In C. Wilder-Mott & J. Weakland (Eds.), *Rigor and imagination* (pp. 230–239). Wesport, CT: Praeger.

Coates, D., Wortman, C. B., & Abbey, A. (1979). Reactions to victims. In I. H. Frieze, D. Bar-tal, & J. S. Carroll (Eds.), *New approaches to social problems.* San Francisco: Jossey-Bass.

Cozby, P. C. (1973). Self-disclosure: A literature review. *Psychological Bulletin, 79*(2), 73–91.

Dabbs, J. M., & Kirscht, J. P. (1971). "'Internal control" and taking of influenza shots. *Psychological Reports, 28,* 959–962.

Davis, M. H. (1983). Measuring individual differences in empathy: Evidence for a multidimensional approach. *Journal of Personality and Social Psychology, 44*(1), 113–126.

Dawson, C., Schirner, M., & Beck, L. (1984). A patient self-disclosure instrument. *Research in Nursing and Health, 7,* 135–147.

Degner, L. F., & Russell, C. A. (1988). Preferences for treatment control among adults with cancer. *Research in Nursing and Health, 11,* 367–374.

Derlega, V. J., & Chaikin, A. (1977). Privacy and self-disclosure in social relationships. *Journal of Social Issues, 33*(3), 102–115.

Deutsch, M. (1958). Trust and suspicion. *Journal of Conflict Resolution, 2,* 265–279.

Deutsch, M. (1960). Trust, trustworthiness, and the F Scale. *Journal of Abnormal and Social Psychology, 61*(1), 138–140.

Drew, N. (1986). Exclusion and confirmation: A phenomenology of patients' experiences with caregivers. *Image, 18*(2), 39–43.

Engel, N. S. (1980). Confirmation and validation: The caring that is professional nursing. *Image, 12*(3), 53–56.

Forsyth, G. L. (1979). Exploration of empathy in nurse–client interaction. *Advances in Nursing Science, 1,* 53-61.

Forsyth, G. L. (1980). Analysis of the concept of empathy: Illustration of an approach. *Advances in Nursing Science, 2*(2), 33–42.

Frankl, V. (1963). *Man's search for meaning: An introduction to logotherapy.* New York: Simon & Schuster. (Originally published 1959.)

Fraser, K., & Gallop, R. (1993). Nurses' confirming/disconfirming responses to patients diagnosed with borderline personality disorder. *Archives of Psychiatric Nursing, 7*(6), 336–341.

Friedman, H. S., & DiMatteo, M. R. (1979). Health care as an interpersonal process. *Journal of Social Issues, 35*(1), 1–11.

Garvin, B. J., & Kennedy, C. W. (1986). Confirmation–disconfirmation: A framework for the study of interpersonal relationships. In P. Chinn (Ed.), *Nursing research methodology.* Rockville, MD: Aspen.

Garvin, B. J., & Kennedy, C. W. (1988). Confirming communication of nurses in interactions with physicians. *Journal of Nursing Education. 27*(4), 161–166.

Gibb, J. R. (1961). Defensive communication. *The Journal of Communication 11*(3),141–148.

Giffin, K. (1967). The contribution of studies of source credibility to a theory of interpersonal trust in the communication process. *Psychological Bulletin, 68,*104–120.

Gladstein, G. A. (1983). Understanding empathy: Integrating counseling, developmental, and social psychology perspectives. *Journal of Counseling Psychology 30*(4), 467–482.

Gotcher, J. M. (1992). Interpersonal communication and psychosocial adjustment. *Journal of Psychosocial Oncology, 10,* 21–39.

Heineken, J. R. (1982). Disconfirmation in dysfunctional communication. *Nursing Research, 31,* 211–213.

Hobart, C. W., & Fahlberg, N. (1965). The measurement of empathy. *American Journal of Sociology, 70,* 595–603.

Hogan, R. (1969). Development of an empathy scale. *Journal of Consulting and Clinical Psychology, 33,* 307–316.

Jezewski, M. A. (1995). Staying connected: The core of facilitating health care for homeless persons. *Public Health Nursing, 12*(3), 203–210.

Johnson, J. E., & Leventhal, H. (1974). Effects of accurate expectations and behavioral instructions on reactions during a noxious medical examination. *Journal of Personality and Social Psychology, 29,* 710–718.

Johnson, J. L., & Morse, J. M. (1990). Regaining control: The process of adjustment after myocardial infarction. *Heart & Lung, 19*(2), 126–135.

Johnson, M. N. (1980). Self-disclosure: A variable in the nurse–client relationship. *Journal of Psychiatric Nursing and Mental Health Services, 18,* 17–20.

Jourard, S. M. (1964). *The transparent self.* Princeton, NJ: Van Nostrand Reinhold.

Jourard, S. M. (1968). *Disclosing man to himself.* Princeton, NJ: Van Nostrand Reinhold.

Jourard, S. M. (1971). *The transparent self* (2nd ed.). New York: Van Nostrand Reinhold.

Jourard, S., & Lasakow, P. (1958). Some factors in self-disclosure. *Journal of Abnormal and Social Psychology, 51,* 91–98.

Kalisch, B. J. (1973). What is empathy? *American Journal of Nursing, 73*(9), 1548–1552.

Kaplan, S. H., Greenfield, S., & Ware, J. E., Jr. (1989). Impact of the doctor–patient relationship on the outcomes of chronic disease. In M. Stewart & D. Roter (Eds.), *Communicating with medical patients* (pp. 228–245). Newbury Park: CA: Sage.

Katon, W., & Kleinman, A. (1981). Doctor–patient negotiation and other social science strategies in patient care. In L. Eisenberg & A. Kleinman (Eds.), *The relevance of social science for medicine* (pp. 253–282). Dordrecht, Holland: D. Reidel.

Klotkowski, D. (1980). Self-disclosure: Implications for mental health. *Perspectives in Psychiatric Care, 18*(3), 112–115.

Laing, R. D. (1967). *The politics of experience.* New York: Pantheon.

Lamb, G. S., & Napodano, R. J. (1984). Physician–nurse practitioner interaction patterns in primary care practices. *American Journal of Public Health, 74,* 26–29.

LaMonica, E. L. (1981). Construct validity of an empathy instrument. *Research in Nursing and Health, 4*(4), 389–400.

Langer, E. J. (1983). *The psychology of control.* Beverly Hills, CA: Sage.

Lazure, L. L., & Baun, M. M. (1995). Increasing patient control of family visiting in the coronary care unit. *American Journal of Critical Care, 4*(2), 157–164.

Lewis, F. (1982a). Research questions and answers: Health locus of control. *Oncology Nursing Forum, 9*(3), 108–109.

Lewis, F. (1982b). Experienced personal control and quality of life in late-stage cancer patients. *Nursing Research, 31*(2), 113–119.

Limandri, B. J. (1989). Disclosure of stigmatizing conditions: The discloser's perspective. *Archives of Psychiatric Nursing, 3*(2), 69–78.

Lipps, T. (1909). *Leitfaden der Psychologie.* Leipzig: Engelmann.

Loveridge, C. E., & Heineken, J. (1988). Confirming interactions. *Journal of Gerontological Nursing, 14*(5), 27–30.

Lowery, B. J. (1981). Misconceptions and limitations of locus of control and the I–E Scale. *Nursing Research, 30*(5), 294–298.

Luce, R. D., & Raiffa, H. (1957). *Games and decisions: Introduction and critical survey.* New York: Wiley.

MacDonald, A. P. (1970). Internal–external locus of control and the practice of birth control. *Psychological Reports, 27,* 206.

Makoul, G., Arntson, P., & Schofield, T. (1995). Health promotion in primary care: Physician–patient communication and decision making about prescription medications. *Social Science and Medicine, 41*(9), 1241–1254.

McIntosh, J. (1974). Processes of communication, information seeking and control associated with cancer: A selective review of the literature. *Social Science and Medicine, 8,* 167–187.

Mehrabian, A., & Epstein, N. (1972). A measure of emotional empathy. *Journal of Personality, 40,* 525–543.

Mitchell, G. W., & Glicksman, A. S. (1977). Cancer patients: Knowledge and attitudes. *Cancer, 40,* 61–66.

Mlott, S. R., & Mlott, Y. D. (1975). Dogmatism and laws of control in individuals who smoke, stopped smoking, and never smoked. *Journal of Community Psychology, 3,* 53–57.

Montbriand, M. J. (1995). Alternative therapies as control behaviors used by cancer patients. *Journal of Advanced Nursing, 22,* 646–654.

Morse, J. M., Anderson, G., Bottorff, J. L., Yonge, O., O'Brien, B., Solberg, S. M., & McIlveen, K. H. (1992). Exploring empathy: A conceptual fit for nursing practice. *Image, 24,* 273–280.

Morton, T. L., Alexander, J. F., & Altman, I. (1976). Communication and relationship definition. In G. R. Miller (Ed.), *Explorations in interpersonal communications* (pp. 105–125). Beverly Hills, CA: Sage.

Moser, D. K., & Dracup, K. (1995). Psychosocial recovery from a cardiac event: The influence of perceived control. *Heart & Lung, 24*(4), 273–280.

Naber, S. J., Halstead, L. K., Broome, M. E., & Rehwaldt, M. (1995). *Communication and control: Parent, child, and health care professional interactions during painful procedures.* Issues in Comprehensive Pediatric Nursing, 18, 79–90.

Northouse, P. G. (1979). Interpersonal trust and empathy in nurse–nurse relationships. *Nursing Research, 28*(6), 365–368.

Northouse, P. G., & Northouse, L. L. (1987). Communication and cancer: Issues confronting patients, health professionals, and family members. *Journal of Psychosocial Oncology, 5*(3), 17–46.

Olson, J. K. (1995). Relationships between nurse-expressed empathy, patient-perceived empathy, and patient distress. *Image, 27*(4), 317–322.

Pearce, W. B. (1974). Trust in interpersonal communication. *Speech Monographs, 41,* 236–244.

Pepler, C. J., & Lynch, A. (1991). Relational messages of control in nurse–patient interactions with terminally ill patients with AIDS and cancer. *Journal of Palliative Care, 7*(1), 18–29.

Peters-Golden, H. (1982). Breast cancer: Varied perceptions of social support in the illness experience. *Social Science and Medicine, 16,* 483–491.

Raudonis, B. M. (1993). The meaning and impact of empathic relationships in hospice nursing. *Cancer Nursing, 16*(4), 304–309.

Rock, D. L., Meyerowitz, B. E., Maisto, S. A., & Wallston, K. A. (1987). The derivation and validation of six multidimensional health locus of control scale clusters. *Research in Nursing and Health, 10,* 185–195.

Rogers, C. R. (1951). *Client-centered therapy.* Boston: Houghton Mifflin.

Rogers, C. R. (1957). The necessary and sufficient conditions of therapeutic personality change. *Journal of Consulting Psychology, 21,* 95–103.

Rogers, C. R. (1958). A process conception of psychotherapy. *American Psychologist, 13,* 142–149.

Rogers, C. R. (1959). A theory of therapy, personality, and interpersonal relationships, as developed in the client-centered framework. In S. Koch (Ed.), *Psychology: A study of a science, Vol. 3. Formulations of the person and the social context* (pp. 184–256). New York: McGraw-Hill.

Rogers, C. R. (1961). Characteristics of a helping relationship. In C. R. Rogers (Ed.), *On becoming a person* (pp. 39–58). Boston: Houghton Mifflin.

Rogers, C. R. (1975). Empathic: An unappreciated way of being. *The Counseling Psychologist, 5*(2), 2–10.

Rotter, J. B. (1954). *Social learning and clinical psychology.* Englewood Cliffs, NJ: Prentice-Hall.

Rotter, J. B. (1966). Generalized expectancies for internal versus external control of reinforcement. *Psychological Monographs, 50*(1) (Whole No. 609).

Rotter, J. B. (1967). A new scale for the measurement of interpersonal trust. *Journal of Personality, 35,* 651–665.

Rotter, J. B. (1975). Some problems and misconceptions related to the construct of internal versus external control of reinforcement. *Journal of Consulting Clinical Psychology, 43,* 56–67.

Seeman, M., & Evans, J. W. (1962). Alienation and learning in a hospital setting. *American Sociological Review, 27,* 772–783.

Seeman, M., & Seeman, T. E. (1983). Health behavior and personal autonomy: A longitudinal study of the sense of control in illness. *Journal of Health and Social Behavior, 24,* 144–160.

Seligman, M. E. P. (1975). *Helplessness.* San Francisco: Freeman.

Sieburg, E. (1969). Dysfunctional communication and interpersonal responsiveness in small groups. (Doctoral dissertation, University of Denver, 1969.) *Dissertation Abstracts International, 30,* 2622A. University Microfilms No. 69-21, 156.

Sieburg, E. (1975). Interpersonal confirmation: A paradigm for conceptualization and measurement. San Diego: United States International University. (ERIC Document Reproduction Service No. ED 098 634)

Sieburg, E., & Larson, C. E. (1971). *Dimensions of Interpersonal Response.* Paper presented at the International Communication Association Annual Conference, Phoenix, AZ.

Spiegel, D., Bloom, J., Kraemer, H. C., & Gottheil, E. (1989). Effect of psychosocial treatment on survival in patients with metastatic breast cancer. *Lancet, 2* (8668), 888–891.

Stotland, E., Matthews, K. E., Jr., Sherman, S. E., Hansson, R., & Richardson, B. Z. (1978). *Empathy, fantasy, and helping.* Beverly Hills, CA: Sage.

Strickland, B. R. (1978). Internal–external expectancies and health-related behaviors. *Journal of Consulting and Clinical Psychology, 46,* 1192–1211.

Sundell, W. (1972). The operation of confirming and disconfirming verbal behavior in selected teacher–student interventions. *Dissertation Abstracts International, 33,* 1838A. University Microfilms No. 72-25, 030.

Tagliacozzo, D. L., & Mauksch, H. O. (1979). The patient's view of the patient's role. In E. G. Jaco (Ed.), *Patients, physicians, and illness* (3rd ed.). New York: Free Press.

Taylor, D. A. (1979). Motivational bases. In G. J. Chelune, *Self-disclosure: Origins, patterns, and implications of openness in interpersonal relationships.* San Francisco: Jossey-Bass.

Taylor, S. E. (1979). Hospital patient behavior: Reactance, helplessness, or control? *The Journal of Social Issues, 35*(1), 156–184.

Thompson, S. C. (1981). Will it hurt less if I can control it? A complex answer to a simple question. *Psychological Bulletin, 90*(1), 89–101.

Thompson, S. C., Sobolew-Shubin, A., Galbraith, M. E., Schwankovsky, L., & Cruzen, D. (1993). Maintaining perceptions of control: Finding perceived control in low-control circumstances. *Journal of Personality and Social Psychology, 64,* 293–304.

Thompson, T. L. (1986). *Communication for health professionals.* New York: Harper & Row.

Thompson, T. L., & Seibold, D. R. (1978). Stigma management in normal-stigmatized interactions: Test of the disclosure hypotheses and a model of stigma acceptance. *Human Communication Research, 4*(3), 231–242.

Vinacke, W. E. (1969). Variables in experimental games: Toward a field theory. *Psychological Bulletin, 71,* 293–318.

Wallston, K. A., Maides, S., & Wallston, B. S. (1976). Health-related information seeking as a function of health-related locus of control and health value. *Journal of Research in Personality, 10,* 215–222.

Wallston, B. S., Wallston, K. A., & DeVellis, R. (1978). Locus of control and health: A review of the literature. *Health Education Monograph, 6*(2), 107–117.

Wallston, B. S., Wallston, K. A., Kaplan, G. D., & Maides, S. A. (1976). Development and validation of the health locus of control (HLC) scale. *Journal of Consulting Clinical Psychology, 44,* 580–585.

Watzlawick, P., Beavin, J., & Jackson, D. D. (1967). *Pragmatics of human communication.* New York: Norton.

Wenburg, J. R., & Wilmot, W. W. (1973). *The personal communication process.* New York: Wiley.

Werner-Beland, J. (1980). *Grief responses to long-term illness and disability.* Reston, VA: Reston Publishing.

Wheeler, K. (1988). A nursing science approach to understanding empathy. *Archives of Psychiatric Nursing, 2*(2), 95–102.

Wheeless, L. R. (1978). A follow-up study of the relationships among trust, disclosure, and interpersonal solidarity. *Human Communication Research, 4*(2), 143–157.

Wheeless, L. R., & Grotz, J. (1975). *Self-Disclosure and Trust: Conceptualization, Measurement, and Inter-relationships.* Paper presented at the annual convention of the International Communication Association, Chicago.

Wheeless, L. R., & Grotz, J. (1976). Conceptualization and measurement of reported self-disclosure. *Human Communication Research, 2*(4), 238–246.

Wheeless, L. R., & Grotz, J. (1977). The measurement of trust and its relationship to self-disclosure. *Human Communication Research, 3*(3), 250–257.

Williams, C. (1979). Empathic communication and its effect on client outcome. *Issues in Mental Health Nursing, 2*(1), 16–26.

Wilmot, W. W. (1979). *Dyadic communication: A transactional perspective* (2nd ed.). Reading, MA: Addison-Wesley.

Wispe, L. (1986). The distinction between sympathy and empathy: To call forth a concept, a word is needed. *Journal of Personality and Social Psychology, 50*(2), 314–321.

Wortman, C. B., Adesman, P., Herman, E., & Greenberg, R. (1976). Self-disclosure: An attributional perspective, *Journal of Personality and Social Psychology, 33,* 256–266.

Wortman, C. B., & Brehm, J. W. (1975). Responses to uncontrollable outcomes: An integration of reactance theory and the learned helplessness model. In L. Berkowitz (Ed.), *Advances in experimental social psychology (Vol. 8.). New York: Academic Press.*

Wortman, C. B., & Dunkel-Schetter, C. (1979). Interpersonal relationships and cancer: A theoretical analysis. *Journal of Social Issues, 35*(1), 120–155.

Communication in 3
Health Care Relationships

Numerous kinds of relationships exist in health care settings. These include physician–patient, nurse–social worker, dietitian–family member, and administrator–clinician, to name just a few. Communication that occurs within these relationships is affected by the roles each person plays within the relationship and by the expectations that they hold of one another. Some roles are clearly established and generally accepted within an organization, whereas others are ambiguous.

Presently, in the health care system, the traditional roles of physician, nurse, and patient, are being challenged and are undergoing considerable change. As a result, the stereotyped rules that previously governed these roles and relationships are no longer valid. For example, it is no longer true that the physician gives the order, the nurse carries it out, and the patient accepts it. Changing roles have increased role ambiguity, stress in relationships, and communication difficulties among participants.

In keeping with the health communication model presented in Chapter 1, the present chapter includes discussions of the four major types of relationships in health care settings: (1) professional–patient, (2) professional–professional, (3) professional–family, and (4) patient–family. We will discuss the nature of these relationships and identify potential barriers to effective communication within each type of relationship.

▶ PROFESSIONAL–PATIENT RELATIONSHIPS

The relationship between the person who provides health care and the person who receives the care has been identified as one of the most crucial components of the entire health care delivery process (Ruben, 1990; Thompson, 1990). The professional–patient relationship has been cited as a major factor in patients' failure to follow treatment regimens, in patients' dissatisfaction with the health care system, and in their increased resort to malpractice suits. However, when positive, caring relationships exist between patients and professionals, patients report a greater ability to cope effectively

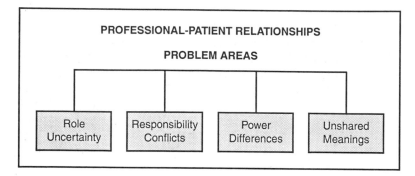

Figure 3–1. Potential barriers to effective communication in professional–patient relationships.

with their illness (Latham, 1996) and greater compliance with health care regimens (Hanna, 1993; Street et al., 1993).

The nature of each professional–patient relationship is influenced by the personal and professional characteristics that both patient and professional bring to the relationship. Characteristics such as an individual's age, sex, ethnic background, personality, and values all impact on the nature of professional–patient communication (Latham, 1996). Professionals' characteristics also have an impact on health communication. The professional's specialty, education, socialization, and aspirations all affect the way in which the professional establishes relationships with patients.

In addition to the unique personal and professional characteristics that influence professional–patient relationships, several other specific factors affect this relationship. Four of these factors that are potential barriers to effective professional–patient communication will be considered in detail: (1) role uncertainty, (2) responsibility conflicts, (3) power differences, and (4) unshared meanings (Fig. 3–1). While there are many other factors that could be identified, these four have been selected because of the central role they play in explaining obstacles to effective professional–patient communication.

Role Uncertainty

One of the key factors affecting communication between the professional and patient involves the expectations that persons hold about their roles in the relationship. To develop an effective relationship, there has to be a fairly high degree of agreement about what the individuals expect of each other, and it also helps if both "sides" are able to revise their expectations. Although it is easy to assume that patients know what is expected of them and what they can expect from health professionals, on closer inspection, it appears that the roles of patient and health professional are not clearly defined.

Patients are often uncertain about what "being a patient" requires. In acute care settings, patients typically enter as loners who are unfamiliar with the physical structure, the organization, and the numerous people with whom they will be dealing. Patients often shed, or at least lose sight of, the familiar roles they occupied before entering the health care agency. Roles of husband, wife, father, mother, employer, employee, sports enthusiast, gardener, and so on are overshadowed by the new role of patient. Although patients may receive brief introductions to their hospital roommates or a quick tour of their immediate surroundings, they are still left on their own to figure out how they fit into the maze of people and places.

Patients' uncertainty about their role is compounded by the fact that they have to interact with a variety of health providers in both community and acute care settings. Considering that a hospitalized patient may be in contact with as many as 30 different people within 1 day, it is not surprising that the patient has some confusion about what is expected of him or her (Taylor, 1979). The following comments of a psychiatric patient indicate how patients try to juggle the expectations of a team of people.

So, what are the things the staff expect? Well, if you are talking about the ward staff, they want you to make life easy for them and to not be unreasonable about the hospital rules. You know, do what you are told and not make demands on them. And of course, be considerate and thankful. . . . Now if you are talking about what the therapist wants, that's a different story. Complete trust in her ability to solve all of my problems in 3 or 4 hours of spilling my guts was what she was after. . . . It's hard to say what the expectations of the doctor were. I guess he had more to do than stand around talking to patients. My contacts with him were too indirect to ever learn what he wanted of me. When I wanted special permission to go to town or something, I would go through the nurse to get it. I suppose doc did the same if he wanted something from me. (Templin, 1982, p. 108)

Having to respond to many different demands from many different providers makes the role of patient problematic. Due to shorter hospital stays with less time for coordinated discharge planning, it is not unusual for a patient to be told by the physician that he or she can go home and take it easy, but be told by the nurse to become more active. Contradictory communication from members of the health team increases the patient's uncertainty about his or her behavior. Not wanting to anger one professional or the other, the patient is often in a double bind as to which person's directives to follow. Sorting out lines of authority or determining which of several conflicting messages is correct presents a complex situation for the patient.

Patients who are uncertain about their role sometimes worry that they are asking for too much time from staff or that they are not functioning independently enough. For example, patients may evaluate their own requests for help and assistance by comparing the severity of their own illness to that of other patients, assuming that the more severe the illness, the more appropriate it is to request help from staff members (Tagliacozzo &

Mauksch, 1979). Role uncertainty makes it hard for patients to know how to act, and their communication with health professionals may contain considerable hesitation and ambivalence as illustrated in the following case situation of a woman with viral pneumonia.

I waited as long as I could before calling the doctor. I know how busy he is and I didn't want to bother him. I was very hesitant to make the call. When I got to his office I saw a whole lot of other people who looked worse off than I and I started to think that maybe I was making a lot out of nothing, and that maybe I should have waited a couple more days before contacting him. I was glad when the nurse took my temperature and it was 102 degrees. Usually what happens is that I have a temperature at home and by the time I get to the doctor's office it's normal—then I really feel foolish, and wish that I hadn't bothered him.

Although patients are uncertain about their own roles, they are even more uncertain about the roles of health professionals. The trend away from traditional professional uniforms, such as a cap with a black ribbon for the registered nurse and a long white lab coat for the physician, and toward street clothes and name tags (with small print) in both community and hospital settings eliminates specific ways of identifying different professionals. Ambiguous introductions further complicate matters. For example, "I am Dr. Jones," does not tell patients whether they are dealing with an intern, a resident, a staff physician, a psychologist, or a nurse scientist. Similarly, the introduction, "I am the person who will be working with you today," does not tell the patient whether the person is an aide, a licensed practical nurse, a registered nurse, a clinical nurse specialist, a respiratory therapist, or an occupational therapist. Health professionals often overlook the fact that the patient is unsure of who they are and what can be expected of them. This uncertainty about *what* to expect from *which* professional can make the patient hesitant to talk with the provider.

One cancer patient who had a tracheostomy felt very uncertain about what to expect from which professionals. He wrote a note to his physician that said, "I want to have the nurse I have now all the time. She understands me and likes me. I like her. She knows what to do for me without asking" (White, 1987, p. 313). Trying to ensure that he would get the same nurse each day was this patient's way of dealing with uncertainty.

One of our students made an interesting observation about role expectation. She said,

---

On hotel doors they tell you what they expect—the price, check-in time, and check-out time. Maybe we need that in health care. We could tell people what they can expect of us and what we will expect of them.

The point she makes is important; patients want and deserve to know what they can expect from others in health care settings. Although the movement toward informing patients of their own rights has done a great deal in letting patients know the specific rights that they have within a health care agency (such as the right to refuse treatment or the right to obtain a second opinion), these guidelines seldom indicate what specific kind of care they can expect from which type of professional. The only professional whose role is discussed in the Patient's Bill of Rights is the physician. None of the roles of the many other professionals who will be providing care are addressed in this document.

What happens when patients are uncertain about their roles and the roles of others?

1. Patients may hesitate to raise health concerns because they are uncertain about which of the many professionals is the appropriate one to approach with a problem.
2. Professionals may interpret the lack of initiation on the patient's part to mean that the patient has no concerns, or else that the patient's concerns are only *minimally* important.
3. Patients may express only *physical* concerns but no emotional concerns, because physical concerns seem more legitimate when asking for a professional's time.
4. Uncertainty about roles and expectations can cause the patient and professional to deal with one another in traditional or stereotyped ways, using only a few of one another's resources. For example, patients who think the nurse only dispenses medication will not seek out the nurse for his or her expertise in health matters. If dietitians are seen only as menu distributors, patients will not ask them about other dietary concerns. Each of these problems occurs as a result of role uncertainty.

Considering the potential problems that can occur in the communication patterns of the patient and professional, it becomes apparent that clarifying expectations, negotiating perceived and actual roles, and dealing with one another in a personalized and individualized manner are essential to effective professional–patient relationships.

Responsibility Conflicts

A second barrier that can emerge in professional–patient relationships is conflict over the issue of responsibility. For example, who is responsible for managing the patient's illness—the patient or the health professional? How much patient participation is optimal in promoting desired health outcomes? What happens when the patient and professional do not agree on areas of responsibility and desired levels of involvement in care? With the growing trend to promote self-care and increase patient responsibility, these questions are being debated more among health professionals and consumers. How these issues are negotiated can have considerable impact on the patient–professional relationship and on desired health outcomes (Northouse & Wortman, 1990).

Responsibility conflicts and the problems they can create in professional–patient relationships have been addressed by Brickman and his associates (1982) in their work on models of responsibility in health care. They named their theoretical framework "models of helping and coping" because they believe that how professionals "help" and how patients "cope" are based on their often unspoken beliefs about responsibility (Fig. 3–2). They contend that problems can occur when a professional and patient are operating from different models that do not fit with one another. The models differ in how much responsibility (high or low) the patient bears for causing health problems, and how much responsibility the patient has for finding solutions to his or her problems. Descriptions of the four models follow.

The *moral* model of helping and coping views people as highly responsible for creating their own problems and, therefore, also highly responsible for changing their situation. For example, a person who believes in the assumptions of the moral model would argue that obese people cause their obesity by overeating and are consequently responsible for correcting their weight problems by mustering up enough willpower to stop overindulging.

The *compensatory model* characterizes people as having little responsibility for causing their problems, but a higher level of responsibility for altering their health problems. For example, a cancer patient would not be held responsible for causing his or her cancer, but would be expected to assume an active role in solving the problems associated with the cancer by attending self-help groups or cancer education groups such as "I Can Cope."

The *medical model,* the third model of helping and coping, has generally been associated with practitioners in the medical profession. However,

		Responsibility for *Solutions*	
		High	Low
Responsibility for *Problems*	High	Moral model	Enlightenment model
	Low	Compensatory model	Medical model

Figure 3–2. Four models of helping and coping. *(Adapted from Brickman, P., Rabinowitz, J., Kuruza, J. Jr., Coates, D., Cohn, E. & Kidder, L. [1982]. Models of helping and coping.* American Psychologist, 37*(4), 370.)*

this model can also characterize nurses, social workers, or others who ascribe little responsibility to the patient. According to the medical model, patients are neither responsible for causing their problems nor responsible for finding solutions to them. For example, the person who develops an intestinal abscess of unknown origin and who has the abscess excised by an expert surgeon would not be held responsible for the onset of the problem or for providing a solution.

The *enlightenment model* is the final combination of levels of responsibility. Patients, according to this model, are held highly responsible for causing their problems but are not as responsible for solving their problems. Responsibility for solving problems is placed into the hands of a powerful "other," such as a religious figure or community group who will provide the solution or "enlighten" people about the real nature of their problems. Alcoholics Anonymous has been identified as a group based on this model of helping and coping (Brickman et al., 1982). Recovering alcoholics are expected to give testimony to their responsibility for having caused their drinking problems rather than blaming problems on outside circumstances. Since responsibility for resolving the drinking problem is viewed as resting outside of the power of the alcoholic, the alcoholic must maintain close ties with a community of supporters, such as Alcoholics Anonymous, whose encouragement and support will help the recovering alcoholic stay on the nondrinking path. Advocates of other groups that are usually outside of the traditional health care setting have also been linked to the beliefs of the enlightenment model. Early practitioners in the natural childbirth movement and "folk healers" of cancer patients have also been identified as basing their practice on the assumptions of the enlightenment model (Cronenwett & Brickman, 1983; Northouse & Wortman, 1990).

Each of the four models of helping and coping has particular strengths and limitations. Brickman and his associates (1982) note that the *moral model*, with its high emphasis on responsibility, is probably most beneficial to those who have the intellectual or behavioral resources to take charge of their lives. The moral model, however, places more blame on patients for causing health problems or for not changing negative health states. The *compensatory model* may be helpful in mobilizing people to work through their problems without being blamed for them. Yet there is a question about how long people can continue to stay motivated to work through problems they have not caused. The *medical model* is criticized for the dependency that it frequently encourages in patients. However, on the positive side, if people are not regarded as responsible for causing or solving their problems, they may feel more justified and willing to seek out health services. Finally, the *enlightenment model* is advantageous because it helps to mobilize a group of supporters for the ill person. On the other hand, this model can lead to abuse of power, illustrated in the classic cases of Jim Jones and Charles Manson whose control over others had negative consequences. Similar to the moral model, the enlightenment model tends to blame the person for causing his or her illness.

Many questions about these four models or ways of viewing responsibility cannot be answered easily. Which of these four models generally guides professional practice with patients? Do professionals change the type of model they use when working with one type of patient versus another, with old versus young patients, or with physically ill patients versus mentally ill patients? When working with a patient who might be described as passive, unmotivated, or noncompliant, could the professional be operating from a moral model while the patient is operating from a medical model? How do the issues of *responsibility* and of varying preferences for involvement affect the relationship between the patient and the professional?

Obviously, the optimal situation is one in which there is a perfect match between the amount of responsibility desired by the patient and the amount encouraged by the professional. Situations in which the patient and professional differ on issues of responsibility are more problematic and require more assessment and negotiation.

Communication assists patients and professionals to work through these issues of responsibility. First, without direct communication, patients and health professionals may be unaware that they are operating from different models of responsibility—a factor that could block the development of a collaborative relationship. Brickman (1982) contends that many of the problems that occur between the help giver and help receiver are due to the fact that the two people's models are "out of sync" with one another. Second, communication provides the means for assessing patients' preferences for involvement in care. Clinicians need to attend closely to patients' verbal requests and nonverbal cues regarding the degree of involvement they prefer (Lepper, Martin, & DiMatteo, 1995). We know very little about what happens when patients are pushed to become more involved in their care when they prefer less involvement, or conversely when patients are prevented from participating when they wish to be more involved. It seems likely, however, that either situation blocks the development of a collaborative role between professional and patient.

A growing body of research has started to examine patients' preferences for involvement in their care and its effect on their health outcomes. For example, Mahler and Kulik (1990) examined the preference for involvement of coronary bypass patients and found that the majority believed that at least part of the responsibility for their recovery rested with them. Patients who indicated preoperatively that they wanted more involvement in their care ambulated more after surgery and were discharged sooner from the hospital. Clearly more research is needed in this area to provide guidelines to clinicians about what level of involvement is optimal for which patient at what time.

Up to now, we have been talking about patients' *preferences* for participating in care and models of perceived responsibility. Orem (1995), a nurse theorist, emphasizes also assessing patients' *abilities* to participate in care. She notes that patients' abilities to engage in self-care vary considerably. For example, a severely depressed patient, a cardiac patient, and a diabetic patient may differ tremendously in their ability to engage in self-care. Both Orem's and Brickman's perspectives are similar in that each highlights the importance of individualizing approaches to patient care depending on patients' abilities (Orem) or preferences for responsibility (Brickman).

Power Differences

It is no surprise that health professionals are generally perceived as the "powerful" and patients as the "powerless." Nor is it unusual that the professional–patient relationship has been characterized as asymmetrical, with the balance of power tipping in favor of the practitioner. What is surprising, however, is that this unequal relationship is so difficult to change in today's health care system and that it still remains a barrier to effective professional–patient relationships. Although the authority of health professionals to make decisions for others is being challenged by a more educated consumer and a more egalitarian society, the change is occuring slowly (Kelner & Bourgeault, 1993).

Sources of the health professional's power are diverse. Health professionals have access to all five sources of power identified in the classic work by French and Raven (1959). Health professionals' knowledge in health matters make their claim to expert power obvious to consumers. However, because consumers are becoming more informed about health matters and taking a more active role in their own care, professionals' claims to legitimate power are being challenged. Equally important, but more subtly exercised, is the health professional's use of reward and coercive power. For example, some patients fear that professionals will provide inadequate care if patients do not follow the prescribed pattern of behavior. In addition, the health professional's power base remains strong because of the patient's faith in professionals and the patient's belief that professionals have nearly mystical powers. Also, people who can "fix bodies" are held in very high esteem by patients who are worried about life and death issues.

Patients have fewer sources of power than health professionals (Beisecker, 1990; May, 1990). Health professionals seldom see the patient as an "expert," even though the patient is the person most familiar with the onset, symptoms, and duration of the distress that he or she is experiencing. Similarly, patients are accorded little legitimate power although they pay high fees for the services they receive from health professionals. Coercive power is available to patients in the form of malpractice suits, aggressive behavior, and negative evaluations. However, patients seldom use this power because of the time and cost involved (malpractice) and because of their fears of retaliation or inadequate treatment if their power tactics fail. Patients will, at times, resort to reward power in the form of "good" patient behavior or praise for the professional's skills. However, as Kritek (1981) suggests, this does not result in any sustained source of power for the patients.

Leary's model of human interaction presented in Chapter 1 is useful for understanding what happens in health care settings when power imbalances occur. According to Leary (1955), communication occurs along dominant–submissive and love–hate dimensions; when one person uses specific communication behaviors, this elicits specific behaviors in another person. Traditionally (Fig. 3–3), the professional has been dominant because of the power attributed to the role of expert and because patients have wanted professionals to act in a dominant manner. In terms of Leary's model, patients have participated in the health communication process from a submissive position. This submissiveness elicits dominant responses from health professionals. So, too, health professionals have communicated in dominant ways toward patients and this has elicited submissiveness from patients. Although there are a few instances in which patients act dominant and professionals act submissive, it is far more common in health care settings for the professional to assume a position of power in an asymmetrical professional–patient relationship.

What happens to relationships in which there is an uneven balance of power? One major problem is that the more powerful person assumes more authority than warranted. Another problem is that the authority of the professional can spill over into making decisions for patients in areas in which patients are perfectly capable of making their own decisions. Health professionals may also make health care decisions based on their own values rather than on patients' values, or they may make life and death decisions for patients that run counter to patients' preferences (Bedell & Delbanco, 1984).

The power clash between professionals and patients is often evident in the issue of patient control over dying. Although in recent years new tech-

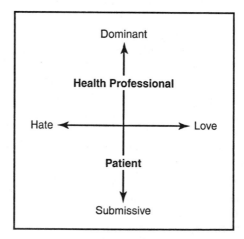

Figure 3–3. Traditional patient–professional relationships.

nologies have enabled terminally ill patients to live longer than ever before, some patients still feel that they have little say in whether or not life-sustaining measures are used. Even greater controversy has surrounded the issue of patient-assisted suicide, raising both power and ethical issues concerning who has the right to decide. Kelner and Bourgeault (1993) interviewed physicians and nurses and found that they were generally in favor of the principle of patient control over dying but had some difficulty accomodating to patients wishes in clinical situations. Some of the health professionals had difficulty with the notion of patient control over dying because it ran counter to their beliefs about themselves as healers, and was perceived as a threat to their authority to make clinical judgments in life and death situations.

To promote effective patient-professional relationships, power needs to be shared more equally between patients and professionals. According to Kelner and Bourgeault (1993), health professionals are struggling to adapt to the increasing demands by patients for more control in decisions affecting their lives. This requires however, that professionals concede some of their power and enter into a partnership with patients. It may be helpful to think of the power relations between professionals and patients on a continuum, with a completely autonomous patient at one end and a completely autonomous professional at the other end. In the middle is shared decision making. It is this middle range of the continuum that patients want to expand (Kelner & Bourgeault, 1993).

Although there will continue to be differences in the professional's and the patient's education, knowledge, and economic background, the opportunity for shared power will allow patients to maintain control over their lives and the decisions affecting their bodies (Beisecker, 1990). In an interesting study, investigators taught women strategies for being more assertive in getting their questions answered and improving their communication with physicians in an obstetric and gynecological clinic (Thompson, Nanni, & Schwankovsky, 1990). Women were randomly assigned to either a control group or to an experimental group. The women in the experimental group were instructed to list three questions they had and to take this list with them into their meeting with the physician. Women in the experimental group asked more questions from their physicians and reported less anxiety during their examinations than women in the control group. The findings of this study suggest that there are fairly straightforward, cost-effective ways that we can use to teach patients to be more assertive in their communication with professionals and to change the power imbalances that exist in patient–professional relationships.

Unshared Meanings

The final barrier to effective professional–patient communication that will be considered here is the issue of unshared meanings—differences in perceptions between the professional and the patient. As we discussed in Chapter 1, it is difficult for effective communication to occur without a common set of meanings between a source and a receiver.

Berger and Luckman, in their classic work, *The Social Construction of Reality* (1967), explain why we often miss or fail to share the same meanings with other people. They believe that what we perceive to be "real" depends on our unique interpretation of events *and* on our different interactions with others—hence our reality is socially constructed. Each person, therefore, carries around a reality that is real to her or him, but that is not necessarily shared with a second person. According to Berger and Luckman, conversation is the most important factor that enables us to maintain our shared perceptions of reality with others as well as to modify our perceptions. Furthermore, they believe that conversation between people must be continued and consistent to be effective.

The professional and the patient often do not see eye to eye on the same issue, partly due to the different perceptual fields from which they are viewing their realities. Danziger (1981) suggests that the professional may be preoccupied with work concerns while the patient is mainly concerned with his or her own well-being. Similarly, Mechanic (1982) suggests that health professionals such as physicians tend to focus on a narrow range of factors when diagnosing disease whereas patients consider a broader range of factors, including their social functioning as well as their overall state of mind.

Although there are many factors that contribute to unshared meanings between professional and patient, two specific sources that will be discussed here are (1) the jargon used by health professionals, and (2) their different interpretations of the same words. The problems that medical jargon creates in communication are well known to health professionals. Words such as *decubitus ulcer, incontinence,* and *alopecia,* are often too technical for patients to understand. Such terms can actually prevent patients from being aware of their health problems or of the side effects of treatments (Sharf, 1984). In one study, investigators asked physicians, health workers, and patients to identify the correct definition for a number of common medical and psychological terms such as depression, schizophrenia, migraine, epilepsy, and stroke (Hadlow & Pitts, 1991). Clear differences were found in the understanding of these terms by these three groups of participants. Of the 12 words tested, correct responses were reported by 70 percent of the physicians, 54 percent of the health workers, and 36 percent of the patients.

Professionals are often educated to use technical terminology so they will be able to communicate more precisely with other professionals. However, when these same words are used in professional–patient interactions, the opposite can occur—communication can be blocked. Although many professionals use medical jargon unintentionally and simply out of habit, overuse of medical jargon can be a way of indirectly withholding information from patients.

Although jargon is a prime cause of unshared meaning, significant problems may arise when professionals and patients have different interpretations or attach different meanings to common words. In our own work with cancer patients, we discovered that several specific words cause problems. *Prognosis*, for example, is a very emotionally charged word to cancer patients; they often think it means *"the chances that I won't make it,"* or *"death."* To practitioners, however, this word is much less negative; it often refers to how long the patient will *live* or *chances of surviving.* Other words like *side effects, weight loss,* and *cure* often carry very different meanings for different individuals.

To illustrate the potential problems that unshared meanings can create, consider the following situation that occurred between a patient and health professional.

A patient, recently diagnosed as having cancer, was just told that she had a "good prognosis." The patient, still feeling threatened and fearful about having a disease like cancer, focused on the word *prognosis* and was struck by the fact that she never thought of life in terms of a shortened life span. The patient overlooked the adjective *good* and responded to the message "good prognosis" with worry and concern.

The staff member was unaware of how the patient was interpreting the words *good prognosis* and did not understand why the patient was pessimistic and not coping better with her illness.

Obviously, if the staff member continued to miss the interpretation that the patient had given to the word *prognosis,* the professional would not be able to assist this patient in working through problems related to her diagnosis.

There are numerous other situations in which meanings are missed and communication between individuals becomes ineffective. For example, to an orthopedic social worker the term *nursing home* probably conjures up a different meaning than it does for the 80-year-old previously independent patient who is being transferred to a nursing home. To a nurse, the word *hospital* may elicit a different meaning than it does from a Spanish-speaking family member in the nurse's community health practice. *Locked ward* means one thing to a psychotic adolescent and something different to a psychologist. The words *God's will* may be interpreted in one way by a 10-year-old leukemic patient, in a different way by his parents, and in yet another way by the hospital chaplain. *Meanings are in people not in words.*

The term "psychosomatic" is a good example of a word that can have multiple meanings and cause misunderstandings among professionals and patients. Although the term was originally used to describe a reciprocal mind–body interaction, over the years it has taken on a more negative connotation, such as "crazy in the head," "imaginary," or "faking it." In a recent study, Courts and Bartol (1996) surveyed approximately 200 adults to determine how they interpreted the meaning of psychosomatic. Only 7 percent of the respondents interpreted the word as it was originally intended—a two-directional, mind–body interaction. The majority of the respondents (60 percent) thought the word meant the mind influencing the body (in one direction only), approximately 14 percent thought it meant an imaginary illness, and the rest of the respondents gave some other negative interpretations such as "psycho" or "complainer." The investigators contend that the term has acquired multiple meanings, some of which can cause patients to feel labeled, discounted, or ignored. They encourage professionals to be aware of the connotative meanings of these words and the powerful effect they have on patients.

Communication is important in facilitating shared meanings between individuals. As Berger and Luckman (1967) noted, we can only understand one another's reality through conversation. Communication is the vehicle through which professionals can develop an understanding of the anxieties and problems experienced by patients. To help patients cope with their situation, health professionals need to understand how patients perceive their world. To illustrate, investigators in one study compared the perceptions of cancer patients and the perceptions of nurses regarding what cancer patients want to learn. Cancer patients and nurses ranked a group of learning needs very differently: Patients said "minimizing side effects of therapy" was a number one learning need, while nurses ranked "dealing with feelings" as the top learning need of the patients (Lauer, Murphy, & Powers, 1982). Obviously, professionals who assume that they know what patients want, rather than assessing patients' actual needs, will miss important areas and be less effective in helping patients. Learning to share common frames of reference is an essential component in effective professional–patient relationships.

Six commonsense ways that professionals can be more aware of previously missed meanings are listed in Table 3–1. Accurate assessment and understanding of the meaning of words and events are an important aspect of communication. Shared meanings do not develop effortlessly. On the contrary, shared meanings develop from an interactional process that takes time, commitment, and a conscious effort. Going through this process, however, will continue to be essential to effective professional–patient interactions.

To summarize, there are four problems areas that disrupt professional–patient communication: (1) role uncertainty, (2) responsibility conflicts, (3) power differences, and (4) unshared meanings. As noted earlier in Figure 3–1, these are potential problem areas that can occur in any type of professional–patient relationship.

TABLE 3–1. SHARING MEANING

1. *Be aware of the multiple meaning of words.* The same word can have more than one meaning. The word *responsibility* may mean "take control" to one patient, while it means "take blame" to another patient.

2. *Be person-minded, not word-minded.* Frequently ask yourself, "This is what it means to me; what does it mean to him or her?"

3. *Paraphrase frequently.* Put the other person's statements in your own words. Restate what they have said to you in similar but different language to check that you have understood.

4. *Be approachable.* Create a personal atmosphere that will invite or encourage the other person to ask questions if he or she does not understand your message.

5. *Use multiple methods of communicating.* Try to use a variety of ways to get your message across to another person. For example, if teaching a psychiatric patient about medications, use pictures and written instructions as well as verbal communication.

6. *Be aware of the contexts (verbal and situational).* Verbal context: How was the particular word used in the sentence? Situational context: What was happening in the environment during the interaction with the patient?

Based on Haney, W. (1979). Communication and interpersonal relations *(4th ed, pp. 284–321). Homewood, IL: Richard D. Irwin.*

▶ PROFESSIONAL–PROFESSIONAL RELATIONSHIPS

Researchers have found that a spirit of collegiality among health professionals is essential to the delivery of quality health care services (Fagin, 1992; Knauss, Draper, Wagner, & Zimmerman, 1986). Health professionals need to collaborate and cooperate with one another in order to help patients resolve complex health care problems. Ironically, this spirit of collegiality and collaboration has not always been present among health care professionals. Although improvements have been made in the past few years, areas of contention and misunderstanding still exist and interfere with professionals' communication with one another.

Focusing on the segment of the health communication model that depicts interprofessional relationships (Fig. 3–4), this section will address three problem areas that have an impact on professional–professional relationships: (1) role stress, (2) a lack of interprofessional understanding, and (3) autonomy struggles. The disruptive effect of professional–professional conflicts is important because ultimately it will affect the quality of patient care.

Role Stress

Facing sick and suffering people every day is no easy task. Health professionals' work constantly places them in contact with patients who are struggling with life crises and who are trying to overcome serious emotional or physical illness. For example, physicians often need to tell patients about

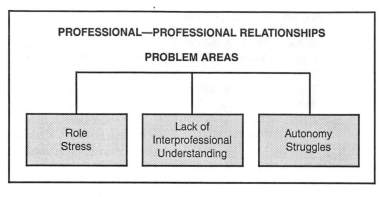

Figure 3–4. Potential barriers to effective communication in professional–professional relationships.

life-threatening diagnoses, social workers need to deal with the resulting family chaos, and nurses need to help patients maintain their courage to live through each day. In acute care institutions, the nature of health care work demands decision making on matters that affect life and death. In community settings, health care work can involve locating scarce resources for patients' long-term health problems. In both settings, the nature of the health care work contributes to the job stress experienced by persons in health care fields.

Yet, the role stress experienced by health professionals is due only in part to the nature of their work. Another major source of work stress and strain is related to problems in carrying out professional roles. We will discuss two types of role stress—role conflict and role overload—as a way to illustrate how they can eventually lead to problems in professional–professional relationships.

A considerable amount of research has been done on *role conflict*, especially as it relates to health professionals who are socialized to fit one role, and yet are expected to fulfill a different role in the work setting. Kramer's classic book, *Reality Shock* (1974), has helped to illuminate the stress created by the gap between education and service. Kramer, studying the stresses experienced by new graduate nurses, coined the term *reality shock* for the shocklike symptoms experienced by nurses who suddenly realize that their education has not adequately prepared them for the work setting. Kramer notes that new graduates learn that their ideals and aspirations are seldom the same as the values that receive praise on the job. Role conflict occurs as new graduates experience the discrepancy between these two very different value systems.

Seasoned professionals also experience role conflict. Nurses often experience frustration about the numerous nonnursing tasks imposed upon them; these tasks interfere with their ability to give more than routine nursing care. The comments of a psychiatric staff nurse illustrate the frustration and role conflict:

I remember the weekend vividly. Most of my time was spent giving medications, charting medications, checking orders, correcting pharmacy errors, playing ward clerk, and assessing dietary needs. I did not do true nursing care. That is, I spent only a little time with each client, so I couldn't assess their individual needs or plan specific care to meet those needs. Many clients' concerns went unmet. I resorted to bringing clients into the nursing station to do one-to-one interactions, so that I could simultaneously supervise the unit, put out crisis fires, and try to tend to their needs.

Role conflict arose as the nurse tried to meet opposing demands in a limited period of time.

Other health professionals are also plagued by role conflicts in their daily work settings. Social workers, for example, often experience stress and burnout carrying out their professional responsibilities. Discharge planning frequently creates problems when institutional efficiency demands that the social worker quickly place a client into a community setting that may not be completely suited to meet the individual's needs. Hurried discharges into less than optimal settings can lead to the client's later rehospitalization. Balancing the professional's desire for better discharge planning with the system's demands for efficiency leads to considerable role stress among these health care providers.

Role overload is a second factor affecting the role stress experienced by professionals. In a recent study, Schaefer and Moos (1996) examined the work stress and job morale among 405 staff members working in 14 long-term care facilities. They found that workload and scheduling stressors had a strong negative effect on staff members' morale and ability to carry out their jobs. Staff members with more workload and scheduling problems reported less satisfaction with their jobs, more depression, and a greater number of physical problems related to job distress (poor appetite, indigestion, etc.) than staff members with less workload and scheduling problems. Due to the nature of health care settings, the health professional is often required to react like an amoeba—constantly expanding or changing to meet the increased demands on his or her time. Emergencies frequently arise in which health professionals need to take on more responsibilities than they can reasonably manage within a given period of time. In addition, health professionals often are expected to wear many hats and to negotiate with numerous other departments or agencies.

Role overload often occurs when a health professional's workload consists mostly of referrals made by others. For example, the number of referrals made to a psychiatric nurse specialist or a clinical social worker may vary considerably from 1 week to another. One social worker's comments illustrate the role overload that she experienced due to an increased number of referrals.

I was supposed to have 12 patients in my caseload, but for some reason a lot of patients came in with family problems and were referred to me. Within a couple of days the number of patients and families in my caseload jumped to 20. I tried to see as many of them as I could, but I wasn't able to see as many as I know I should have seen. I tried to give some of my cases to another social worker, but she was overloaded herself and was not familiar with the agencies to which my patients needed referrals. I felt in a real bind: if I kept all of the cases, the patients would not get adequate care; if I transferred them to other caseworkers, they would be more overloaded and ticked off at me for not managing the patients myself.

The social worker is frustrated by the role overload that she is experiencing. The mental energy that she is expending to try to resolve the situation also adds to her job stress.

Assuming that role stress (e.g., role conflict and role overload) is common among health professionals, what effect does role stress have on the interpersonal relationships among health care providers? We believe that role stress is often the underlying source of professional–professional tensions. Role stress leaves the professional in a vulnerable position, more easily stressed by minor conflicts with co-workers. The social worker mentioned previously also described the following situation:

At 4:30 p.m. I got a telephone call from the physician working with the K. family. He wanted to discharge Mrs. K. as soon as possible and he wondered if I had the nursing home placement worked out. I suddenly felt my anger rising—I don't know why; it was a legitimate question on his part. I snapped back that I had a million other things to do that were more important, so I did not have one spare minute to see her. He didn't sound too pleased about the situation. . . . I don't know if he realized it but he took the brunt of my feelings about a missed lunch break, my physical exhaustion, and my general frustration.

In this situation, the social worker felt tense and irritable as a result of her role stress. As the social worker's tension increased, it eventually spilled over into her interaction with the physician. With less role stress, the social worker would probably have been able to handle the physician's inquiry with less exasperation.

The role overload of one professional may interfere with the role functioning of another. Nurses who work in hospital settings sometimes experience stress caused by workload spillover from different shifts. For example, nurses who are unable to meet role demands during a day shift may leave these tasks undone, adding to the work responsibilities of the nurses working the evening shift. Interpersonal conflicts emerge between nurses on different shifts as they struggle to cope with the role overload.

A second effect of role stress is that professionals may withdraw from one another as a means of coping with role conflicts and role overload. As role stress increases, the health professional may shift priorities from process functions to task functions. The professional under stress may become unwilling to invest energy in maintaining professional relationships and instead may direct all of his or her energies into getting the job done. For example, a nurse feeling very stretched by role demands may resolve role overload by skipping an interdisciplinary team meeting and by focusing solely on finishing other tasks (e.g., passing medications). This nurse's absence from the meeting removes one opportunity for important professional–professional relationship building and also limits the nurse's input into important patient care decisions.

Obviously the effect of role conflict and overload will eventually have an impact on the patient. Professionals who are physically and mentally exhausted by these role stresses will have less energy remaining to attend to patients' needs.

Lack of Interprofessional Understanding

Another factor that influences professional–professional relationships is a lack of interprofessional understanding. We would expect health providers, of all people, to understand the many professional roles in health care settings. Amazingly, this is not the case. Although some progress has been made in understanding one another's role, much confusion about the unique expertise of each professional still remains. This lack of understanding has been cited as a cause of role confusion and territorial disputes among the various disciplines (Fagin, 1992; Laschinger & Weston, 1995).

Why do health professionals know so little about one another's roles? Professional education that takes place in virtual isolation from other health disciplines is a major cause of this problem. A health professional can spend between 2 and 8 years in an educational program and yet get little exposure to the roles and skills of the other professionals. However, as soon as these new graduates enter health care settings, they are suddenly expected to collaborate with one another in a collegial manner—without any understanding of the other professionals' roles. For example, the distinctly separate educational experiences of nurses and physicians often lead to a lack of insight into one another's roles and responsibilities. Laschinger and Weston (1995) studied the perceptions that nursing students and medical students held regarding one another's areas of expertise. The two groups of students differed considerably in their understanding of one another's roles. In general, medical students were less clear about areas of nursing expertise than were nursing students about areas of medical expertise. The investigators found that the greater the gap in students' understanding of one another's roles, the more negative they were toward collaborative decision making.

Another factor that contributes to a lack of awareness of the various professional roles is the limited amount of contact that exists between health professionals on a daily basis. Katzman and Roberts (1988) studied nurse–physician communication in a hospital setting and found that there was surprisingly little interaction between these health professionals on a regular basis. Over a 3-month period of time, the investigators observed that a majority of the physicians came to the unit and left without ever interacting with nursing staff. Similarly, Lamb and Napodano (1984) reported little interaction between nurse practitioners and physicians in a primary care setting. The rapid tempo in health care settings and the busy schedules of professionals leave little time for professionals to sit down and discuss patient problems, much less to learn more about one another's role responsibilities.

How does lack of knowledge of one another's roles contribute to the problems in professional–professional relationships? First of all, health professionals may make demands on other professionals that are not compatible with others' perceptions of their own responsibilities. These discrepancies in role expectations can lead to professional–professional conflicts. Nurses, for example, are often frustrated that other professionals expect them to carry out nonnursing tasks, especially on evening and night shifts when other services are limited. Nurses are expected to absorb the work of others as well as carry out their own responsibilities (Prescott, Phillips, Ryan, & Thompson, 1991). One nurse shared with us her frustrations about being asked to do nonnursing tasks:

....

One day when a ward clerk was not assigned to the unit, I remember the phone constantly ringing and interrupting my plans for nursing care. The physician who entered the unit station never answered the phone. Yet during this very busy time he asked me to write down a couple of verbal orders for him. Noting no overt sign of hand paralysis in the physician, I cheerfully responded that I would write his physician notations if he would write my nursing notes for me. . . . Why should I interrupt my professional responsibilities to be unit control clerk or stenographer?

....

Here the physician erroneously assumes a nurse's role includes answering the phone, keeping the unit in order, and transcribing orders (nonnursing tasks). As the staff nurse's comments show, tensions and misunderstandings can occur when health professionals relate to each other in stereotyped ways or are unaware of one another's *real* areas of responsibility.

A second problem created by a lack of interdisciplinary understanding is an increase in territorial disputes among health professionals. In recent years, health professionals' roles have expanded considerably, leading to confusion as to which professional has expertise in a particular area (Fig. 3–5). For example, many of the tasks formerly regarded as primarily the

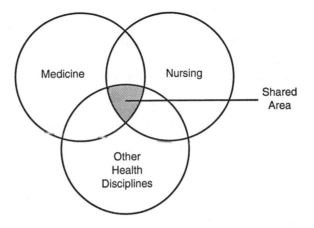

Figure 3–5. Areas of shared knowledge among health professionals.

tasks of physicians, such as monitoring cardiac arrhythmias and drawing blood gases, are now tasks commonly shared with nurses. Lister (1980), reporting on a survey of 13 types of health professionals, found numerous areas in which health professionals' roles overlapped or conflicted with one another. Lister noted that role overlap occurred especially in those areas that were outside of the more traditional role of a particular discipline. Weiss (1983) reported that when subjects in her study (nurses, physicians, and consumers) were asked to place 417 health-related behaviors into the domain of the physician, nurse, or both, the respondents placed 82 percent of the items into the area considered common to both groups. In other words, the respondents reported a large amount of overlap between the role of the nurse and the role of the physician.

When health professionals' roles overlap considerably, it is not unusual for one professional to think that the other person is trying to take over his or her power and responsibilities. This can result in unproductive competition. For example, in recent years many hospitals have created a position called a discharge planning nurse to facilitate the early discharge of hospitalized patients. This position, however, has angered many hospital social workers who contend that discharge planning and referral is their area of responsibility and not the primary role of a nurse. Role overlap and a lack of understanding of one another's areas of expertise has led to interprofessional conflict between discharge planning nurses and medical social workers in many hospital settings.

Several innovative approaches have been proposed to deal with the lack of awareness of one another's professional roles. One innovative approach (yet least practical in terms of wide usage by others) was reported by Staver (1983). A physician worked alongside intensive care nurses for 1 week in order to get a firsthand understanding of the nurses' work experiences. He said:

- Although everyone talks about the high level of stress among intensive care nurses, I realized that despite all of my medical training, I really had little idea of what a nurse's day-to-day experience was really like. . . .
- Physically, the work is exhausting, I can't remember ever being as tired, even during my days as an intern or resident. . . .
- And I didn't even have the usual patient care responsibilities since I was always working with one of the nurses rather than having the full load the way a nurse actually would. . . .
- I think more physicians would be more receptive to the nursing staff if they observed first hand as I did. The doctors are so busy with their own responsibilities that they may not stop to think how valuable the nursing staff is in improving patient care. . . . Although few health professionals would be willing to take 1 week to work alongside another health professional, the value of such an activity is unmistakably clear. (Staver, 1983, p. 13)

Hoping to achieve similar interprofessional understanding, other approaches such as sharing common core courses during educational experiences, increased contact with one another during the clinical rotations, and interdisciplinary seminars have been proposed to increase role knowledge among professionals. In addition, Fagin (1992) contends that faculty members in nursing and medicine need to develop stronger collegial relationships so that they can model collaborative relationships to their students.

As health professionals increase their familiarity with one another's roles, they will be able to make better use of one another's expertise and be less threatened by areas of role overlap. Increased interdisciplinary understanding will enhance professional–professional relationships.

Autonomy Struggles

A final problem that threatens harmony in professional–professional relationships is the issue of autonomy—the freedom to be self-governing or self-directing. The importance of autonomy is underscored by Conway (1988), who states that the capacity to exercise autonomy is crucial in order for professionals to fulfill their professional roles. In today's continually changing health care system, health professionals need autonomy so that they can shape changes rather than just respond to them (Schutzenhofer & Musser, 1994). Higher degrees of professional autonomy are related to better job morale and job performance among staff members in health care settings (Schaefer & Moos, 1996).

The degree of autonomy experienced by a health professional depends on three factors:

1. The permissible scope of practice for that group contained in state licensing laws.

2. The ability of that group to secure access to necessary health facilities, such as hospitals.
3. The ability of that group to obtain reimbursement from private and governmental third-party payers (Latanich & Schultheiss, 1982, p. 421).

Looking more closely at these three factors, it is evident that the various health disciplines differ considerably on these criteria for autonomy.

To illustrate, the medical profession generally scores well on all three criteria. Physicians have considerable latitude in their actions in professional practice; they have ready access to admit and discharge patients from health care settings, and can easily obtain third party reimbursement for the services they render to patients.

Other health professionals do not compare as favorably on these three criteria. Nurse practitioners, for example, complain that restrictive state licensing laws limit their ability to practice at the level for which they have been educationally prepared. Social workers, nurses, and physical therapists often are limited in their access to health organizations. Although nurse midwives and psychologists continue to contest their perceived professional rights to obtain hospital privileges, their ability to fully exercise this second criterion for autonomy remains limited. The third criterion, reimbursement for third-party payments, is becoming more available to some nurse practitioners but is still blocked in some states.

While the medical profession has been influential in making physicians dominant throughout history, characteristics of the other health professions have played a role in maintaining their submissive position. Kalisch and Kalisch contend that professions such as nursing with larger female memberships have been deferent (due to their socialization as women) to the predominantly male medical profession (1977). Other factors such as unassertive approaches in the physician–nurse game or unequal ways of addressing other professionals (e.g., *Dr.* physician versus *First-name* health professional) have continued to perpetuate submissive roles (Katzman & Roberts, 1988; Mauksch, 1983).

How do discrepancies in professional autonomy affect professional–professional relationships? The dominant profession tends to underestimate the professionalism or competence of other professionals. In other words, the members of the dominant profession tend to rate themselves higher in such areas as autonomy of judgment or evaluative skills than they would rate other health professionals (Silva, Clark, & Raymond, 1981).

Discrepancy in degrees of autonomy among the professionals can also lead to interpersonal tension. Nurses, for example, often express frustration that they lack the authority to make the simple decisions that are necessary for the safety and comfort of their patients, such as changing inappropriate diets or deciding on the frequency of vital sign monitoring. Nurses are often expected to defer to medical authority even though, in many settings such as nursing homes or extended care facilities, physicians are seldom present and nurses have the primary responsibility for the ongoing care and well-being of the patient. Considerable debate has raged over the prescriptive authority of nurse practitioners. While politicians and physicians have argued for limiting nurse practioners' prescriptive authority, some studies have indicated that nurse practitioners are well qualified to prescribe medications and make more appropriate prescriptive decisions with certain clients than physicians (Mahoney, 1994). Professionals need the authority to make decisions and practice within their sphere of expertise and competence. Dominance of one professional group can lead to erroneous assumptions about control over other professions or to an exaggerated sphere of influence.

Finally, the dominance of one profession can interfere with the flow of communication between the higher- and lower-status professionals. Wessen (1958) found that in a hierarchical hospital organization, hospital personnel tended to interact only with members of their own group; as the social distance between the various occupational groups increased, their interactions with one another decreased. Wessen found that rigid status roles and limited intergroup communication can be disruptive to professional relationships.

There are reports that the old hierarchical ways of communicating, especially between nurses and physicians, are changing. The early images of nurses as handmaidens are giving way to new views of nurses as independent, specialty-trained, certified advanced practitioners with separate responsibilities and areas of expertise (Stein, Watts, & Howell, 1990). Physicians are increasingly depending on nurses' expertise and skill in critical care settings and emergency departments, as well as in community settings, such as rural health care centers, residential care settings, and home care services. Complex patient care, whether provided inside or outside of acute care institutions, necessitates strong collaborative relationships among a variety of health professionals.

Organizations need to take a more active role in developing organizational structures that facilitate better working relationships among health professionals. Good working relationships and team building efforts are needed to empower health professionals to deal with the demanding, resource-scarce environments that typify today's health care organizations (Schaefer & Moos, 1996). Knauss and associates (1986) compared 13 intensive care units with regard to various organizational characteristics and patient care outcomes. The investigators found that the hospital with the best performance in terms of patient outcomes had better nurse–physician communication than the other hospitals, and it also had an atmosphere of mutual respect among the health professionals. The hospital that received the lowest ranking in terms of patient care outcomes had no established routine for discussing patient care plans, exhibited poor physician–nurse communication, and manifested an atmosphere of distrust. This study highlights that a multifaceted approach is needed to facilitate effective relationships among health professionals and to ensure optimal patient care.

As the provision of health care continues to move toward community-based settings, there is a need for better communication between professionals in acute care and community-based settings and between professionals in various community agencies. Anderson and Helms (1993) studied the transfer of information between hospitals and home health care organizations and found that only half of the essential information was transferred from one agency to another. Most of the information transmitted was either background or medical data. For the most part, little nursing care data and almost no psychosocial information was communicated between the hospital and home health care agencies. More information was transferred when standardized written referral forms were used, when the information was provided by smaller hospitals, and when the home care agency was affiliated with the hospital. The results of this study point out that professionals will need to focus greater attention on ways to foster interprofessional communication in order to provide "seamless" continuity of care from one health care setting to another. Greater understanding of each agency's and each professional's contribution to the health care of patients will help to enhance the continuity of care provided.

In summary, this section of Chapter 3 has addressed three potential barriers of communication among health professionals: (1) role stress, (2) a lack of interdisciplinary understanding, and (3) autonomy struggles. In order to solve complex patient problems, health professionals need to invest energy into collaborative efforts with one another, using each professional's unique expertise, so that territorial problems and role stress do not interfere with patient care.

▶ PROFESSIONAL–FAMILY RELATIONSHIPS

In contrast to the vast amount of literature describing professional–patient relationships and professional–professional relationships, there is relatively little literature describing relationships between health professionals and family members. This lack of systematic study of professional–family interaction is symptomatic of the lack of importance that health professionals have traditionally attributed to this relationship in health care. The emphasis in health care has generally been on the provider–patient relationship with all other relationships assigned lesser importance.

During recent years, however, health professionals have become increasingly aware that family members play an important role in promoting positive health outcomes for the ill person. Research on social support has helped to highlight the role of significant others in mediating various life stresses and serious illnesses (Bloom, 1996). Family members, for example, have been identified as the first line of defense to support other family

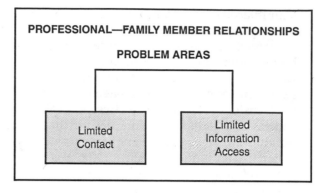

Figure 3–6. Potential barriers to effective communication in professional–family member relationships.

members during crisis. Family members and other significant individuals affect patients' health behaviors, their ability to cope with illness, and their compliance with treatments (Aaronson, 1989; Mannes et al., 1993).

   If family members are to maintain their supportive role in health care, they need to have effective communication with health professionals. Family members have traditionally faced two problems: (1) they have limited contact with health professionals, and (2) their access to information about the patient's status is limited or "managed." These two problems are shown in Figure 3–6.

Limited Contact with Professionals

Serving as primary support persons for the patient produces considerable stress for family members. In spite of the stress that family members experience, they generally receive little support from professionals. Hampe's early study of the needs of grieving spouses (1975) revealed that only 15 percent of the spouses felt that they had received support from health professionals. Similarly, in a study of mastectomy patients and their husbands, Northouse (1988) found that husbands experienced as much distress as their wives but received considerably less professional support. Breu and Dracup (1978) noted that spouses of cardiac patients were reluctant to "bother" the hospital staff and as a result tended not to voice their concerns.

   In light of the stress experienced by family members, why have health professionals directed so little attention to their needs? From a transactional perspective, we believe both family members and staff have contributed to the problem. Family members at times act in ways that hinder professionals from learning about their needs. Typically, family members have been hesitant to ask for help, thinking that they do not have a legitimate right to take up professionals' time because they are not really "sick" (in the sense of being physically ill). Also, family members have feared that if they use the professional's time, valuable resources would be diverted away from the primary needs of the ill family member. Studies have indicated that family members rank the needs of patients higher than their own needs (Ryan, 1992). Intuitively, this seems reasonable. But it also means that family members and their needs are thrust into a position of secondary importance. In trying to place the ill patient's needs first, family members give messages to health professionals that their own needs are not important when, in fact, this is not the case. Family members have real needs just as the sick person has needs, as illustrated in the following example.

M̲rs. F., a 72-year-old woman, was hospitalized for transient periods of confusion and disorientation. Prior to her hospitalization she had been living independently in her own home. During her hospitalization, it became apparent that she could no longer manage by herself at home. When Mrs. F. was approached about an alternative living situation, she adamantly stated that she would not go to a nursing home since "those were places where they put people to be forgotten and to die." Mrs. F. said that she would much rather move in with her son.

Mrs. F.'s son Robert was 50 years old and operated a small microcomputer business. He lived alone and spent many hours working at the office. Robert felt considerable conflict about his mother's situation. On the one hand, he felt he should have his mother move in with him—he had a large house, adequate income, and no other family responsibilities. He was also receiving a great deal of pressure about the situation from out-of-town relatives. On the other hand, he felt that the added responsibility of his mother living at his house would be emotionally exhausting. She was a very religious woman and could be quite domineering at times. He was also convinced that his work schedule and lifestyle would change drastically if she started living in his house.

Robert felt that there was no one with whom he could discuss his ambivalence and guilt. He was hesitant to talk these worries over with the staff. He was afraid that they would think he was self-centered and that he did not care about his mother. When it became clear that his mother would have to leave the hospital within the week, he finally shared his worries with one of the evening nurses. When the health care team became aware of his feelings, a family conference was scheduled to discuss discharge plans.

Health professionals have also contributed to the problems faced by family members. In a recent study of family caregivers of patients undergoing bone marrow transplants, Stetz, McDonald and Compton (1996) found that communication with health professionals was a major problem. Caregivers said they felt invisible to health professionals, received little acknowledgment from them, and were often excluded from discussions and decision making regarding the patient's welfare. Street (1992) analyzed the interactions between physicians and parents of pediatric patients and found that physicians rarely made partnership-building statements or encouraged them to express opinions or ask questions. In the few instances in which physicians actively elicited parents' comments, parents responded by asking more questions and becoming more involved in the visit. Until recently, health professionals have been fairly unattentive to family members' needs for information or have left the responsibility for obtaining information up to the family members. Bond (1982), for example, studied the communication between nurses and family members and found that in all but one instance the family members reported that they had initiated the interaction with the professional. Furthermore, the attitudes of professionals toward family members have not always been positive. At times staff members have considered family members a nuisance, as getting in the way of patient care or as a source of the patient's problem, especially in psychiatric settings. Sometimes health professionals simply rank family members' need lower than the patient's because they realize their own resources are limited and that nearly all resources need to be directed toward the ill patient.

With the emergence of family systems theory (Bowen, 1971; Minuchin, 1974), it is becoming more apparent that the "healthy" family member versus "sick" family member dichotomy is more of a myth than a reality. According to family theorists, the stress of illness reverberates throughout the entire family system (Minuchin, 1974). Although objective signs of illness are more obvious in the "sick" person, the mental anguish is often high in all family members who are affected in one way or another by the illness.

There is increasing evidence that family members are an integral part of the overall treatment process. However, as family members experience more stress, they will be less effective in providing ongoing support to the ill family member. Rigid boundary lines between who is sick and who is "only a family member" are limiting because they lessen family members' access to care or support. Family members who feel they have no "rights" to professionals' time will hesitate to initiate interactions or to express concerns to staff members. On the other hand, professionals who are unaware of family members' needs will not actively try to support the whole family system.

Overall, an overstressed, undersupported family network will have a negative effect on patient care goals. Yet if more attention is given to the needs of family members and friends, they will be able to join forces with staff to support the patient and achieve health care goals. Labreque and colleagues (1991) studied the effect of a family member's presence on physi-cian–patient interactions in outpatient settings. When a family member was present, physicians spent more time with patients and provided more infor-mation than when family members were absent. Similarly, Beisecker and Moore (1994) reported that when companions accompanied patients to medical appointments the visits lasted longer, patients asked more ques-tions, and physicians obtained more information.

In a qualitative study of nurse–family member interaction, Robinson (1996) asked family members what the nurse working with them did that was helpful. To the surprise of the investigator, it was not a particular inter-vention per se, but relationship-building that was most helpful. Family members appreciated the active listening and useful questions asked by nurses. They found the nurse's nonjudgemental approach useful because it allowed them to share their concerns without feeling blamed or criticized. Finally, they found it helpful when the nurse identified family strengths be-cause it fostered their sense of competence as a family. The findings from this study emphasize the important nature of professional–family member relationships and the powerful role they can play in helping family mem-bers adjust to an illness. Overall, these studies indicate that when family members have greater contact with professionals, it has a positive effect on patient and family outcomes.

Access to Information

A second problem that surfaces in professional–family relationships is ac-cess to information. In a study by Thorne and Robinson (1988), family members reported that their involvement in the care of the patient was hin-dered by the difficulty they encountered in obtaining information from health professionals. Forty-nine percent of the family members in another study reported difficulty in getting information (Wright & Dyck, 1984). Spe-cific problems they encountered included getting concrete answers from physicians, getting in touch with physicians, getting information over the telephone, and getting information about the patient's progress from nurses on a daily basis. Access to information from health care providers often takes one of two forms: *privileged* communication and *filtered* communica-tion. Privileged communication occurs when family members are given in-formation that has not been made available to the patient (Fig. 3–7). Filtered communication, in contrast, is "secondhand" information that family mem-bers obtain after it has been filtered indirectly through the patient or some-one else.

Privileged communication was more common in earlier years when health professionals did not disclose information or diagnoses to patients. Okun (1961), for example, reported that 90 percent of the physicians in his study did not tell cancer patients their diagnoses. In some of these situa-tions, family members were given this privileged information so that they

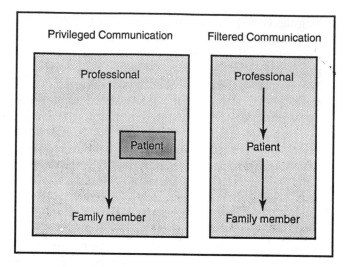

Figure 3–7. Common channels of communication used in information management.

could get financial or business matters arranged before the death of the patient (Okun, 1961). Although studies indicate that the majority of physicians now tell patients their diagnoses, remnants of this practice still remain (Gould & Toghill, 1981). For example, it is not unusual for family members to be told the diagnosis either sooner than the patient or in more detail than is given the patient. Comments from the daughter of a cancer patient illustrate this problem.

Dad was admitted to the hospital for a growth in his lung. It turned out to be cancer, but the doctor decided not to tell Dad for a few days. The doctor did tell Mom and me about the cancer but wanted Dad to regain his strength before he got the bad news. It was hard for us—especially Mom—to know Dad had cancer when he didn't know. Mom became a nervous wreck. She finally called the family doctor for a nerve pill. A few days later they told Dad. It wasn't easy, but at least we all knew about it.

Another type of privileged information takes the form of family members' knowing more detailed information than is given to the patient. This situation is illustrated in the comments of a patient's wife:

The doctor was at the nursing station when he called me aside and said, "Your husband has cancer and it's hopeless." I was shocked and didn't know what to say. I asked him if there was a place where we could go and talk about it and he said, "There's really nothing more to talk about." I asked him to tell my husband and he said that he would. When he told my husband about the cancer he soft-pedaled my husband's prognosis. He did not use the word *hopeless* which he had used with me.

These two situations illustrate how privileged information can create problems for family members. Privileged information is often given on the assumption that family members are "healthy" while patients are "sick" and less able to take the truth. Although some family members may encourage these practices by asking professionals not to tell the patient a particular type of information or to give them more specific details than are given to the patient, information management of this type can eventually lead to problems in professional–family and in patient–family communication.

Family members not only have problems of dealing with privileged communication but also with interpreting *filtered communication*, which is relayed to them by the patient or other nonprofessionals (see Fig. 3–7). The family members of hospitalized patients often receive only filtered information because they usually are not in the hospital during the times in which health professionals give reports to patients. Similarly, family members of outpatients remain in the waiting room during examinations and receive only secondhand information. In nursing homes the same problem occurs. Family members are frequently not present for status reports on patients and therefore have to rely heavily on the patients or other residents for feedback on the patient's status.

Problems that arise from filtered information are analogous to the problems that arose from the telephone game that many of us played as children. As you may recall, during the telephone game the first person whispers a message to the second person and so on down the line until the last person announces the message. As children we would laugh with amusement that the message changed so drastically from the first person to the last person. In the same way, but without the amusement, family members often receive information that is incorrect—especially if the patient who is transferring the information is hard of hearing, has transient periods of confusion, or is highly anxious and unable to attend closely to detailed information. Receiving information in a roundabout way prevents family members from asking for clarification, correcting misassumptions, and developing a rapport with health professionals. All in all, filtered communication is a problem because it is one-way communication that does not allow for direct feedback between family members and professionals.

The need for direct communication is expressed by the woman in the following example.

I told my mother that I wanted to talk with the doctor after her examination. At the end of the examination Mother told him that I wanted to hear from him about what he thought was wrong. He told her, "I don't need to talk to your daughter, I'd just tell her the same thing that I told you."

Mother was insistent that he talk to me—I guess she knew how worried I was—but when he saw me he acted sort of put out and briskly glossed over her problems. I felt like I was wasting his time.

....

This example illustrates the problems that confront family members in their attempts to communicate directly with the health professional, rather than rely on filtered information. Family members' requests for information that has already been given to the patient may be brushed off as unnecessary by professionals or seen as needlessly taking up professionals' time.

It is true that communicating with family members or significant others involves professionals' time, but giving direct communication to family members can assist them to cope better and more realistically. Welch (1981), in a study of the families of cancer patients, reported that a majority of the spouses in the study "strongly agreed" with the statement that if a doctor or nurse were to talk to them and provide explanations about treatments, these events would be easier to "cope with" (p. 367). The point is that family members often have a strong need for information. If professionals can help family members to satisfy their needs, family members will be strengthened and better able to help the ill family member.

Some attempts have been made to attend to the needs of family members and to enhance their relationships with health professionals. Among these approaches have been family support groups, joint patient–family educational groups, family conferences, and family involvement in interdisciplinary team meetings. Interventions such as these can give professionals the opportunity to assess family needs and to provide a forum for more direct and open communication as illustrated in the following case study.

....

Mr. Mason had a stroke and was admitted to an acute care hospital. The family was very concerned about Mr. Mason and felt frustrated by the lack of information that they were able to obtain from staff members about his condition.

Three weeks later, Mr. Mason was transferred to a rehabilitation center. The family was amazed at the sharp contrast between the two settings. In the rehabilitation setting, family members were viewed by staff members as important participants in the patient's recovery. In addition, family members were also viewed as having their own emotional concerns and needs for information.

The staff held weekly progress conferences on Mr. Mason's condition. The meetings were attended by Mr. Mason's primary nurse, physician, social worker, occupational therapist, and physical therapist. Mr. Mason and his wife and children were also encouraged to attend the weekly conferences. At these sessions, each professional described their own assessment of Mr. Mason's progress and offered their own recommendations for treatment. Mr. Mason and his family were encouraged to ask questions or share comments throughout these conferences.

The family members found the conferences extremely helpful. Mrs. Mason said, "It really helped me to understand how my husband was progressing and gave me the opportunity to talk directly with some of the staff members whom I seldom saw during visiting hours. I also had the feeling that my comments were important to them—even helpful."

In summary, in this section two barriers to effective professional–family relationships were identified: (1) family members have limited contact with health professionals, and (2) they have difficulty with information management (privileged or filtered communication). By recognizing the needs of family members, health professionals can assist family members to feel involved, supported, and less isolated from the health care environment.

Increasingly, patients are leaving acute care settings earlier and are moving out into settings in the community (family homes, nursing homes, extended care facilities, and hospices) where family members are being asked to assume active roles in the patient's care. Recognizing this trend, health professionals can direct more attention to professional–family relationships.

▶ PATIENT–FAMILY RELATIONSHIPS

The fourth set of relationships that we believe are central to the communication process in health care settings are the relationships between patients and their families. When the traditional focus of health care has been on the sick individual, health professionals have frequently overlooked the many ways in which patients affect family members and vice versa. This two-way interaction affects patients' and family members' ability to cope with health crises and influences their interactions with other members of the health care team (Northouse, Dorris, Charron-Moore, 1995).

Family systems theorist Salvador Minuchin (1974) contends that the family is an open system, and that changes in one part of the system are accompanied by compensatory changes in another part of the system. The onset of a stress such as serious illness can disrupt the family system and force each family member to make adaptive changes. Family goals, income level, role relations, communication patterns, and family lifestyles can all be disrupted by the onset of an illness (Gotcher, 1995; Minuchin, 1974). Two major

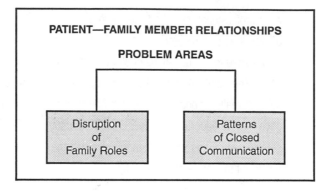

Figure 3–8. Potential barriers to effective communication in patient–family member relationships.

problems that affect the relationship between patients and family members are (1) the disruption of family members' roles, and (2) the closed patterns of communication used by family members (Fig. 3–8).

Disruption of Family Member Roles

Some families are able to adapt to change, but other families find change difficult and disruptive. Oftentimes disruption in families is primarily due to problems of role adaptation. Problems with role adaptation can occur in two extremes: (1) role ambiguity, in which family roles become too loose and undefined; and (2) role rigidity, in which family roles become too rigid and narrowly defined (Ackerman, 1966; Jones, 1980). Each of these patterns will be discussed in the next section.

Family members normally assume various roles within the family. Each member knows what needs to be done and who will be responsible to do it. However, with the onset of serious illness, old roles and patterns of relating to each other may undergo drastic alteration, leaving family members uncertain as to who will do what to maintain family functioning. As roles change, individuals become unsure of their own roles as well as the roles of others. *Role ambiguity* creates confusion and then stress in the family system, as illustrated in the following example:

Helen, a 34-year-old woman, fractured her femur during a motorcycle accident and was hospitalized for several weeks. Her husband, Keith, and four young school-aged boys were totally unprepared for the abrupt shift in their home life. Keith tried to keep their home life running smoothly in Helen's absence by making weekly chore lists for the boys and by using the help of family and friends. In spite of these attempts, considerable chaos still occurred in the family, especially around mealtimes and bedtimes. These were the specific times when Helen normally oversaw the activities in the home.

The amount of confusion and role change accompanying an illness may depend on a number of factors. More prolonged and complicated illnesses have a greater impact on family role relations than acute temporary illnesses (Northouse, 1996). Temporary illnesses are easier to cope with because family members realize that the disruption will be short lived and that they will soon be returning to their traditional family roles. In addition, the amount of role change is also affected by which family member becomes ill. If the wife-mother becomes ill, this disrupts the family more than if the father falls ill (Litman, 1979). Also, illness in a child will influence family functioning differently than illness in a parent. Taken together, these various factors influence the amount of role confusion experienced by family members.

The other role pattern that can be disruptive to families is *role rigidity*, which occurs when individuals are inflexible or are unable to change their roles to meet the demands of a new situation. Role rigidity can limit a family's adaptive potential. A form of role rigidity is typified by a pattern in which one family member consistently assumes an overfunctioning role and another family member consistently assumes an underfunctioning role. Either pattern can be detrimental to family functioning.

In families where the stress of illness is present, the overfunctioning role is frequently assumed by the spouse or significant other who does not have the illness, while the underfunctioning role has often been assumed by the ill family member. When a husband or wife becomes ill, the other spouse often takes on new responsibilities in addition to previous ones. These overfunctioning and underfunctioning roles are very natural and appropriate as long as individuals do not remain fixed within the role. However, over an extended period of time, the shifts required of well family members can lead to overwhelmed or angry family caregivers (Johnson, Baird, Malone, & McCorkle, 1993) and negatively affect the quality of marital relationships (Lewis, Hammond, & Woods, 1993). The following example illustrates how these roles can develop and interfere over time with family relationships.

M r. W., a 52-year-old man, developed severe back problems after an automobile accident. He underwent several back surgeries and was unable to return to his previous job. Also, due to his back injury, he was told to stop doing heavy lifting and yard work. After Mr. W.'s accident, his wife took on a full-time job to help defray the medical costs and to maintain the family income. She also took on many of the household and yard tasks that he previously did while she continued doing the cooking, laundry, and shopping.

After several months, Mr. W. was told that he could return to work and resume some of his previous activities. He was not able to find a new job, primarily because employers were hesitant to hire a man of his age with back problems. Over the next few months he became more and more depressed. He did not resume the yard work, something he enjoyed previously, because he was afraid he would reinjure his back. He spent most of his day watching TV.

Mrs. W. was frustrated that her husband helped so little around the house and "wasted so much time." However, she hesitated to make demands on him because of his despondency at not being able to find a job and his anger about facing a life of chronic pain. She continued in her many activities but found herself becoming increasingly tense and irritable around her husband.

The circumstances surrounding the accident and Mr. W.'s surgeries led to Mrs. W. taking an *over*functioning role and Mr. W. an *under*functioning role. Over a short period of time this could assist the family through the crisis; however, over a long period of time, especially when the original health problem subsides, this form of role functioning can lead to interpersonal conflicts between the family members.

How do rigid overfunctioning and underfunctioning roles get perpetuated in families during a health crisis? Both the patient and the family members can contribute to the development of these role patterns. For example, the anxiety that some patients experience while recovering from a health crisis such as a heart attack can cause them to feel apprehensive about assuming an active role. Family members of these patients, on the other hand, may worry that the patient will have another heart attack and may discourage the patient from assuming more responsibilities. To compensate for the patient, family members take on overfunctioning roles. In addition, new roles may be perpetuated because individuals find them to be more satisfying than their roles before the illness. Finally, the directives from health professionals can perpetuate overfunctioning and underfunctioning: Vague instructions (e.g., "use in moderation" or "a few times a day") may contribute to underfunctioning roles (Wishnie, Hackett, & Cassem, 1971), and instructions such as "do as much as you can" may add to overfunctioning roles.

Although role disruption and brief periods of overfunctioning and underfunctioning are likely, families need to maintain role flexibility. Researchers in one study found that families of cancer patients who were able to maintain role flexibility following the onset of illness were more effective in carrying out family and household tasks (Vess, Moreland, & Schwebel, 1985). Health professionals can assist families through the turmoil of role disruption by providing empathic understanding and by assisting them in working through difficult role changes. When planning interventions, health professionals need to take into account the reality of the home situation and the multiple role demands that confront patients and family members (Green, 1986). For example, not all families have the caretaking capacities or emotional resources to participate with a hospice team and to provide care for a dying family member in the home setting. For these families, a hospice in an institutional setting may fit better with the patient's and family's needs and resources. Although many families show great resiliency in the face of stressful illnesses, other families will need additional assistance from professionals to cope with family disruption due to role changes.

Closed Communication Patterns

A second potential barrier to effective patient–family relationships occurs in the area of family communication. During stress, family communication can either become closed or it can remain open with interactions continuing throughout the period of stress. Closed patterns of communication are often less constructive for family members. Closed communication hinders effective relationship building among family members at a time when supportive relationships are needed the most.

Family members' tendencies to engage in closed communication have been reported by several researchers. Vachon and her associates (1977) reported on the communication between cancer patients and their spouses during the final stage of illness; they found that only 29 percent of these couples "discussed the possibility of the husband dying of his illness" (p. 1152). Of those couples who did not discuss death, 61 percent said that they consciously avoided the topic, not wanting to upset their partner. Stern and Pascale (1979) also reported decreased communication between cardiac patients and their spouses. Some people refused to even participate in the study because they believed that the "less said about it [the heart attack] the better" (p. 84).

In a more recent study of children (aged 6 to 16) whose parents had advanced cancer, Siegel, Raveis, and Karus (1996) found that most children (92 percent) discussed their parent's illness with at least one of the parents. Of those who discussed the topic, 71 percent did so with the well parent and 35 percent did so with the ill parent. Unlike discussions of the illness, discussions of the possibility of death were more limited. Even though all of the ill parents eventually died, only 56 percent of the children reported having discussed that possibility with one of their parents. For most of these children the discussion took place less than two months' prior to the parent's death. Only 10 percent of the children indicated having had a discussion regarding death with the dying parent. The investigators contend that when ill parents do not discuss the possibility of death, their children are deprived of the opportunity to work through their feelings and come to closure on important or unresolved issues.

Given the fact that patterns of communication are sometimes closed, what factors contribute to closed communication? How do closed communication patterns get perpetuated? Two factors that can foster closed communication among family members are (1) family rules and (2) family protectiveness.

Family communication theorists develop the concept of *family rules* (Jackson, 1965; Satir, 1972). Family rules are a set of unwritten guidelines that indicate how family members will and "ought" to behave toward one another. These implicit ground rules for the family's operations are usually based on the family's values. When family members violate family rules or when family rules are ambiguous, problems can surface. To open up family communication family rules need to be altered.

Satir (1972) lists a rule inventory that family members can use to determine what rules are operating in their family (Table 3–2). Not all families operate under family rules that give family members permission to comment on feelings or thoughts. For example, some families have the rule that "angry feelings are not discussed," while in other families, "sad feelings are not shared with Dad." Although some of these rules may be effective when families are experiencing little stress or disruption, they may become ineffective when families face major stresses such as serious illness. Satir states that some families operate on the basis of outdated family rules. During illness, families need to adjust old rules to fit alterations in the family system.

Satir believes that a first step for some families is just to become aware of the unwritten, unspoken family rules that exert a powerful influence on their family communication. Once they are able to define the rules, family members may better understand the difficulties that they experience in communicating with particular family members or in discussing a specific topic. Satir notes that some families may need to update rules that are no longer useful so that family communication can be more supportive of family members' needs.

TABLE 3–2. RULE INVENTORY

1. What are your rules?
2. What are they accomplishing for you now?
3. What changes do you now see you need to make?
4. Which of your current rules fit?
5. Which have to be discarded?
6. What new ones do you have to make?

Adapted from Satir, V. (1972). Peoplemaking *(p. 111). Palo Alto, CA: Science and Behavior Books.*

In addition to family rules that hinder open communication, the *protectiveness of family members* toward one another can also lead to closed communication. Family theorist Bowen (1976) states that family communication can become constricted when one member faces a life-threatening illness. Family members try to protect themselves as well as others from the anxiety they are experiencing. Parents with a fatal illness, for example, are often reluctant to discuss the nature of their illness with their children because they fear they will break down in front of their children or have difficulty dealing with their children's concerns (Siegel, Raveis, & Kraus 1996). Stern and Pascale (1979) report that spouses of cardiac patients not only limit their discussion about medical problems but also about their concurrent family stress. They report that family members often become "preoccupied with their husband's health, feeling that a 'wrong move' or 'bad move' on their part would produce another infarct" (p. 84). As a result, these spouses often reported trying to solve family problems by themselves, a task that at times was overwhelming. Families of psychiatric patients also worry about the amount of stress an ill family member can tolerate, and at times, this can limit the person from involvement in family decision making. For example, the wife of a man who was hospitalized for depression decided not to tell him about the financial problems that she and the children were facing at home. She said, "He's just starting to feel better, more hopeful; if he finds out about the money problems he may start going downhill again."

Some family members think that they are protecting the patient when in fact they are also really trying to protect themselves from facing painful experiences. Hearing and accepting information about a family member's deteriorating health can be especially difficult for family members, and something that family members may not be willing to acknowledge. The following excerpt from the play *The Shadowbox*[1] illustrates the unwillingness of the wife of a cancer patient to accept and communicate openly about her husband's failing health. The wife (Maggie) is trying to get her husband (Joe) to leave the hospice setting and to return home with her. Joe wants Maggie to accept the reality of his illness.

Maggie: Come home, that's all. Come home.

Joe: I can't, Maggie. You know I can't.

Maggie: No, I don't know. I don't.

Joe: I can't.

Maggie: You can. Don't believe what they tell you. What do they know? We've been through worse than this. You look fine. I can see it.

----

[1] Excerpt from *The Shadowbox* by Michael Cristofer, copyright 1979 by the author. Used by permission of the author. All rights reserved. New York, NY: Avon.

Joe: No, Maggie.

Maggie: You get stronger every day.

Joe: It gets worse.

Maggie: No. I can see it.

Joe: Every day, it gets worse.

Maggie: We'll go home, tomorrow. I got another ticket. We can get a plane tomorrow.

Joe: Don't do this, Maggie.

Maggie: I put a new chair in the apartment. You'll like it. It's red. You always said we should have a big red chair. I got it for you. It's a surprise.

Joe: No! It won't work.

Maggie: We'll get dressed up. I'll get my hair done. We'll go out someplace. What do we need? A little time, that's all.

Joe: It's not going to change anything.

Maggie: No. It's too fast. Too fast. What'll I do? I can't remember tomorrow. It's no good. We'll look around. Maybe we can find a little place. Something we like.

Joe: No. This is all. This is all we got.

Maggie: No. Something farther out. Not big. Just a little place we like. All right, a farm, if you want. I don't care. Tomorrow!

Joe: *(Angry and frustrated):* Tomorrow is nothing. Maggie! Nothing! It's not going to change. You don't snap your fingers and it disappears. You don't buy a ticket and it goes away. It's here. Now.

Maggie: No.

Joe: Look at me, Maggie.

Maggie: No.

Whether closed family communication is due to unspoken family rules or protectiveness on the part of family members, problems can arise in family communication as a result of these patterns. Closed communication can lead to unnecessary estrangement in relationships. Persons confronting illness are often already experiencing some aloneness and isolation in their relationships with others. Concealment and closed communication perpetuate these feelings of separateness from others. In addition, closed communication can lead to distortions of information and erroneous assumptions. Finally, when family members attempt to protect one another, they limit their ability to support one another and assist each other to work through emotional pain.

Gotcher (1995) compared the family communication patterns of well-adjusted and maladjusted cancer patients and found that they differed in four aspects of communication. In communicating with their families, well-adjusted patients discussed their illness more frequently, perceived more encouragement to interact, were more honest in their discussions, and discussed unpleasant topics more often than did maladjusted patients. In an extensive study of families, Pratt (1976) found that regular and varied communication among family members was linked to sound health practices among family members. Open communication not only assisted them in reducing stresses associated with illness, but also in negotiating with others within the health care system. Pratt believes that open communication does not have to be intrusive; it can respect the autonomy of individual family members within the complex family setting.

Although the importance of open communication among family members has been emphasized in this section, it is important to add that for some families closed patterns of communication may be more comfortable and adaptive. In other words, for some families, it may be unrealistic and undesirable to try to quickly change longstanding patterns of family communication. It may also be unrealistic to expect that family members' patterns of communication during a crisis will be better than their communication during stable, preillness times. In a study of couples facing breast cancer, couples raised in families with closed communication tended to persist in using closed communication during the illness, whereas couples from families with more open communication tended to interact more openly (Hilton, 1994).

One additional issue that needs to be considered in assessing family communication needs is the degree to which family members' preferences for open communication are similar or different. Hilton (1994) found that the more discrepant the views of family members (i.e., one family member wanted open and the other wanted closed communication) the greater the distress they experienced in managing illness. Conversely, when couples viewed communication openness in the same way, they reported greater satisfaction with their relationships, greater support from others, and better adjustment to their illness. To best help family members, professionals need to determine their needs. Assessment is essential. What are the typical patterns of communication in the family? Are these patterns helpful during a health crisis? What alterations, if any, would family members like to make? Answers to questions such as these will give professionals an indication of the ways in which they can assist family members.

In summary, in this section two barriers to patient–family relationships were identified: (1) disruption in family member roles, and (2) closed patterns of family communication. Health care workers can assist families to cope with the stress of role disruption and to maintain open channels of communication. Although many families are able to cope well with the stress of illness and are brought closer together during the stress, other families will need the help and assistance of health professionals. Providing empathic understanding of role disruption, encouraging role flexibility, refraining from overloading an already overfunctioning family member, and communicating with family members in a way that will enhance their supportive communication with one another will facilitate patient–family relationships and also relationships with members of the health care team.

► SUMMARY

Four major types of relationships that exist in health care are professional–patient, professional–professional, professional–family, and patient–family relationships. In each type of relationship there are factors that have the potential for hindering effective communication.

Four factors that can affect the quality of professional–patient relationships are role uncertainty, responsibility conflicts, power differences, and unshared meanings. Role uncertainty hinders patients' understanding of their own role as well as the role of the many health care providers with whom they will be working. Responsibility conflicts may arise when professionals and patients do not adhere to the same models of responsibility (moral, compensatory, medical, or enlightenment). Power differences are problematic in this relationship since professionals have traditionally held more power and influence than have patients. Finally, the differing perceptions or unshared meanings that professionals and patients have about various words may block effective professional–patient communication.

Three factors that affect professional–professional relationships are role stress, a lack of interprofessional understanding, and autonomy struggles. Due to the nature of health care settings, professionals experience considerable role stress. This role stress can lead to the interpersonal tensions among health professionals as they attempt to cope with role conflict or it can lead to withdrawal from one another as they attempt to cope with role overload. A lack of interprofessional understanding can cause professionals to underuse one another's unique areas of expertise or to become embroiled in "turf" negotiations. Finally, friction due to autonomy struggles can lead to professional–professional competition and decreased collaboration.

The professional–family relationship is one that has not received much attention in health care until recently. A potential problem in this relationship is that family members have little contact with health professionals. Family members have felt uninvolved in health care and often have not made their needs known to professionals. Professionals, on the other hand, have not always been attuned to the special needs of family members, or to the importance of a collaborative relationship with family members. Access to information is another problem area. Family members have often received privileged or filtered communication, with both patterns creating potential problems.

In patient–family relationships, coping with the disruption of family roles is a major problem for both patients and family members. In the face of such disruption, too much role ambiguity may lead to confusion, while

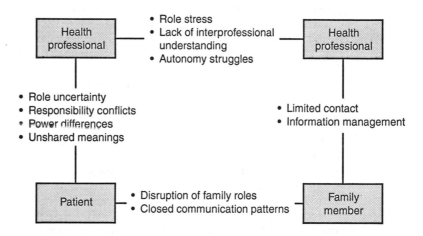

Figure 3–9. Potential barriers to effective communication among participants in health care settings.

too much role rigidity may inhibit appropriate adaptation to the circumstances of the illness. Closed communication is another problematic area for patients and family. Closed communication, whether due to family rules or to family members' desire to protect one another, can limit supportive communication among family members during the stress of illness.

The four major relationships and potential barriers to effective health communication are summarized in Figure 3–9. As noted throughout the chapter, problems in one set of relationships, for example, professional–professional, can lead to problems in another set, such as professional–patient relationships. Ways to alter these potential problem areas were discussed throughout the chapter.

► REFERENCES

Aaronson, L. (1989). Perceived and received support: Effects on health behavior during pregnancy. *Nursing Research, 38*(1), 4–9.

Ackerman, N. (1966). *Treating the troubled family.* New York: Basic Books.

Anderson, M. A., & Helms, L. (1993). Home health care referrals following hospital discharge: Communication in health services delivery. *Hospital & Health Services Administration, 38*(4), 537–553.

Bedell, S. E., & Delbanco, T. L. (1984). Choices about cardiopulmonary resuscitation in the hospital. *New England Journal of Medicine, 310,* 1089–1093.

Beisecker, A. E. (1990). Patient power in doctor–patient communication: What do we know? *Health Communication, 2*(2), 105–122.

Beisecker, A. E., & Moore, W. P. (1994). Oncologists' perceptions of the effects of cancer patients' companions on physician–patient interactions. *Journal of Psychosocial Oncology, 12,* 23–29.

Berger, P., & Luckman, T. (1967) *The social construction of reality*. New York: Anchor Books.

Bloom, J. R. (1996). Social support of the cancer patient and the role of the family. In L. Baider, C. L. Cooper, & A. Kaplan De-Nour (Eds.), *Cancer and the family* (pp. 53–70). New York: Wiley.

Bond, S. (1982). Communicating with families of cancer patients: 2. The nurses. *Nursing Times, 78*(24), 1027–1029.

Bowen, M. (1971). The use of family theory in clinical practice. In J. Haley (Ed.), *Changing families: A family therapy reader*. New York: Grune & Stratton.

Bowen, M. (1976). Family reaction to death. In P. Guerin (Ed.) *Family therapy*. New York: Gardner Press.

Breu, C., & Dracup, K. (1978). Helping spouses of critically ill patients. *American Journal of Nursing, 78*(1), 50–53.

Brickman, P., Rabinowitz, V., Karuza, J., Jr., Coates, D., Cohn, E., & Kidder, L. (1982). Models of helping and coping. *American Psychologist, 37*(4), 368–384.

Conway, M. (1988). Organizations, professional autonomy and roles. In M. Hardy & M. Conway (Eds.), *Role theory*. E. Norwalk, CT: Appleton & Lange.

Courts, N. F., & Bartol, G. M. (1996). Psychosomatic: Connotations for people who are neither nurses nor physicians. *Clinical Nursing Research, 5*(3), 283–293.

Cristofer, M. (1977). *The Shadowbox*. New York: Avon Books.

Cronenwett, L., & Brickman, P. (1983). Models of helping and coping in childbirth. *Nursing Research, 32*(2), 84–88.

Danziger, S. (1981). The uses of expertise in doctor–patient encounters during pregnancy. In P. Conrad & and R. Kern (Eds.), *The sociology of health and illness*. New York: St. Martin's Press.

Fagin, C. (1992). Collaboration between nurses and physicians: No longer a choice. *Nursing and Health Care, 13*(7), 354–363.

French, R. P., & Raven, R. (1959). The bases of social power. In D. Cartwright (Ed.), *Studies in social power*. Ann Arbor, MI: Institute of Social Research.

Gotcher, J. M. (1995). Well-adjusted and maladjusted cancer patients: An examination of communication variables. *Health Communication, 7*(1), 21–33.

Gould, H., & Toghill, P. (1981). How should we talk about acute leukemia to adult patients and their families? *British Medical Journal, 282*, 210–212.

Green, C. P. (1986). Changes in responsibility in women's families after the diagnosis of cancer. *Health Care for Women International, 7*, 221–239.

Hadlow, J., & Pitts, M. (1991). The understanding of common health terms by doctors, nurses and patients. *Social Science and Medicine, 32*(2), 193–196.

Hampe, S. O. (1975). Needs of the grieving spouse in a hospital setting. *Nursing Research, 24*(2), 113–120.

Haney, W. (1979). *Communication and interpersonal relations* (4th ed.). Homewood, IL: Irwin.

Hanna, K. M. (1993). Effect of nurse–client transaction on female adolescents' oral contraceptive adherence. *Image: Journal of Nursing Scholarship, 25*(4), 285–290.

Hilton, B. A. (1994). Family communication patterns in coping with early breast cancer. *Western Journal of Nursing Research, 16*(4), 366–391.

Jackson, D. D. (1965). The study of the family. *Family Process, 4*, 1–20.

Johnson, E. T., Baird, S. B., Malone, D., & McCorkle, R. (1993). Factors associated with anger in cancer patients and their caregivers. *Cancer Practice, 1*, 101–109.

Jones, S. (1980). *Family therapy*. Bowie, MD: Brady.

Kalisch, B., & Kalisch, P. (1977). An analysis of the sources of physician–nurse conflict. *Journal of Nursing Administration, 7*(1), 51–57.

Katzman, E. M., & Roberts, J. I. (1988). Nurse–physician conflicts as barriers to the enactment of nursing roles. *Western Journal of Nursing Research, 10*(5), 576–590.

Kelner, M. J., & Bourgeault, I. L. (1993). Patient control over dying: Responses of health care professionals. *Social Science and Medicine, 36*(6), 757–765.

Knauss, W. A., Draper, E., Wagner, D., & Zimmerman, J. E. (1986). An evaluation of outcomes from intensive care in major medical centers. *Annals of Internal Medicine, 104,* 410–418.

Kramer, M. (1974). *Reality shock.* St. Louis: Mosby.

Kritek, P. B. (1981). Patient power and powerlessness. *Supervisor Nurse, 12*(6), 26–34.

Labreque, M S., Blanchard, C. G., Ruckdeschel, J. C., & Blanchard, E. B. (1991). The impact of family presence on physician–cancer patient interaction. *Social Science and Medicine, 11,* 1253–1261.

Lamb, G. S., & Napodano, R. J. (1984). Physician–nurse practitioner interaction patterns in primary care practices. *American Journal of Public Health, 74*(1), 26–29.

Laschinger, H. K. S., & Weston, W. (1995). Role perceptions of freshman and senior nursing and medical students and attitudes toward collaborative decision making. *Journal of Professional Nursing, 11*(2), 119–128.

Latanich, T., & Schultheiss, P. (1982). Competition and health manpower issues. In L. Aiken (Ed.), *Nursing in the 1980's: Crises, opportunity, challenges.* Philadelphia: Lippincott.

Latham, C. P. (1996). Predictors of patient outcomes following interactions with nurses. *Western Journal of Nursing Research, 18*(5), 548–564.

Lauer, P., Murphy, S., & Powers, M. (1982). Learning needs of cancer patients: A comparison of nurse and patient perceptions. *Nursing Research, 31*(1), 11–16.

Leary, T. (1955). The theory and measurement methodology of interpersonal communication. *Psychiatry, 18,* 147–161.

Lepper, H. S., Martin, L. R., & DiMatteo, M. R. (1995). A model of nonverbal exchange in physician–patient expectations for patient involvement. *Journal of Nonverbal Behavior, 19*(4), 207–221.

Lewis, F. M., Hammond, M. A., & Woods, N. F. (1993). The family's functioning with newly diagnosed breast cancer in the mother: The development of an exploratory model. *Journal of Behavioral Medicine, 16*(4), 351–371.

Lister, L. (1980). Role expectations of social workers and other health professionals. *Health and Social Work, 5*(2), 41–49.

Litman, T. (1979). The family in health and health care: A social behavioral overview. In E. G. Jaco (Ed.), *Patients, physicians, and illness* (3rd ed.). New York: Free Press.

Mahler, H. I. M., & Kulik, J. A. (1990). Preferences for health care involvement, perceived control and surgical recovery: A prospective study. *Social Science and Medicine, 31*(7), 743–751.

Mahoney, D. F. (1994). Appropriateness of geriatric prescribing decisions made by nurse practitioners and physicians. *Image: Journal of Nursing Scholarship, 26*(1), 41–46.

Mannes, S. L., Jacobsen, P. B., Garfinkle, K., Gernstein, F., & Redd, W. H. (1993). Treatment adherence difficulties among children with cancer: The role of parenting style. *Journal of Pediatric Psychology, 18,* 47–62.

Mauksch, I. (1983). An analysis of some critical contemporary issues in nursing. *Journal of Continuing Education in Nursing, 14*(1), 4–6.

May, C. (1990). Research on nurse-patient relationships: Problems of theory, problems of practice. *Journal of Advanced Nursing, 15,* 307–315.

Mechanic, D. (1982). Nursing and mental health care: Expanding future possibilities for nursing services. In L. Aiken (Ed.), *Nursing in the 1980's: Crises, opportunity, challenges.* Philadelphia: Lippincott.

Minuchin, S. (1974). *Families and family therapy.* Cambridge, MA: Harvard University Press.

Northouse, L. L. (1988). Social support in patients' and husbands' adjustment to breast cancer. *Nursing Research, 37*(2), 91–95.

Northouse, L. L. (1996). Sharing the cancer experience: Husbands of women with initial and recurrent breast cancer. In L. Baider, C. L. Cooper, & A. Kaplan De-Nour (Eds.). *Cancer and the family* (pp. 305–320). New York: Wiley.

Northouse, L. L., Dorris, G., & Charron-Moore, C. (1995). Factors affecting couples' adjustment to recurrent breast cancer. *Social Science and Medicine, 41,* 69–76.

Northouse, L. L., & Wortman, C. (1990). Models of helping and coping in cancer care. *Patient Education and Counseling, 15,* 49–64.

Okun, D. (1961). What to tell cancer patients: A study of medical attitudes. *Journal of the American Medical Association, 175,* 1120–1128.

Orem, D. (1995). *Nursing: Concepts of practice.* St. Louis: Mosby.

Pratt, L. (1976). *Family structure and effective health behavior.* Boston: Houghton Mifflin.

Prescott, P. A., Phillips, C. Y., Ryan, J. W., & Thompson, K. O. (1991). Changing how nurses spend their time. *Image: Journal of Nursing Scholarship, 23*(1), 23–28.

Robinson, C. A. (1996). Health care relationships revisited. *Journal of Family Nursing, 2*(2), 152–173.

Ruben, B. D. (1990). The health caregiver–patient relationship: Pathology, etiology, treatment. In E. B. Ray & L. Donohew (Eds.), *Communication and health: Systems and applications* (pp. 51–68). Hillsdale, NJ.: Erlbaum.

Ryan, P. Y. (1992). Perceptions of the most helpful nursing behaviors in a home-care hospice setting: Caregivers and nurses. *American Journal of Hospice & Palliative Care, 9*(5), 22–31.

Satir, V. (1972). *Peoplemaking.* Palo Alto, CA: Science and Behavior Books.

Schaefer, J. A., & Moos R. H. (1996). Effects of work stressors and work climate on long-term care staff's job morale and functioning. *Research in Nursing & Health, 19,* 63–73.

Schutzenhofer, K. K., & Musser, D. B. (1994). Nurse characteristics and professional autonomy. *Image: Journal of Nursing Scholarship, 26*(3), 201–205.

Sharf, B. F. (1984). *The physician's guide to better communication.* Glenview, IL: Scott, Foresman.

Siegel, K., Raveis, V. H., & Karus, D. (1996). Patterns of communication with children when a parent has cancer. In L. Baider, C. L. Cooper, & A. Kaplan De-Nour (Eds.), *Cancer and the family* (pp. 109–128). New York: Wiley.

Silva, D., Clark, S., & Raymond, G. (1981). California physicians' professional image of physical therapists. *Physical Therapy, 61*(8), 1152–1157.

Staver, S. (1983). M.D. learns firsthand about nurses' duties. *American Medical News, 25*(1), 13.

Stein, L. I., Watts, D. T., & Howell, T. (1990). The doctor–nurse game revisited. *Nursing Outlook, 38*(6), 264–268.

Stern, M., & Pascale, L. (1979). Psychosocial adaptation post-myocardial infarction: The spouse's dilemma. *Journal of Psychosomatic Research, 23*(1), 83–87.

Stetz, K., McDonald, J. C., & Compton, K. (1996). Needs and experiences of family caregivers during marrow transplantation. *Oncology Nursing Forum, 23*(9), 1422–1427.

Street, R. L., Jr. (1992). Communicative styles and adaptations in physician–parent consultations. *Social Science and Medicine, 34*(10), 1155–1163.

Street, R. L., Jr., Piziak, V. K., Carpentier, W. S., Herzog, J., Hejl, J., Skinner, G., & McLellan, L. (1993). Provider–patient communication and metabolic control. *Diabetes Care, 16*(5), 714–721.

Tagliacozzo, D., & Mauksch, H. (1979). The patient's view of the patient's role. In E. G. Jaco (Ed.), *Patients, physicians, and illness* (3rd ed.). New York: Free Press.

Taylor, S. (1979). Hospital patient behavior: Reactance, helplessness or control? *Journal of Social Issues, 35*(1), 156–184.

Templin, E. (1982). The system and the patient. *American Journal of Nursing, 82*(1), 108–111.

Thompson, S. C., Nanni, C., & Schwankovsky, L. (1990). Patient-oriented interventions to improve communication in a medical office visit. *Health Psychology, 9*(4), 390–404.

Thompson, T. L. (1990). Patient health care: Issues in interpersonal communication. In E. B. Ray & L. Donohew (Eds.), *Communication and health: Systems and applications* (pp. 27–50). Hillsdale, NJ: Erlbaum.

Thorne, S., & Robinson, C. A. (1988). Health care relationships: The chronic illness perspective. *Research in Nursing and Health, 11*, 293–300.

Vachon, M., Freedman, K., Formo, A., Rogers, J., Lyall, W., & Freeman, S. (1977). The final illness in cancer: The widow's perspective. *Canadian Medical Association Journal, 117*(10), 1151–1153.

Vess, J. D., Moreland, J. R., & Schwebel, A. I. (1985). A follow-up study of role functioning and the psychological environment of families of cancer patients. *Journal of Psychosocial Oncology, 3*(2), 1–13.

Weiss, S. (1983). Role differentiation between nurse and physician: Implications for nursing. *Nursing Research, 32*(3), 133–139.

Welch, D. (1981). Planning nursing interventions for families of adult cancer patients. *Cancer Nursing, 4*(5), 365–370.

Wessen, A. (1958). Hospital ideology and communication between ward personnel. In E. G. Jaco (Ed.), *Patients, physicians, and illness* (3rd ed.). New York: Free Press.

White, A. B. (1987). I'm not letting you go. *American Journal of Nursing, 87*(3), 312–313.

Wishnie, H., Hackett, T., & Cassem, N. (1971). Psychological hazards of convalescence following myocardial infarction. *Journal of the American Medical Association, 215*(8), 1292–1296.

Wright, K., & Dyck, S. (1984). Expressed concerns of adult cancer patients' family members. *Cancer Nursing, 7*, 371–374.

Nonverbal Communication in Health Care Settings

4

In recent years, the area of nonverbal communication has received a great deal of attention. People today are interested in being able to understand and to explain their own as well as other people's nonverbal behavior. Health care professionals are also taking an equally strong interest in nonverbal communication, (Buller & Street, 1992; Derlega, 1995; DiMatteo, Hays, & Prince, 1986; Friedman, 1979; Hall, Roter, & Rand, 1981; Street & Buller, 1988).

So much attention is being given to nonverbal behavior because individuals recognize that it plays a key role in the overall communication process. Birdwhistell (1970), for example, who studied the area of body movement, suggests that 65 to 70 percent of the social meaning of an interaction is transmitted by nonverbal behavior. Mehrabian (1971), another well-known authority on nonverbal communication, estimates that 93 percent of the meaning of a message can be accounted for by nonverbal communication (p. 43). Although these percentages are only estimates, they do indicate that nonverbal behavior is a central aspect of human communication.

To understand the complexities of health transactions among professionals, clients, and family members, one needs to be aware of the contribution made by the nonverbal dimension of the communication process. Health transactions, as depicted in the health communication model (see Chap. 1), are comprised of both verbal and nonverbal components. The emphasis in this chapter is on the nonverbal component. In this chapter, we define nonverbal communication, describe how it functions in the human communication process, and dispel several myths about nonverbal behavior. In addition, we describe specific dimensions and examples of nonverbal communication.

▶ THE IMPORTANCE OF NONVERBAL COMMUNICATION IN HEALTH CARE

Nonverbal communication has special relevance in health care primarily because patients pay close attention to the nonverbal communication of professionals, and professionals, likewise, rely heavily on the nonverbal communication of patients.

Patients' Attentiveness to Nonverbal Communication

Patients and family members are very sensitive to professionals' nonverbal communication for a variety of reasons (Friedman, 1979; Lepper, Martin, & DiMatteo, 1995). First, health care settings evoke considerable fear and uncertainty in patients and family members. To lessen their uncertainty, patients and family members become especially alert to information in their environment and to the nonverbal cues emitted by practitioners. For example, when patients cannot understand the complex medical jargon being used, they focus instead on the professionals' nonverbal behavior as a way of understanding the situation.

Second, patients sometimes believe that health professionals are not completely honest with them. Patients may think that health professionals are trying to protect them from bad news or are hiding their real feelings from them. Nonverbal communication becomes increasingly important during times of illness because many people believe that the truth is often "leaked" through nonverbal channels (Friedman, 1979). For example, even though a clinician may tell the parents of a young child with a birth defect that the defect is minor, the parents will usually scrutinize the clinician's facial expression carefully for some clue as to how serious the clinician *really* thinks the birth defect is for the child.

Third, patients and family members will sometimes rely on nonverbal observations as a rapid means of gaining information even before any verbal interaction takes place. For example, parents who are anxiously awaiting the results of their child's bone marrow test may quickly scan the clinician's face as he or she enters the room to get a clue to whether they will be receiving good or bad news. This rapid preinteraction observation may help the parents "get ready" for the verbal interaction that will follow.

Finally, patients often rely heavily on nonverbal communication if they perceive that the practitioner is too busy or is unapproachable. In these situations the patient will use nonverbal cues to supplement the information that is either missing or not understandable from the verbal interaction. These are a few of the main reasons why patients and family members are so attentive to health professionals' nonverbal communication.

Professionals' Attentiveness to Nonverbal Communication

It is not surprising that professionals are usually attentive to patients' nonverbal communication. During their educational experiences, most students are taught about the importance of assessing such things as facial expression, body posture, and gestures. Nursing students, for example, are often required to write extensive process recordings that provide information about *patients'* nonverbal communication as well as their *own* nonverbal communication.

In clinical practice, the practitioner becomes very aware of the need to assess nonverbal communication. In fact, in some cases, nonverbal assessment is the only means of gaining information about the patient's experience. In mental health settings, for example, the psychotically depressed client may be unable to find the words to express the loss, pain, or aloneness that he or she is experiencing. In medical settings, the patient on a respirator will not be able to express concerns to staff members in words. In neonatology units, infants cannot verbally communicate their needs to the nurses. In these situations the health professional needs to rely primarily on the expressions, gestures, and other modes of nonverbal communication to understand and assess the client's needs.

Professionals also need to be attentive to nonverbal communication because it plays a critical role in the degree to which patients become involved in their own care. For example, Lepper, Martin, and DiMatteo (1995) contend that medical encounters between physicians and patients deal mostly with asking questions and giving information, and give less attention to the direct expression of feelings or expectations. Feelings and expectations about medical encounters are often transmitted and understood nonverbally by means of nonverbal cues such as voice tone, touch, gaze, and body movement. Providers and patients mutually effect each other through these nonverbal cues and in so doing negotiate how involved the patient will be in the health care encounter. Lepper, Martin, and DiMatteo suggest that health care professionals should be trained to interpret patients' nonverbal cues more accurately. Greater attention to nonverbal cues will make providers more senstive to patients' feelings and will help the participants negotiate their role in the health care process.

In light of its importance, understanding the nature, function, and dimensions of nonverbal communication is essential for effective health communication.

▶ THE NATURE OF NONVERBAL COMMUNICATION

Nonverbal Communication Defined

What is nonverbal communication? Is it simply communication without words? Is it communication without sound? Does it include behaviors that have unintended meanings for others? Answers to questions such as these have been the subject of much controversy among researchers of nonverbal communication, because nonverbal communication covers a wide range of overlapping human behaviors.

Nonverbal communication represents a smaller portion of the communication process—that portion which is free of words. In essence, nonverbal communication is *communication without words* and it includes messages created through body motion, the use of space, the use of sounds, and touch.

Although nonverbal communication does not encompass language, nonverbal communication can be either vocal or nonvocal. This may sound surprising, because nonverbal communication is usually thought of as silent. However, vocal sounds that do not involve language or words fall within the category of nonverbal communication. For example, a groan or a scream of pain by a patient under stress would be *vocal nonverbal* communication, whereas a smile or frown on a health professional's face would be *nonvocal nonverbal* communication.

In addition, nonverbal communication can be either intentional or unintentional. If a person is communicating an important message to others, she or he will most probably use a facial expression that notes the seriousness of the situation. A community health nurse who maintains a serious facial expression while telling a client about the potential side effects of a new hypertensive drug is using *intentional* nonverbal communication. *Unintentional* nonverbal communication would be characterized by a client at a reproductive health center who appears to be carrying on a pleasant, relaxed conversation with the intake clerk but whose facial expressions show fear and uncertainty at the same time. In this situation the client is not aware of her facial expression; it is unintentional nonverbal behavior.

Purposes of Nonverbal Communication

The overriding purpose of nonverbal communication is the effective sharing of information between participants in an interaction. Nonverbal communication performs several identifiable functions in the process of communication, including (1) the expression of feelings and emotions, (2) the regulation of interaction, (3) the validation of verbal messages, (4) the maintenance of self-image, and (5) the maintenance of relationships. At any time in an interaction, one or several of these functions may be operating.

Expression of Feelings and Emotions

Through nonverbal behavior, individuals express their joy, anger, despair, and fear. Clients and professionals, alike, reveal aspects of their inner states to others by using nonverbal communication. Nonverbal communication allows clients to tell health professionals that they feel helpless, they are uncertain, they feel powerless, or they feel anxious. The elderly woman who stands in front of a health professional, nervously rubbing her hands together, is communicating some of her inner feelings of anxiety and agitation. Nonverbal communication is a channel for venting and releasing pent-up feelings as well as an avenue for expressing day-to-day feelings.

Regulation of Interaction

A second function of nonverbal communication is that of regulating the flow of messages between people. Nonverbal cues, such as a tilted head, intense eye contact, raised eyebrows, a lowered voice, a shift in body posture, or a movement toward or away from someone, all regulate the flow of messages. Nonverbal cues regulate an interaction by indicating to others whether individuals want to talk, when they want to talk, whether they want to listen, how long they want to listen, and when a conversation is over. For example, in a home visit, nonverbal communication is used by both the health professional and the client to establish when a formal interview is to begin, how long the interview is to last, whose turn it is to ask or answer questions, and when the interview is completed. The clinician who glances frequently at a wristwatch near the end of a conversation may be indicating (intentionally or not) that the interaction is concluding. On the other hand, the client who stands up and starts to take coffee cups to the kitchen may be suggesting to the home care nurse that it is time for the conservation to stop. In each of these instances nonverbal messages are used to regulate the flow of the interaction.

Validation of Verbal Messages

It could be argued that of all the functions of nonverbal communication, the main function is validating the verbal dimensions of an interaction. When the words match the individual's expressed feelings and emotions, communication is most effective. If a client says, "I feel great," but looks troubled and angry, the nonverbal dimension of the client's message is incongruent with the verbal dimension. This makes it difficult for others to know how to respond to the client. Or consider the health care administrator who says, "I'm very pleased with how things are going," but has an extremely disgruntled and rather angry facial expression. It is difficult to interpret the administrator's meaning because the nonverbal expressions do not match or correspond with the words. Communication is most effective when the nonverbal dimensions of messages validate the verbal dimensions.

Maintenance of Self-Image

A fourth function of nonverbal communication is maintaining the self-image of the communicator. Although this function of nonverbal communication may not seem as obvious as the other functions just described, it does play an important role in self-preservation, or in assisting us to convey an image of ourselves to others. Goffman (1959, 1963, 1967) has theorized that interaction is much like a stage performance in which individuals assume various roles and act them out. Nonverbal communication assists individuals in performing their roles appropriately in front of others and helps individuals to present the image they want to project to others.

In any interaction, individuals have images of themselves they want to maintain. For example, in an extended care facility, an 80-year-old resident who was a banker for 40 years before his retirement may want to be dressed daily in a coat and tie because that is the way bankers dress. His clothes communicate to others that he wants to be seen as a respectable banker. Or consider the newly graduated nurse who wears a stethoscope around her neck during breaks in the coffee shop because she wants to be seen by others as a qualified professional. In both of these examples, the individuals are using nonverbal cues to maintain a role that communicates to others a part of their self-image. Although the nonverbal cues in these examples are obvious to illustrate the point, in many interactions there are subtle and not so subtle nonverbal cues present that individuals give to establish a self-image.

Maintenance of Relationships

Finally, nonverbal communication serves the function of defining relationships; nonverbal cues help individuals describe to each other how they feel about their relationship. In Chapter 1, we discussed how communication has both a content and a relationship dimension, and that the meaning in a message emerges as a result of *what* is said (the content) in conjunction with *how* it is said (the relationship). The "how it is said" aspect of a message depends primarily on the nonverbal cues that accompany a message. Nonverbal cues give individuals information about their interpersonal relationship and, therefore, about how they should interpret the content of a particular message. For both patients and providers, nonverbal cues play a key role in negotiating aspects of the provider–patient relationship (Buller & Street, 1992).

Through nonverbal communication, individuals convey relational messages to others about such things as inclusion, status, control, or affection. For example, a health professional can often determine his or her level of inclusion in a meeting by looking at the way chairs are set up in the room. A nurse educator told us about a treatment planning session at a psychiatric facility where she worked with her students. Staff members sat directly at the oval table in the room and students were asked to sit in chairs behind the staff, away from the table. Although it was never verbally indicated, the larger padded chair at the end of the table was always left vacant for the psychiatrist who ran the treatment planning meetings.

In professional–professional relationships, relational messages concerning status differences can sometimes be observed in how people dress. In some health care settings, a long white laboratory coat may indicate high status while a short laboratory coat indicates low status. In other settings, professionals who wear street clothes may be viewed as having higher status than personnel required to wear uniforms.

Relational messages about control can also be indicated by nonverbal cues. When a professional sits next to a client, a feeling of shared control is expressed; but if the professional hovers over the client, it implies dominance. Warmth or hostility are also relational messages communicated through nonverbal communication channels. A kind look or caring expression communicates to others a good relationship while an angry look or harsh tone of voice can express to others a cold and more distant relationship. Although one particular nonverbal behavior does not always indicate a particular relationship message, a combination of nonverbal behaviors can often be taken together to provide information about characteristics of the relationship.

Myths About Nonverbal Communication

Several myths have been identified concerning the scope and importance of nonverbal elements in the human communication process (Knapp, 1980). These myths have developed as a result of widespread popular interest in nonverbal communication. It is important to dispel some of these myths so that they do not provide an inaccurate picture of the role that nonverbal communication plays in human communication. The four myths Knapp identifies are (1) the isolation myth, (2) the key to success myth, (3) the transparency myth, and (4) the single meaning myth (p. iv).

The Isolation Myth

The isolation myth suggests that nonverbal communication is separate and discrete from other aspects of the communication process. It implies that we can treat nonverbal messages in isolation. The problem with this notion is that it fails to see the interrelatedness between nonverbal and verbal communication. Meaning emerges from the interaction between nonverbal and verbal elements in the communication process. To isolate one part of the process from the rest may be appropriate for purposes of teaching or research, but in reality nonverbal communication is *closely bound* to verbal communication.

The Key to Success Myth

The key to success myth suggests that nonverbal communication is the key to successful interpersonal communication. Implied within this myth is the notion that individuals will indeed be effective communicators if only they stand in certain ways, sit appropriately, and wear the right clothes. This idea overemphasizes nonverbal communication, and regards it as a cure-all for effective communication. Although the potency of nonverbal communication should not be underestimated, neither should nonverbal communication be viewed as the only element contributing to success in human interaction. Nonverbal communication is just one of a multitude of elements comprising the human communication process. To focus on one element as the "key" can distort and misrepresent the overall process of human interaction.

The Transparency Myth

In many ways the popular newstand-type books about nonverbal communicaton are directly responsible for the transparency myth—the conception that our nonverbal behavior makes us fully transparent to others. These books purport to provide "quick and guaranteed" ways of accurately assessing people's personalities by focusing on specific nonverbal cues. The faulty assumption made in these books is that an individual's clothes, posture, or stance can totally reveal his or her inner thoughts, feelings, and personality. In reality, each of us gives off a multitude of nonverbal cues in addition to our verbal cues. We can control many of these cues, which means that we can influence how we want to be seen by others. Thus, it is not true that nonverbal cues allow others to "read us like a book." Nonverbal communication is such a complex and often intentional process that no single nonverbal cue or group of cues makes individuals transparent to others.

The Single Meaning Myth

It is also a myth to assume that every nonverbal cue has a single, specific meaning. Nonverbal cues are like words; they can have multiple meanings. It must be recognized that there are many ways to interpret the nonverbal expressions of patients and professionals alike. A scowl can mean an individual is questioning someone else or it can mean an individual is angry. Similarly, a questioning tone of voice can mean an individual is confused or it can mean that an individual disagrees with another person. People who cross their arms in front of their chest may not be trying to shut themselves off from others—they may only be trying to retain a little body heat in a cold room. The point is that the nonverbal communication process is intri-

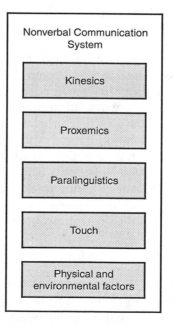

Figure 4–1. Dimensions of the nonverbal communication system.

cate, and each nonverbal behavior can have several meanings depending on the participants and the context in which they are communicating.

▶ DIMENSIONS OF NONVERBAL COMMUNICATION

Nonverbal communication is a complex and multifaceted phenomenon. Researchers have commonly divided the nonverbal communication area into five distinct categories: (1) kinesics, (2) proxemics, (3) paralinguistics, (4) touch, and (5) environmental and physical factors (Fig. 4–1). Taken together, these categories of nonverbal communication provide a framework for understanding the intricacies of the nonverbal process, and they provide the basis for discussing the clinical implications of sending and receiving nonverbal messages.

Kinesic Dimensions of Nonverbal Communication

Kinesics is the study of body motion as a form of communication. It is the most familiar type of nonverbal communication and it includes such areas as gestures, facial expressions, and gaze or eye movement (Fig. 4–2).

Gestures

Gestures are one of the most obvious and common forms of nonverbal communication, and they are often used in place of words. For example, putting your first finger perpendicularly across your lips is a way of telling others

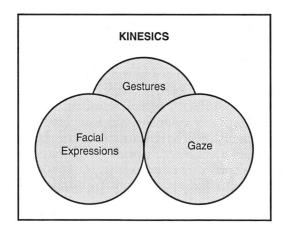

Figure 4–2. Major types of kinesic nonverbal communication cues.

"shhh." Similarly, putting your hand out straight up with an open palm facing outward is a way of saying "stop."

Gestures are also used to illustrate or pictorialize what is being communicated. Giving a patient directions for how to get to the X-ray department, or showing a patient how to change a dressing are examples of situations in which individuals would employ gestures in their communication with others.

In addition to illustrating, gestures play a major role in regulating the flow of conversations between two individuals. They help to establish the pace by regulating the back-and-forth speaking and listening of the individuals. For example, through a simple head nod we tell another person, "Go ahead and finish what you have to say," or, by raising an eyebrow, we can let them know that "When you're finished, I'd like to respond to your comments." Gestures such as these serve an important role in making conversations flow smoothly.

Facial Expressions

The human face provides a complex but rich source of information for health professionals and clients alike. For the most part, facial expressions are used to display emotions, either intentionally or unintentionally. However, they are also used by individuals to punctuate conversations or regulate the flow of interaction between two communicators.

It is essential for health professionals to understand clients' emotions and facial expressions because some clients are reluctant at times to express their feelings verbally. Health professionals need to learn to interpret nonverbal facial expressions accurately, but this is no simple task, especially when one considers that facial expression is often controlled by clients and that the human face is extremely complex (Prkachin & Craig, 1995). Researchers have found, in the laboratory setting, that the muscles of the face are so complex that in only a few hours time the actions of the facial muscles can express as many as 1000 different facial expressions (Ekman, Friesen, & Ellsworth, 1972).

Generally, researchers agree that the expression of some emotions by facial appearances is a universal phenomenon. The position, first proposed by Darwin (1872) in *The Expression of the Emotions in Man and Animals*, has been supported by recent research; facial expressions of some emotions (e.g., happiness, sadness, and fear) are biologically determined, universal, and learned similarly across cultures (Ekman & Friesen, 1975). Although these emotions are universally expressed, there are cultural differences in when a particular facial expression is shown; that is, the rules for displaying a particular emotion are not the same in all cultures (Ekman & Friesen, 1975).

Researchers also agree on a system to categorize the major emotional expressions of the face. Nearly all of the studies in the last 40 years that

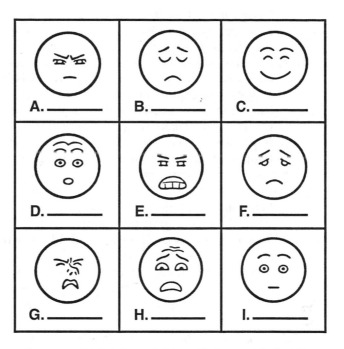

Can you match the above sketches with the correct affects?
(1) happy, (2) sad, (3) surprise, (4) fear, (5) anger, (6) disgust.

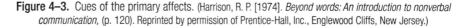

Answers: A–5, B–2, C–1, D–3, E–5, F–2, G–6, H–4, I–3.

Figure 4–3. Cues of the primary affects. (Harrison, R. P. [1974]. *Beyond words: An introduction to nonverbal communication*, (p. 120). Reprinted by permission of Prentice-Hall, Inc., Englewood Cliffs, New Jersey.)

have focused on emotions expressed by the face have identified the following six emotions: happiness, sadness, surprise, fear, anger, and disgust (Ekman & Friesen, 1975). Figure 4–3 illustrates a simplified and somewhat exaggerated depiction of the six emotions that was created by Harrison (1974).

The task of reading other individuals' nonverbal facial cues becomes difficult and confusing because individuals may simultaneously express different emotions with different parts of their face (e.g., eyes, brows, forehead, mouth). Facial expressions that combine two or more emotions are called *affect blends* (Knapp, 1978a). A person who simultaneously expresses feelings of either anger and fear, or disgust and surprise, fear and sadness, or happiness and contempt is portraying a blend of affects.

In their book, *Unmasking the Face*, Ekman and Friesen (1975) provide an elaborate guide based on research findings for recognizing emotions and affect blends from facial clues. They describe distinct styles that characterize individuals' facial expressions (pp. 155–157). Perhaps you can recognize your own style or someone else's in one or more of the following categories.

- *Withholders*: These are individuals whose faces rarely signal how they feel. The muscles of their face do not move a great deal, and their faces are unexpressive.
- *Revealers*: These individuals express their feelings readily, and their emotions are shown all over their face. It is difficult for revealers to control their expressions.
- *Unwitting expressers*: These people show their feelings (usually one or two particular feelings) to others, but they are unaware that they have done so. For example, individuals who show anger or contempt on their faces without knowing it.
- *Blanked expressers*: These are individuals who think their faces are expressing a particular feeling or emotion when, in fact, they are blank and neutral. For example, some people say they are happy while their faces show no emotion.
- *Substitute expressers*: These are individuals who display one emotion while they are feeling another. They look mad although they say that they are feeling sad; or they look happy when, in fact, they say they are feeling afraid. These people are usually unaware of the fact that their faces give cues that are incongruent with their real feelings.
- *Frozen affect expressers*: These are persons whose faces consistently express a trace of a particular emotion. They are individuals whose faces always look a bit sad, mad, or glad.

The fact that Ekman and Friesen have been able to delineate so many styles of facial expressions with subtle differences between the styles helps to point out the difficulty in assessing the nonverbal messages in facial appearances. Regardless of the complexity of the face, however, there is strong evidence that facial expression is a useful source of fairly accurate information and that a person can improve his or her skill in assessing nonverbal facial cues (Rosenthal et al., 1979).

Facial expression of pain is one area that should be of particular importance to health care providers. In a review of research on how pain is communicated through facial cues, Prkachin and Craig (1995) reported that there are real differences in how individuals exhibit pain during painful events. They point out that grimaces of pain are not observed in individuals until an individual's threshold of pain is reached, and this threshold level varies from individual to individual. From their studies, Prkachin and Craig concluded that (1) pain is expressed by a discrete set of recognizable facial cues, (2) when pain is expressed it is likely that patients' experience of pain is already pronounced, (3) the absence of a display of pain does not mean pain is not present, and (4) observers of pain tend to underrate the facial expression of pain. People vary in their abilities to make observations of pain expressions. Prkachin and colleagues (1995) found that people who live with patients suffering from chronic illness made better assessments of pain than people who had not had that experience. However, for clinicians this was not the case. Clinicians who routinely worked with patients who were chronic pain sufferers made exaggerated underestimates of pain expressions when compared to clinicians who did not have the same experience. Although these findings about how clinicians underestimate pain expressions are counterintuitive, they highlight the importance of understanding nonverbal pain expressions as a transactional communication process that must take into account both the patient's expression of pain and the provider's ability to observe these expressions.

Gaze

Gaze is the last type of kinesic nonverbal communication we will consider. Gaze, which is closely linked with facial expressions, refers to how individuals use their eyes in the communication process to give information to others, receive information from others, and establish relationships. Gaze plays a central role in nonverbal communication and is an important form of social behavior.

How does gaze function in social interaction? What is a normal pattern for individuals who attempt to establish eye contact? How should individuals use their eyes when talking with others? These are the types of questions that have been addressed in research on the functions of gaze and on the normal patterns of gaze.

FUNCTIONS OF GAZE. Individuals use their eyes to perform primarily three functions: (1) monitoring, (2) regulating, and (3) expressing (Kendon, 1967, p. 52). *Monitoring* involves assessing or checking out how others appear and how others are responding to us. Both clients and professionals often use their eyes in this way. In a psychiatric setting, a suspicious patient may isolate himself or herself in the corner of a day room and carefully use his or her eyes to monitor the people and events in the room. Health professionals often use monitoring as a primary source of information about the client's condition and response to treatment. In intensive care settings, for example, a nurse may gaze closely at a patient to monitor respiratory rates or signs of increasing restlessness that give clues to a change in the patient's condition.

Regulating refers to how individuals use gaze to synchronize their conversation. They use gaze to signal information about whose turn it is to talk and whose turn it is to listen. The regulatory function of gaze allows the speaker and listener to give feedback to each other about how they are proceeding. Hardin and Halaris (1983) reported on the differences in gaze between patients and nurses in videotaped interaction. Although their sample was small, they found that nurses maintain longer and more direct gaze toward patients, whereas patients tend to look at and away from the nurse more often during the interaction. Cipolli and associates (1989) compared the gaze behavior of anorexic teenagers with a control group. The anorexic teenagers made less eye contact and maintained eye contact for shorter periods of time than subjects in the control group. The way in which gaze helps to regulate interaction between people is described straightforwardly by Harrison (1974):

In conversation, the speaker is likely to catch the listener's attention. But then, before launching into a long utterance, the speaker will drop his eyes. He will make periodic checks, to see if his listener is still there—and still a listener. But he will avoid eye contact at pauses when, for example, he is trying to think of how to complete his thought. When he is finished, however, he will return his gaze to the listener and prepare to give up the floor. (p. 126)

A third function performed by our eyes is *expressing* to others feelings about affiliation, intimacy, and a range of common emotions. Ekman and Friesen (1975) point out that individuals' eyes vary while expressing the basic emotions: surprise, fear, disgust, danger, happiness, and sadness. They contend that these variations in eye expression can be recognized by others.

Some unique research on the role of gaze in health communication has been conducted by researchers in the Netherlands who studied over 300 videotaped consultations between general practitioners and patients (Bensing, Kerssens, & van der Pasch, 1995). They found that length of gaze by general practitioners was directly related to their correct identification of patients' mental health problems. Patients who received longer gaze from providers seemed to talk more freely about health concerns, present more health problems, and give more information about psychosocial issues. These findings underscore the importance of considering gaze and its functions in health care interviews.

NORMAL PATTERNS OF GAZE. All of us are familiar with the advice, "When talking to others, it is important for one to establish *good eye contact.*" Although this principle is helpful because it stresses the importance of nonverbally acknowledging and confirming others, this advice does not actually describe what is meant by *good* eye contact. Researchers have studied how individuals use eye contact in their ongoing relationships, and several rather interesting findings have been made.

First, researchers have found that, contrary to what one might think, individuals in a typical conversation do not look at one another all the time. In fact, the best estimate of the time individuals spend in direct eye contact in a normal conversation is about 50 to 60 percent (Argyle & Ingham, 1972; Cook, 1977). Second, the average length of each gaze is usually less than 3 seconds, and the average length of mutual gazes has been reported to be less than 2 seconds (Argyle & Ingham, 1972). Third, speakers spend about 40 percent of their time gazing at the listener and listeners spend about 75 percent of their time looking at the speaker (Arglye & Ingham, 1972). Mutual eye contact occurs during 31 percent of the time in a conversation (Argyle & Ingham, 1972). Fourth, there are differences in how the sexes tend to employ gaze. During interaction, females tend to look more at the other person than males do (Argyle & Cook, 1976).

Given these findings, it becomes easier to interpret the advice to "make good eye contact." Good eye contact means that an individual should look directly at others, but not necessarily 100 percent of the time. Some people seem to operate from the position of "more is better" in regard to eye contact and never shift their gaze from a person during an interaction. Good eye contact does not require long gazes or lengthy mutual gazes. Basically, individuals should try to establish the amount of eye contact with which both participants in an interaction are comfortable. Eye contact, like other kinds of human communication, is a transactional process. Each person affects the other and is affected by the other. Too much eye contact can be uncomfortable and interfere with the normal ebb and flow of an interaction. Too little eye contact may make the other individual feel impersonal, or it may lead to one or both participants feeling disconfirmed or unimportant. "Good" eye contact requires moderate amounts of gazing which are appropriate to the situation.

Before concluding this discussion of kinesics, we would like to consider two additional questions: (1) How can we measure our own or other people's skills in the area of nonverbal communication? and (2) Are some people better at sending and receiving nonverbal messages than others?

A considerable amount of work in finding answers to these questions has been done by Rosenthal and his associates at Harvard University. The majority of their work has centered on developing and testing a tool called the Profile of Nonverbal Sensitivity, or the PONS (Rosenthal et al., 1979). This instrument measures a person's ability to decode nonverbal behaviors. The PONS consists of a 45-minute black-and-white film that illustrates various forms of nonverbal behavior. A person views the film and tries to identify types of nonverbal behavior depicted. After completing the PONS test, a person receives a specific score on reading nonverbal cues as well as an overall score for nonverbal accuracy.

Using the PONS test in many different studies, Rosenthal and his associates identified a number of factors that were related to accuracy in interpreting nonverbal cues. They found that (1) in general, females were more accurate decoders of nonverbal cues than males; (2) accuracy appeared to increase with age and started to level off when people reached 20 to 30 years of age; (3) intelligence played only a small role in a person's nonverbal accuracy; and (4) the personality profiles of accurate decoders described them as better adjusted, more interpersonally democratic, more extroverted, and more interpersonally sensitive people (Rosenthal et al., 1979). These findings provide an interesting starting point for understanding factors that influence nonverbal accuracy.

Proxemic Dimensions of Nonverbal Communication

Proxemics is a second major component in the nonverbal communication system (see Fig. 4–1). *Proxemics* refers to how individuals use and interpret space in the communication process. Unlike kinesics, which focuses on the individual and the individual's body motion, proxemics is concerned with the space and environment surrounding the individual. Proxemics is an area of nonverbal communication that deals with questions such as, How much personal space do clients usually want when talking with a health professional? How close should one be to others in a personal conversation? How does furniture arrangement affect the meaning of messages? The areas of proxemics that address questions of territoriality, personal space, and distance are particularly relevant to health communication.

Territoriality and Personal Space

In studying animal life, scientists first observed what has now come to be called *territoriality*—the behavioral process of laying claim to an area of space and then protecting it from intrusion by outside forces. For animals, territoriality provides protection and a place for a species to learn, to play, to hide, and to engage in group activities (Hall, 1966). Studies of animal behavior have provided the background for understanding how the concept of territoriality functions in human communication.

It is generally believed that humans also show territoriality, although there is debate over whether humans learn territorial behaviors or possess them instinctively. Personal space, or one's own territory, is important because it provides people with a sense of identity, security, and control. Individuals feel threatened when others invade their territory because it disrupts their psychological homeostasis, creates anxiety, and produces feelings of loss of control (Allekian, 1973; Stillman, 1978).

When people enter health care settings, they are required to give up the personal space and privacy provided by their own homes. They must reside in an entirely new setting and often must establish living arrangements with strangers whom they have never seen before. In addition, patients often have to undergo many diagnostic procedures that further compromise their sense of privacy and personal space. Stillman (1978) vividly points out the intrusions experienced by patients:

Into [the patient's] territory will come a parade of intruders who seem to exhibit more of a right to be there than he does. These trespassers enter often without knocking, carry out activities often without introduction or explanation, and depart, seldom leaving the patient's territory as it was before they arrived. The sick person is often too weak due to his physical and psychological condition to repel the intruders; lack of territory may render him less assertive and unsure of his rights. The patient, in a strict sense, becomes the trespasser on the territory of those health professionals legitimized by society to be within the hospital's walls. (p. 1671)

Stillman's comments portray the difficulty patients have in establishing territorial boundaries or in maintaining them if they have been assertive enough to establish them in a health care setting. Patients in extended care facilities also experience intrusions. F. L. P. Johnson (1979) found that 68 percent of the residents in one nursing home had high anxiety about intrusions into their personal territory.

How do these intrusions into patient's personal space affect patients? Allekian (1973) reported that moving chairs out of patients' rooms, rearranging bedside tables, or looking through their personal belongings without asking permission were all intrusions of patients' territory and events to which patients responded with annoyance. Allekian also noted that patients reacted with more annoyance when objects specifically identified with them (e.g., their belongings in the drawer) were involved versus objects less personalized (e.g., a chair in the room).

Minckley (1968) also observed the reactions of postoperative patients to territoriality issues. She noted that patients often indicated a desire to leave the recovery room and return to "their own" rooms. In addition, many patients reported less tension when they eventually returned to "their own" beds. Reporting on the problems of obtaining personal space in nursing homes, Tate (1980) reported that residents often share bedrooms, dining areas, lounge areas, and even bathrooms, and for the most part have little space to call their own. As a result, she contends, many residents may engage in aggressive behavior or social withdrawal as a means of coping with an environment that offers them no space to call their own.

Although health professionals may not be able to eliminate these problems of territoriality, there are some fairly straightforward ways to assist patients in lessening the anxiety created by intrusions and loss of space. Stillman (1978) has suggested the following approaches.

- *Give the patient respect.* Recognize his or her hospital territory, belongings, and rights to privacy.
- *Give the patient control.* Allow the patient to make decisions about his or her territory. Let the patient have control over whether the door should be open or closed, whether the shades should be up or down, and where the bedside table should be placed.
- *Give the patient information.* Recognize the patient's individuality and provide explanations for activities and procedures that directly or indirectly affect the patient.
- *Give attention to patients' privacy needs.* If possible, protect against leaving the patient's body exposed and minimize the discomfort involved in procedures that require the invasion of privacy. (p. 1672)

Distance

A second subarea of proxemics is concerned with how distance affects interpersonal communication. The flow and shift of distance between people as they interact with each other is a major part of the communication process, and it plays a significant role in how individuals interact.

In a classic study of distance zones, Hall (1966) attempted to answer the question of whether human beings have a uniform way of handling distance and whether distance could be delineated into specific zones. His study involved interviews and observations of a sample of middle-class adults from the northeastern seaboard of the United States. Although his research cannot be generalized to other classes, racial groups, or cultures, his results provided the basis for a typology of distance zones in human interaction that has become the accepted framework for analysis of this area.

According to Hall, individuals in social situations use essentially four distance zones: (1) intimate, (2) personal, (3) social, and (4) public. For each zone, Hall has provided a description of what commonly occurs.

INTIMATE DISTANCE. For individuals, this distance includes the area in which people are able to touch one another to the area in which they are approximately 1 1/2 feet apart. Talking in this area is usually soft or at a whisper, and topics are usually very personal. Individuals are selective about allowing others within this distance; it is usually reserved for very close friends. Being forced into intimate distance in public places such as in a bus or in an elevator can produce anxiety.

Due to the types of interventions and activities carried out in health care settings, clinicians often need to enter the patient's intimate distance zone. Providing mouth care or perineal care to a patient who is unable to carry out these hygiene measures requires close distance and contact between the clinician and patient. Some patients will accept and appreciate clinicians' willingness to provide needed care within these close distances. However, those situations in which the clinician enters the intimate distance zone by accident or with little attentiveness to the patient may produce discomfort.

PERSONAL DISTANCE. Personal distance ranges between 1 1/2 and 2 1/2 feet between individuals—about arm's length. This is the distance at which individuals can carry on personal conversations with intimates or close friends using soft to moderate voice levels. Significant variations often exist between cultures in the use of personal distance. For example, individuals from one culture may require less space in informal dialogue at this distance than individuals from another culture.

The personal distance zone is commonly used in health care settings in which the practitioner is explaining a procedure to a patient, reading over preoperative instructions, or discussing a matter of personal concern to the patient.

SOCIAL DISTANCE. When individuals are 4 to 12 feet apart, they are establishing social distance. Communication in business and work settings or at casual social events such as parties is typically carried out at this distance.

Social distance in health care settings would be characterized by the nurse or physician who stands in the doorway of the patient's room to carry on a conversation. This distance is also common in work areas where professionals are writing progress notes or health assessments.

PUBLIC DISTANCE. When people are from 12 to 25 feet or more apart, they are at public distance. Lectures, public speeches, and presentations at large events are examples of places where individuals use public distance. In health care, the community health nurse who is presenting a public seminar on hypertension to a group of senior citizens would most likely be using public distance.

Questions that frequently arise regarding distance zones are, how do people choose spatial distance or what accounts for the distance selections people make? According to Hall (1966), individuals choose distance zones according to their feelings, what they are doing, the nature of their relationships, and the communicative transaction itself (p. 120). Personal distance will also vary depending on such things as race, culture, sex, status, age, personality, and the psychological predispositions of the individuals (Burgoon & Jones, 1976). For example, Street and Buller (1988) found that age was a key factor that influenced personal distance between physicians and patients. Physicians in their study maintained a closer interpersonal distance with middle-aged patients than with younger patients.

We probably become most aware of distance zones in our interactions when the distance used does not seem appropriate for the particular situation. For example, some of us might feel uneasy if a stranger walked up to us, stood 6 inches away, and started a conversation. Awareness of distance zones is also illustrated by the following example.

A friend of ours who had recently been diagnosed as having cancer was attending a public lecture being given by a former professor of his. At the end of the lecture as people were leaving the audience, the professor happened to glance up into the audience where he saw his former student. The professor yelled out into the audience, "Hi—it's nice to see you. . . . Say, I hear you have cancer. . . . Are you OK?" The former student smiled and yelled back that he was fine. While retelling this story, however, our friend said that he was quite surprised that the professor yelled such a personal question in a public setting with an audience. He also said that he was tempted to yell back to the professor, "By the way, how did your hemorroidectomy turn out?" as a way of humorously sensitizing the professor to the situation.

This rather extreme example of imbalance between distance and content of the interaction helps to point out the need for health professionals and others to keep in mind the distances we use with others and how distance plays a role in the comfort and effectiveness of our communication with others.

There are no strong rules that can be set for health professionals to follow in every health care situation. Nevertheless, it is possible for health professionals to be sensitive to the distance norms for different situations, and to try to allow patients to participate in establishing distance zones when possible. Sensitivity and awareness will enhance the possibility of creating a situation in which effective interaction can take place.

Paralinguistic Dimensions of Nonverbal Communication

A third dimension of the nonverbal communication process is paralinguistics (see Fig. 4–1). *Paralinguistics* refers to the vocal sounds such as "ah" and "um" that accompany spoken verbal communication. These voice sounds run alongside our use of language. Paralinguistics focuses on how the voice plays a role in the interpretation of messages. Each individual's voice is unique and varies in regard to paralinguistics. For example, some individuals have voices that are deep, thick, and resonant while others' voices are high, thin, and nasal. Our voice quality is a physical characteristic that often makes us recognizable to others.

In paralinguistics, three vocal qualifiers have been identified: intensity, pitch height, and extent. *Intensity* refers to the degree of energy or power behind a person's voice—like the volume of a radio. A highly intense voice is overloud; its opposite is oversoft. *Pitch height* has reference to how high or low an individual's voice is perceived to be. *Extent* is the length of time a voice carries and includes voices with long drawling or a short clipping quality.

Earlier in this chapter we discussed how facial cues affect the expression of emotions. Similarly, vocal cues also affect emotional expressions. In studying the relative impact of vocal cues, facial expressions, and words on perceived feelings, Mehrabian (1972) found that vocal cues accounted for 38 percent of the effect, while words contributed 7 percent and facial expressions accounted for the remaining 55 percent. Although Mehrabian's research findings cannot be generalized to all messages in all situations, they do point to the importance of the paralinguistic (or vocal) component in human communication.

Paralinguistics is an area of nonverbal communication to which health professionals need be closely attuned. According to Ray and Ray (1990), paralinguistic cues, such as rate and pitch, can affect the health professional's communication with patients. The paralinguistic cues expressed by professionals influence patients' perceptions of professionals. These cues also affect patients' abilities to recall various kinds of information that is verbally transmitted to them.

Touch: A Special Type of Nonverbal Communication

Touch is a particular type of nonverbal communication. Touch can take a variety of forms and it can convey a variety of meanings. A firm handshake, a gentle squeeze, a sharp pinch, or an enveloping hug are all forms of touch. The meaning of the message conveyed by each of these forms of touch can vary considerably. In this section we will discuss the importance of touch in health care, the factors that influence an individual's degree of comfort or discomfort with touch, and clinical considerations regarding touch.

Importance of Touch in Health Care

Touch has particular relevance to health communication (Bottorff, 1993; Frankel, 1983), and health professionals use touch for many different purposes. Touch can ease a patient's sense of isolation and can enhance a patient's reality orientation. Touch is an important tool for diagnosing health problems, as well as for showing nurturance (McCorkle, 1974; Weiss, 1988).

TOUCH AND HUMAN DEVELOPMENT. Historically, it has been found that touch plays an important role in growth and development. Harlow, in his well-known experiments with infant monkeys, demonstrated the importance of soft contact during the developmental process (Harlow & Zimmermann, 1959). Harlow constructed two types of surrogate mothers for infant monkeys. One type, made of molded wire, provided nourishment to the infant. A second type was made of the same wire, covered with a soft terrycloth fabric, but it did not provide nourishment. The infant monkeys showed a strong preference for the cloth-covered mother over the wire-covered mother, even though they were not able to receive food from this surrogate mother. Harlow also found that the infant monkeys with cloth mothers formed stronger attachments and had fewer behavioral problems than the infants with the wire mothers. These experiments contradicted earlier beliefs that the infant–mother bond is based primarily on receiving food, and highlighted the importance of contact comfort to the mother–infant relationship and to the infant monkey's normal development.

The early work of Spitz (1946) also underscores the importance of contact to normal growth and development. Spitz studied human infants who were institutionalized and whose lives were devoid of human contact. He observed that these infants had a number of behavioral problems, which he attributed to their lack of consistent contact with significant others. There is strong evidence that touch is the earliest and most basic form of human communication for infants and the primary means of communication between the infant and the environment. Early and ongoing tactile experiences appear to be strongly related to an adult's emotional and intellectual development.

TOUCH AND HUMAN RELATIONSHIPS. Touch is also valuable in enhancing relationships with others. Aguilera (1967), a psychiatric nurse, studied the usefulness of touch with psychiatric patients. Patients in one group received both touch and verbal communication, while patients in a second group received only verbal communication. Aguilera reported that patients who were touched had more verbal interaction and more rapport with the nurse than those patients who were not touched. In counseling relationships, the therapist's touch contact with the client has been related to increased amounts of self-exploration by the client (Pattison, 1973) and to more positive client evaluations of the counseling session (Alagna, Witcher, Fisher, & Wicas, 1979). Touch, together with verbal communication, was found to quiet distressed children more than verbal comfort alone. (Triplett & Arneson, 1979). Similarly, premature infants on ventilators who received planned intermittent touch were more relaxed over time (Jay, 1982). These studies are only a few of many that indicate that touch has a positive effect on human relationships. Touch is an important intervention that can be used to supplement verbal communication and to show care and concern toward others.

TOUCH AND HEALING. In the last 20 years there has been an increase in research on the relationship of touch and healing. For example, a touching technique similar to the ancient healing practice in which practitioners would use a laying on of hands was identified by Krieger (1975). Krieger's touch intervention, called "therapeutic touch," involves the healer's becoming aware of his or her own energies, and directing the energy from this "centered" state toward helping the ill person. The clinician places his or her hands on or close to the ill person's body for approximately 10 to 15 minutes (Krieger, 1975). During this time the clinician's energy is directed or "transferred" to the ill person, who is believed to be in a less than optimal state of energy (Krieger, Peper, & Ancoli, 1979). In various experiments, Krieger and her associates have reported that this touch intervention has altered patients' hemoglobin rates (Krieger, 1975) and decreased preoperative patients' anxiety levels (Heidt, 1981). In an experimental study of patients with tension headaches, Keller and Bzdek (1986) found that patients who received a therapeutic touch intervention reported significantly less headache pain than patients in the control group. Simington and Laing (1993) reported that therapeutic touch in the form of a back rub reduced the state anxiety for the institutionalized elderly. Although more in-depth study is needed on the mechanism underlying the effectiveness of touch intervention, these results highlight the potential of touch as a special clinical intervention.

Although some research points to the effectiveness of therapeutic touch, researchers are not in agreement regarding the efficacy of this type of nonverbal behavior. For example, Oberst (1995) argues that "the research [on therapeutic touch] is flawed and that there is, therefore, no empirical evidence to support its effectiveness" (p. 383). She argues further that therapeutic touch must be considered experimental until data exist that can verify its effectiveness.

Before leaving our discussion of the importance of touch, it is interesting to note that touch interventions have not always been positively received by patients. On the contrary, there are situations in which touch is perceived negatively or at least as not helpful. For example, when touch was used with nursing home residents, some of the residents reported feelings of discomfort at being touched by the nurse (DeWever, 1977). Similarly, when the effect of touch on preoperative male patients was studied, patients who were touched responded more negatively on the outcome measures than the men who did not receive the touch intervention (Whitcher & Fisher, 1979). In another study, a majority of postpartum women reported positive feelings about being touched, but 37 percent of the women reported either neutral reactions or negative reactions to the touch that they received (Penny, 1979). In light of these reports, it seems clear that touch will not always be perceived in the same way by each person. Some patients will regard touch as positive and helpful, while others will view it as negative and not helpful.

Factors Influencing Touch

There are a number of factors that influence not only our comfort with being touched but also our comfort in touching others. Factors such as our gender, sociocultural background, the type and location of touch used, and the nature of our relationship with the other person can all contribute to our comfort with touching others or with their touching us.

GENDER. Gender is an important component of our receptivity to touch. In health care settings, the gender of the patient and the gender of the health professional can affect receptivity to touch (Weiss, 1988). For example, male surgical patients in one study were more receptive than female patients to being touched by nurses (Lane, 1989). In another study, however, female patients reacted favorably to a touch intervention by a female nurse, while male patients reacted negatively to the intervention (Whitcher & Fisher, 1979). Although these studies in no way provide guidance on whether to touch women and not to touch men or vice versa, they do suggest that the gender of the toucher and the person being touched are important factors influencing not only receptivity to touch but also the meaning given to it.

SOCIOCULTURAL FACTORS. A second factor that influences our reaction to touch is our sociocultural background. Some people are born into families in which a great deal of touching occurs among family members. Other people are raised in families in which touch is more inhibited among family members or limited to task situations. Family environment and early experiences thus influence our preferences and comfort with touch as adults.

In addition to family environment, the cultural environment also influences a person's receptivity to touch. Some cultural groups have been referred to as "contact" cultures, whereas others have been referred to as "noncontact" cultures, depending on how much touch they encourage among people (Knapp, 1978a). Montagu (1978) has suggested that there is a continuum of varying preferences for touch among different cultural groups. It is important to note, however, that individual differences still exist within each culture, even though similarities among people within the cultures have been identified. Taken together, our early family experiences and our sociocultural characteristics are both factors influencing our receptivity to touch.

TYPE AND LOCATION. Although a touch gesture seems relatively uncomplicated and straightforward, each gesture can be characterized by finer discriminations, such as the type of touch, the duration of the touch, and the location of the touch. These specific characteristics influence how a person interprets a particular gesture and whether or not the person will be comfortable with the touch.

The type of touch can also be distinguished by the message that it conveys. Heslin (1974) identified five types of messages that were transmitted through touch (Table 4–1). The functional–professional type of touch is probably the most common type of touch used in health care, followed by either the friendship–warmth type of touch or the social–polite type of touch. The love–intimacy and the sexual arousal types of touch are probably the least *intentionally* used types of touch, although there are instances in which the touch used by a clinician to a patient or by a patient to a clinician has been interpreted in this manner.

Receptivity to touch depends on both the specific characteristics of the touch gesture (e.g., form, duration, and location) as well as on the message conveyed by the particular type of touch. This is illustrated in the following anecdote told by a nurse who was hospitalized for infectious hepatitis. While she was in room isolation, a nurse's aide entered and offered to return later in the evening to give the nurse a back rub. The aide appeared later wearing a pair of rubber gloves to carry out the procedure. The

TABLE 4–1. MESSAGES CONVEYED BY TYPES OF TOUCH

1. *Functional–professional.* This type of touch usually involves task completion such as touching a patient's arm to take a blood pressure or holding a patient's hand to assist him or her with ambulation. The professional using this type of touch sends the message, "I will assist you."

2. *Social–polite.* This type of touch is exemplified by a handshake used to greet a new patient who has just been introduced to you. This type of touch characterizes a fairly superficial involvement between two people.

3. *Friendship–warmth.* This type of touch conveys a liking for the other person. If a patient tells a social worker a humorous story and the social worker laughs and squeezes the patient's arm, the social worker is using a type of touch that conveys the message, "I like you."

4. *Love–intimacy.* This type of touch signifies a close attachment between two people. It could be characterized by an enveloping hug between two people that transmits the message, "I care deeply for you."

5. *Sexual arousal.* This form of touch conveys a physical attraction between two people and may be evident in a close physical embrace or a stroking touch. This type of touch sends the message, "I am very attracted to you."

Adapted from Heslin, R. (1974, May). Steps Toward a Taxonomy of Touching, (p. 1). Paper presented to the Midwestern Psychological Association, Chicago.

nurse–patient said that although the massage was technically done well, it offered her little soothing comfort because the message she kept being reminded of as the aide's rubber gloves touched her skin was, "You are infected and I am afraid of getting your germs." In other words the negative message conveyed by the gloves contradicted the positive intention of the touch.

NATURE OF PARTICIPANTS' RELATIONSHIP. The last factor influencing receptivity to touch is the nature of the relationship between the participants. Touch is often a subtle factor that can be used to characterize the nature and boundaries of a relationship. Estabrooks (1989) found that when the relationship between a nurse and patient was positive, when it "clicked," more touch occurred. However, when the form of touch used is seen as incongruous with the nature of the relationship or if the norms of the relationship are violated, then discomfort can occur.

The following example illustrates the discomfort that occurs when a touch seems to violate relationship norms.

A young female nursing student was talking to a young male psychiatric patient who was diagnosed as having an acute schizophrenic reaction. A nursing instructor, who observed the interaction from a distance, noticed that the student touched the patient a couple of times during the interaction. This was not surprising since the student was a warm, caring person who frequently touched people when she conversed with them. However, later in the interaction when the young male patient touched the student's knee, the student appeared uncomfortable and terminated the interaction.

This incident illustrates the interrelationship between type of touch, message conveyed, and nature of the relationship. The nursing student believed that she was using a functional–professional form of touch with the client, which was compatible with her perception of the relationship. However, she perceived the patient's touch as associated with an intimate or sexual message that was not within the guidelines of the relationship. Although the gesture was the same, the message was interpreted differently according to who touched whom and the context of the relationship.

Touch can also signify lines of power and authority within a relationship. Henley (1973) observed that it is more common for the higher-status person in a relationship to touch a lower-status person, and for men to touch women. The following example may illustrate the relationship between touch and status.

A young female staff nurse was carrying on a discussion with a middle-aged male hospital administrator about the value of nurses having advanced educational preparation. The administrator, who believed that advanced preparation was unnecessary and too costly, frequently touched the nurse during the discussion. He would touch the nurse's shoulder, make a point, and then withdraw his hand. In addition, he would often touch her shoulder to interrupt her when she made a point to counter his arguments. The conversation continued for some time and became quite heated.

Later when retelling the story, the nurse said, "I felt as if he was treating me like a little girl—touching and interrupting me. When he started touching me less, he seemed to be hearing me out more as an equal." Then with a glint in her eye she said, "When he stopped touching me altogether, I knew that either I had won the argument, totally infuriated him, or changed how he perceived me and our relationship.

In this case, touch was seen as a way to define the power and authority within the relationship. The male administrator, who perceived himself as having more status and authority than the staff nurse, frequently touched the nurse and also used touch to control the flow of the interaction. He thought his position gave him the power to touch the nurse. The nurse, however, defined their relationship differently. She did not want to be touched and did not feel the administrator's position gave him the power to touch her. In effect, the nurse and administrator saw status—exhibited through touch—differently. Overall, receptivity to touch is influenced by many factors. We have identified gender, sociocultural background, type and location of touch, and the nature of the participants' relationship as factors influencing the degree of individuals' comfort and discomfort with touch.

Clinical Considerations Regarding Touch

Unfortunately there is no precise formula for determining when to touch or not to touch patients, and there is no universally accepted meaning that can be given to a single touch. Interpretation and receptivity to touch will depend on many factors.

Although some uncertainty surrounds our understanding of when touch will be most effective with clients, the following statements are general guidelines that can be used to increase the likelihood that touch will be perceived positively in therapeutic relationships.

USE A FORM OF TOUCH THAT IS APPROPRIATE TO THE PARTICULAR SITUATION. There are many forms of touch that can be used in a variety of ways. Using a touch gesture that seems compatible with the context will most likely have positive outcomes. For example, a person who has just been told distressing information (e.g., that a son has been injured in an automobile accident) may respond positively to the clinician who places his or her hand on the distressed person's arm. On the other hand, this touch may not be well received by a young male patient who is venting anger about having diabetes. The angry patient needs to vent his feelings in this situation. Letting him get the anger out is better than using consoling gestures.

DO NOT USE A TOUCH GESTURE THAT IMPOSES MORE INTIMACY ON A PATIENT THAN HE OR SHE DESIRES. To some people certain gestures may imply a level of intimacy or a degree of closeness. When the gesture suggests a degree of closeness that is not equally shared or implicitly agreed upon by both parties, discomfort may result (Fisher, Rytting, & Heslin, 1976). Touch gestures need to be monitored in order to adapt to the intimacy needs of patients.

OBSERVE THE RECIPIENT'S RESPONSE TO THE TOUCH. Touch will be most effective when the toucher assesses the impact of the touch on the other person. Assessment is especially important when touch is used in initial meetings with patients and the clinician has no prior knowledge of how the person will respond. Moy (1981) identified behaviors such as the person's pulling away, appearing frightened, or displaying tense facial muscles or other anxious body gestures as negative responses to touch. On the other hand, if the person appears to relax or to seem more comfortable after a touch gesture, then it is likely that the touch is being received positively.

In summary, touch is an effective mode of human communication. However, too often touch is used in relationships without attention being paid to what the touch conveys. Health professionals need to be aware of potential negative responses to touch, of situations in which the meaning of touch can be misunderstood, and of situations in which the message conveyed by a type of touch is not compatible with the nature of the relationship. In health care situations in which both the clinician and the client are comfortable with touch, and the use of touch is assessed for its therapeutic effects, touch can be a very valuable means of communication.

Environmental and Physical Factors

Nonverbal communication also includes environmental factors that impact on interpersonal relationships. Environment includes such things as lighting, noise, color, room temperature, furniture arrangement, and building structure. According to Williams (1988), environmental factors can have a major impact on people in health care settings, especially the seriously ill, frail, and mentally handicapped. These individuals, Williams contends, have more difficulty than their healthy counterparts in entering, leaving, and controlling their environments. Environmental and physical factors actually influence the types of messages that professionals send to patients; and these factors also influence the degree of comfort or discomfort patients feel with the messages (Sharf, 1984).

Perception of the Environment

Knapp (1978b) has identified six dimensions that people use to assess the environment: formality, warmth, privacy, constraint, distance, and familiarity. Although Knapp does not attempt to apply these dimensions to health care settings, these characteristics are useful in describing health care settings as well.[1]

FORMALITY. According to Knapp, people react to their surroundings based on how formal or informal the setting appears. To some people, large health care institutions in university settings seem more formal, while smaller satellite clinics in rural settings seem informal. Knapp notes that the more formal the setting, the more likely that communication will be more superficial, "less relaxed, more hesitant, and generally more difficult" (1978b, p. 73).

WARMTH. Environments can also be perceived in terms of their warmth or coolness. The color of the room and the texture of the upholstery contribute to these perceptions. In health care settings, stark white examination rooms and bright fluorescent lights give an impression of coldness. Knapp believes that psychologically warm environments "encourage us to linger, to feel relaxed, and to feel comfortable" (1978a, p. 88).

PRIVACY. Partitioned or enclosed environments, where interactions cannot be easily overheard by others, are associated with privacy. In health care settings, six-bed wards offer little personal privacy whereas single-bed rooms do. Curtains pulled around patients' beds offer visual privacy but the next door patient can hear everything. Situations that provide more privacy probably foster more personal communication (Knapp, 1978b).

CONSTRAINT. The freedom to enter and leave an environment influences our perceptions of constraint. A patient who can move freely about his or her room would probably perceive the environment as less constricting than the patient who is anchored to a bed because of monitors and equipment. Patients in one study ranked being "tied to the bed with tubes" as the most stressful factor in their intensive care unit environment (Ballard, 1981). Knapp suggests that in environments where physical and psychological constraint is perceived as high, people will be slower to share and to initiate personal disclosures (1978b, p. 75).

---

[1]The following section is adapted with permission from M. L. Knapp, *Social Intercourse: From Greeting to Goodbye.* Boston: Allyn and Bacon, Inc., 1978.

DISTANCE. Environmental distance can involve physical distance as well as psychological distance. Hospital rooms at the end of a long hallway may seem both physically and psychologically distant from other patient rooms and the nursing station. Before the recent efforts to sensitize health care personnel to the needs of patients facing death, dying patients were often placed at the end of hallways where they had little attention or communication from others.

FAMILIARITY. A visit from a clinician in the home would be perceived as a familiar environment by patients and family members, whereas visiting a clinician in a psychiatric setting would be regarded as an unfamiliar environment—especially for patients and family members who have never been in a psychiatric setting. Cautious and hesitant behaviors often occur in new or unfamiliar settings (Knapp, 1978b, p. 74).

Although these six dimensions represent only some of many possible dimensions, they offer a way to look at environments and see how they affect our communication with others. While Knapp (1978a) notes that many of these dimensions overlap and interrelate with one another, in general, more personal communication is often associated with "informal, unconstrained, private, familiar, close and warm environments" (p. 89). Future research is needed to determine more specifically how environmental perceptions affect communication.

Hospital and clinic staff in some specialized areas have worked toward developing comfortable and relaxing environments for patients. In pediatric settings, for example, there have been successful attempts to create an atmosphere of familiarity and warmth; bleak walls have been covered with brightly colored murals of children's favorite cartoon figures, and staff members have replaced sterile white uniforms with more casual and colorful shirts and smocks. The nursing station in one pediatric setting was constructed with lower walls so that small children or children in wheelchairs could talk more easily with staff members (Johnson, M., 1979). In addition, the nursing station was renamed the "communication station" to eliminate boundaries created by the name "nursing" station.

Family birthing centers are now being constructed in some hospitals, with comfortable furniture, lighting, and homelike atmospheres, as an alternative to the formal and impersonal labor and delivery areas. In oncology clinics, comfortable recliner chairs are replacing desklike chairs and hospital beds as a way of fostering a warmer and more casual environment for receiving chemotherapy. In each of these settings, health professionals are demonstrating an awareness of the environment's impact on patient care and interpersonal relationships.

Sound

The clatter of trolleys, the beep of monitors, the click of respiratory equipment, and the rattle of dietary carts all contribute to the sounds of health care facilities. To health care personnel accustomed to this environment, these sounds often go unnoticed. But these sounds often cause patients and family members distress, and they can interfere with rest and recovery. According to Williams (1988), patients who are most vulnerable to the effects of loud sounds are premature infants in incubators, seriously ill patients in high-tech critical care areas, and patients on ototoxic medications.

Several research studies have focused on the possible negative effects of sound in health care. Minckley (1968), for example, studied the relationship between noise and the amount of discomfort experienced by patients in a recovery room. She found more pain medication was given to patients during times in which noise levels were very high in the recovery room than during periods of low noise levels. Minckley points out that noise acts as another irritant to the person who is already in pain. Keefe (1987) compared the amount of noise during the night in a neonatal nursing area with the noise in a rooming-in environment. She found that infants in the nursery were exposed to higher noise levels for a much longer period of time (146 minutes) than infants in the rooming-in environment (20 minutes). Baker (1992) has reported that the heart rates of postoperative surgical intensive care patients were significantly higher when others were talking inside their room than when their rooms were quiet or had background sound. However, Baker and associates (1993) found that equipment sounds did not significantly affect the heart rate or blood pressure of coronary care patients.

Noise is an environmental factor that can cause sensory overload and can interfere with effective professional–professional communication as well as with professional–patient interactions. It is important that health professionals be sensitive to the negative impact of noise, and that they find ways to reduce noise in health care environments.

Furniture Arrangement and Structural Design

A vivid image comes to mind when considering the importance of furniture arrangement and human communication. If you had visited a large, old psychiatric hospital 30 years or more ago, the most noticeable feature would not have been the high-gloss waxed floors or the cagelike screened porches or the long corridors stretching from one side of the building to the other—but the long rows of rocking chairs placed one behind the other outside the patients' rooms so that a patient sitting in one chair looked at the back of the head of another patient, who looked at the back of someone else, and so on. With this arrangement of chairs, it was not difficult to understand why so little social interaction took place on these wards.

The importance of arranging furniture and designing structures to encourage interaction has received some attention by health professionals. Sommer and Ross (1958) studied the effect of room arrangement on a group of geriatric residents. The researchers found that staff members were reluctant to alter previously established seating patterns because of potential housekeeping problems and because they did not believe it would change ward communication. Patients were also reluctant to have their environment changed and at times would return moved furniture to previous arrangements. In spite of initial resistance, Sommer and Ross found that interactions nearly doubled among the residents when furniture was rearranged to facilitate communication. The authors suggest that staff members who do not arrange furniture to encourage interaction are, in effect, allowing *furniture* to arrange the *patients* and possibly to discourage interactions (p. 133).

Seating arrangements have also been analyzed in other settings. In some types of family therapy settings, family therapists often alter who sits next to whom during a session (Minuchin, 1974). For example, two parents with poor communication are often directed to move their chairs closer to one another so that they can converse more directly. The assumption is that altering seating arrangements will also change interaction patterns in a positive way (Minuchin, 1974). In other settings, such as treatment planning sessions, circular arrangements of chairs are used to facilitate the team members' ability to observe and to interact with one another. Using long tables in these settings has sometimes limited the dialogue among members at different ends of the table and prevented them from reading one another's nonverbal expressions.

The structural design of health care settings also influences communication patterns. The design of various nursing stations, for example, can affect nurses' travel time to patients' rooms and ultimately can affect the ease and frequency of interaction among nurses, patients, and family members (Williams, 1988). In some of the newer hospitals, nurses stations with rooms forming a circle around them have replaced older designs in which the nursing station was the midpoint between two long wings. Other structural changes have included more lounge areas for patients and family members, and various kinds of open and closed areas in the units in which staff can interact with patients as well as other staff members.

Environmental factors do have an impact on our communication with others. The preceding discussion briefly touches on some factors—environmental perception, sound, furniture arrangement, and structural design—that affect human relations and communication in health care settings. Environment does not have a neutral role in health communication. It can facilitate or inhibit communication within a particular setting, and environmental components require close attention by health professionals.

▶ SUMMARY

This chapter has focused on the role of nonverbal communication in the total health communication process. Nonverbal communication is communication without words, a process that can be vocal or nonvocal as well as intentional or unintentional. Nonverbal communication fulfills several purposes in the communication process: to express feelings, to regulate interactions, to validate verbal messages, to maintain self-image, and to maintain relationships. Despite certain myths that frequently surround people's perceptions of nonverbal behavior, nonverbal communication is closely bound to verbal communication; it is one of a multitude of elements comprising the human communication process; it does not make individuals transparent; and nonverbal behavior has multiple rather than single meanings.

Five major dimensions of nonverbal communication are kinesics, proxemics, paralinguistics, touch, and environmental and physical factors. Kinesics is the study of body motion and includes gestures, facial expression, and gaze.

The second major dimension of nonverbal communication is proxemics, the study of how people use and interpret space in their interactions. Proxemics focuses on how people deal with territorial issues and invasions of personal space, and how various types of distance (e.g., intimate, personal, social, and public) affect communication.

Vocal sounds and cues that accompany spoken verbal communication are part of paralinguistics, the third dimension of nonverbal communication. Paralinguistics assist individuals in understanding and interpreting messages. They supplement the words and gestures that are used in health interactions.

The fourth dimension, touch, plays a special role in human growth and development, in the development of interpersonal relationships, and in healing. Among the factors that can influence the meaning of touch and a person's receptivity to touch are gender, sociocultural characteristics, type and location of touch, and the nature of the participants' relationships.

The fifth dimension of nonverbal communication, environmental and physical factors, can be analyzed according to the types of perceptions that people form about their environment (e.g., formal or private) and how these perceptions affect interaction in those settings. The effects of sound, object arrangement, and structural design are important factors in creating or detracting from an effective environment for health communication.

▶ REFERENCES

Aguilera, D. (1967). Relationship between physical contact and verbal interaction between nurses and patients. *Journal of Psychiatric Nursing, 5*(1), 5–21.

Alagna, F., Whitcher, S., Fisher, J., & Wicas, E. (1979). Evaluative reaction to interpersonal touch in a counseling interview. *Journal of Counseling Psychology, 26*(6), 465–472.

Allekian, C. I. (1973). Intrusions of territory and personal space: An anxiety-inducing factor for hospitalized patients—An exploratory study. *Nursing Research, 22*(3), 236–241.

Argyle, M., & Cook, M. (1976). *Gaze and mutual gaze*. Cambridge: Cambridge University Press.

Argyle, M., & Ingham, R. (1972). Gaze, mutual gaze, and proximity. *Semiotica, 6*, 32–49.

Baker, C. F. (1992). Discomfort to environmental noise: Heart rate responses of SICU patients. *Critical Care Nursing Quarterly, 15*, 75–90.

Baker, C. F., Garvin, B. J., Kennedy, C. W., & Polivka, B. J. (1993). The effect of environmental sound and communication on CCU patients' heart rate and blood pressure. *Research in Nursing & Health, 16*, 415–421.

Ballard, K. (1981). Identification of environmental stressors for patients in a surgical intensive care unit. *Issues in Mental Health Nursing, 3*(1–2), 89–108.

Bensing, J. M., Kerssens, J. J., & van der Pasch, M. (1995). Patient-directed gaze as a tool for discovering and handling psychosocial problems in general practice. *Journal of Nonverbal Behavior, 19*(4), 223–242.

Birdwhistell, R. L. (1970). *Kinesics and context*. Philadelphia: University of Pennsylvania Press.

Bottorff, J. L. (1993). The use and meaning of touch in caring for patients with cancer. *Oncology Nursing Forum, 20*(10), 1531–1538.

Buller, D. B., & Street, R. L., Jr. (1992). Physician–patient relationships. In R. S. Feldman (Ed.), *Applications of nonverbal behavioral theories and research* (pp. 119-142). Hillsdale, NJ: Erlbaum.

Burgoon, J. K., & Jones, S. B. (1976). Toward a theory of personal space expectations and their violations. *Human Communication Research, 2*, 131–146.

Cipolli, C., Sancini, M., Tuozzi, G., Bolzani, R., & P. Mutinelli (1989). Gaze and eye contact with anorexic adolescents. *British Journal of Medical Psychology, 62*(4), 365–369.

Cook, M. (1977). Gaze and mutual gaze in social encounters. *American Scientist, 65*, 328–333.

Darwin, C. (1872). *The expression of the emotions in man and animals*. London: John Murray. (Reprinted 1965, University of Chicago Press.)

Derlega, V. J. (1995). Health, health care, and nonverbal behavior: An issue overview. *Journal of Nonverbal Behavior, 19*(4), 189–190.

DeWever, M. (1977). Nursing home patients' perception of nurses' affective touching. *The Journal of Psychology, 96*, 163–171.

DiMatteo, M. R., Hays, R. D., & Prince, L. M. (1986). Relationship of physicians' nonverbal communication skill to patient satisfaction, appointment noncompliance, and physician workload. *Health Psychology, 5*(6), 581–594.

Ekman, P., & Friesen, W. V. (1975). *Unmasking the face: A guide to recognizing emotions from facial clues*. Englewood Cliffs, NJ: Prentice-Hall.

Ekman, P., Friesen, W. V., & Ellsworth, P. (1972). *Emotion in the human face: Guidelines for research and an integration of findings*. New York: Pergamon.

Estabrooks, C. A. (1989). Touch: A nursing strategy in the intensive care unit. *Heart & Lung, 18*(4), 392–401.

Fisher, J., Rytting, M., & Heslin, R. (1976). Hands touching hands: Affective and evaluative effects of an interpersonal touch. *Sociometry, 39*(4), 416–421.

Frankel, R. (1983). The laying on of hands: Aspects of the organization of gaze, touch, and talk in a medical encounter. In S. Fisher & A. Todd (Eds.), *The social organization of doctor–patient communication* (pp. 19–54). Washington, DC: Center for Applied Linguistics.

Friedman, H. S. (1979). Nonverbal communication between patients and medical practitioners. *Journal of Social Issues, 35*(1), 82–100.

Goffman, E. (1959). *The presentation of self in everyday life.* Garden City, NY: Doubleday & Co.

Goffman, E. (1963). *Behavior in public places.* New York: Free Press.

Goffman, E. (1967). *Interaction ritual: Essays on face-to-face behavior.* New York: Anchor Books.

Hall, E. T. (1966). *The hidden dimension.* Garden City, NY: Doubleday.

Hall, J. A., Roter, D. L., & Rand, C. S. (1981). Communication of affect between patient and physician. *Journal of Health and Social Behavior, 22,* 18–30.

Hardin, S., & Halaris, A. (1983). Nonverbal communication of patients and high and low empathy nurses. *Journal of Psychosocial Nursing and Mental Health Services, 21*(1), 14–19.

Harlow, H., & Zimmermann, R. (1959). Affectional responses in the infant monkey. *Science, 130,* 421–432.

Harrison, R. P. (1974). *Beyond words: An introduction to nonverbal communication.* Englewood Cliffs, NJ: Prentice-Hall.

Heidt, P. (1981). Effect of therapeutic touch on anxiety level of hospitalized patients. *Nursing Research, 30*(1), 32–37.

Henley, N. (1973). The politics of touch. In P. Brown (Ed.), *Radical psychology.* New York: Harper & Row.

Heslin, R. (1974, May). *Steps Toward a Taxonomy of Touching.* Paper presented to the Midwestern Psychological Association, Chicago.

Jay S. S. (1982). The effects of gentle human touch on mechanically ventilated very-short-gestation infants. *Maternal Child Nursing, 11,* 199–256.

Johnson, F. L. P. (1979). Response to territorial intrusion by nursing home residents. *Advances in Nursing Science, 1*(4), 21–34.

Johnson, M. (1979). Toward a culture of caring: Children, their environment, and change. *Maternal Child Nursing, 4*(4), 210–214.

Keefe, M. (1987). Comparison of neonatal nightime sleep–wake patterns in nursery versus rooming-in environments. *Nursing Research, 36*(3), 140–144.

Keller, E., & Bzdek, V. M. (1986). Effects of therapeutic touch on tension headache pain. *Nursing Research, 35*(2), 101–105.

Kendon, A. (1967). Some functions of gaze-direction in social interaction. *Acta Psychologica, 26,* 22–63.

Knapp, M. L. (1978a). *Nonverbal communication in human interaction* (2nd ed.). New York: Holt, Rinehart & Winston.

Knapp, M. L. (1978b). *Social intercourse: From greeting to goodbye.* Boston: Allyn & Bacon.

Knapp, M. L. (1980). *Essentials of nonverbal communication.* New York: Holt, Rinehart & Winston.

Krieger, D. (1975). Therapeutic touch: The imprimatur of nursing. *American Journal of Nursing, 75*(5), 784–787.

Krieger, D., Peper, E., & Ancoli, S. (1979). Therapeutic touch: Searching for evidence of physiological change. *American Journal of Nursing, 79*(4), 660–662.

Lane, P. L. (1989). Nurse–client perceptions: The double standard of touch. *Issues of Mental Health Nursing, 10,* 1–13.

Lepper, H. S., Martin, L. R., & DiMatteo, M. R. (1995). A model of nonverbal exchange in physician–patient expectations for patient involvement. *Journal of Nonverbal Behavior, 19*(4), 207–221.

McCorkle, R. (1974). Effects of touch on seriously ill patients. *Nursing Research, 23*(2), 125–132.

Mehrabian, A. (1971). *Silent messages.* Belmont, CA: Wadsworth.

Mehrabian, A. (1972). *Nonverbal communication.* Chicago: Aldine-Atherton.

Minckley, B. (1968). Study of noise and its relationship to patient discomfort in the recovery room. *Nursing Research, 17*(3), 247–250.

Minuchin, S. (1974). *Families and family therapy.* Cambridge, MA: Harvard University Press.

Montagu, A. (1978). *Touching.* New York: Harper & Row.

Moy, C. (1981). Touch in the counseling relationship: An exploratory study. *Patient Counselling and Health Education, 3*(3), 89–94.

Oberst, M. T. (1995). The naked emperor revisited. *Research in Nursing & Health, 18,* 383.

Pattison, J. (1973). Effects of touch on self-exploration and the therapeutic relationship. *Journal of Consulting and Clinical Psychology, 40*(2), 170–175.

Penny, K. (1979). Postpartum perceptions of touch received during labor. *Research in Nursing and Health, 2*(1), 9–16.

Prkachin, K. M., & Craig, K. D. (1995). Expressing pain: The communication and interpretation of facial pain signals. *Journal of Nonverbal Behavior, 19*(4), 191–205.

Prkachin, K. M., Solomon, P. S., Hwang, T., & Mercer, S. R. (1995). Does experience affect judgements of pain behavior?: Evidence from relatives of pain patients and health-care providers. Manuscript submitted for publication.

Ray, E., & Ray, G. (1990). The relationship of paralinguistic cues to impression formation and recall of medical messages. *Health Communication, 2*(1), 47–57.

Rosenthal, R., Hall, J. A., DiMatteo, M. R., Rogers, P. L., & Archer, D. (1979). Sensitivity to nonverbal communication: The PONS test. Baltimore: Johns Hopkins University Press.

Sharf, B. F. (1984). *The physician's guide to better communication.* Glenview, IL: Scott, Foresman.

Simington, J. A., & Laing, G. P. (1993). Effects of therapeutic touch on anxiety in the institutionalized elderly. *Clinical Nursing Research, 2*(4), 438–450.

Sommer, R., & Ross, H. (1958). Social interaction on a geriatrics ward. *International Journal of Social Psychiatry, 4*(2), 128–133.

Spitz, R. (1946). Hospitalism. In A. Freud (Ed.), *The psychoanalytic study of the child* (Vol. 2). New York: International University Press.

Stillman, J. J. (1978). Territoriality and personal space. *American Journal of Nursing, 78*(10), 1670–1672.

Street, R. L., & Buller, D. B. (1988). Patients' characteristics affecting physician–patient nonverbal communication. *Human Communication Research, 15*(1), 60–90.

Tate, J. W. (1980). The need for personal space in institutions for the elderly. *Journal of Gerontology Nursing, 6*(8), 439–449.

Triplett, J., & Arneson, S. (1979). The use of verbal and tactile comfort to alleviate distress in young hospitalized children. *Research in Nursing and Health, 2*(1), 17–23.

Weiss, S. (1988). Touch. *Annual Review of Nursing Research, 6,* 3–27.

Whitcher, S. J., & Fisher, J. D. (1979). Multidimensional reaction to therapeutic touch. *Journal of Personality and Social Psychology, 37,* 87–96.

Williams, M. A. (1988). The physical environment and patient care. *Annual Review of Nursing Research, 6,* 61–84.

Interviewing in the 5
Health Care Context

The health care interview plays a pivotal role in clinical practice because acquiring information, discussing results with patients, and monitoring the effects of treatments all depend on interviewing. From intake interviews and initial nursing assessments to discharge planning interviews and home visits, much of the interpersonal communication that takes place in health care settings is carried out through the interview process. In general, interviews play a primary role in the communication of health professionals in all contexts.

Given the prevalence of interviewing in health care, the questions this chapter will address are: What is the nature of interviewing? How can it be used most effectively by professionals in health care settings? In essence, we will take the position that interviewing is simply a special type of interpersonal communication. Concepts and theories that apply to interpersonal communication can also be applied to explanations of interviewing. Our discussion in this chapter will focus on the communication dynamics of the interview process.

Based on the communication assumptions, models, and variables discussed in Chapters 1 and 2, this chapter focuses on the communication dimensions of interviews as they occur in health care relationships. At the outset of the chapter, we define interviewing and describe several common types of interviews that occur in health care settings. Next we discuss what actually goes on during the preparation, initiation, exploration, and termination phases of an interview. In the final section of the chapter, we discuss a series of communication techniques that can be used by professionals to make health care interviews more effective.

► INTERVIEWING DEFINED

Interviewing is a process that has the same transactional and multidimensional characteristics we discussed earlier in regard to interpersonal communication (Fig. 5–1). An interview usually takes place between two people in face-to-face interaction and as a rule it involves both verbal and nonver-

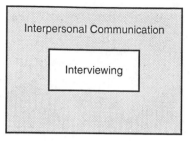

Figure 5–1. Interviewing as a subset of interpersonal communication.

bal messages. Like the communication process, the interview process involves sharing information through a common set of rules. Although all interviews involve interpersonal communication, not all interpersonal communication in health care involves interviewing.

How does an interview differ from other forms of interpersonal communication? What are the specific characteristics of an interview? Interviewing has been defined by Benjamin (1981) as "a conversation between two people, a conversation that is serious and purposeful" (p. xxii). As this

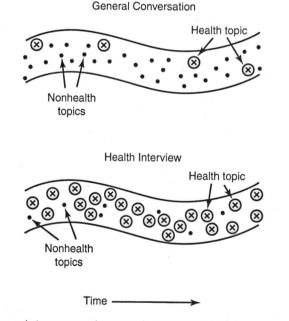

Figure 5–2. Difference between general conversation and health interviews in regard to the focus of interaction. (Adapted from Kahn, R. L. & Cannell, C. F. [1957]. *The dynamics of interviewing: Theory, technique, and cases* (p. 15). New York: Wiley.)

definition suggests, one major characteristic of interviewing that differentiates it from other types of interpersonal communication is that it has a specific purpose. Because interviews are intentional, they usually require the participants to keep their conversation focused on particular topics. Figure 5–2 illustrates that the number of different topics brought up for discussion in a general conversation is far greater than the number of topics that are typically discussed in a health interview. In a health interview, the range of topics is restricted primarily to health-related issues.

A second distinguishing characteristic of interviews is that they usually involve the use of questions and answers. Most of the information written about interviewing centers on how to use communication techniques to ask appropriate questions. Later in the chapter, we will discuss how different kinds of questions result in different kinds of answers—and how questions, if used properly, can make interviews more effective.

Based on the preceding discussion, we will approach interviewing in this chapter using the following definition: Interviewing is a special type of interpersonal communication which is purposeful and serious, usually involving questions and answers, with the goal of sharing information or facilitating therapeutic outcomes.

▶ TYPES OF INTERVIEWS IN HEALTH CARE SETTINGS

Traditionally, interviews have been divided into *information-sharing interviews* and *therapeutic interviews*. In health care organizations there is an overlap between these two major types of interviews because one of the overriding goals of communication in health care is to be therapeutic. Because of this, it is difficult to say that one type of interview is therapeutic and one type is not. For example, a "good" admissions interview focuses on information sharing, but it can also have therapeutic benefits for the client (Stoeckle & Billings, 1987). Although there is some overlap between the major types of interviews, the two categories—information sharing and therapeutic—are used in this chapter to distinguish between interviews that are content focused and of brief duration (information sharing) and interviews that are relationship focused and of longer duration (therapeutic). We now turn to a closer examination of the specific characteristics and dynamics that are distinctive to each type of interview.

Information-Sharing Interviews

Much of what health professionals do involves sharing information through interviews. Information-sharing interviews are designed for the purpose of requesting and providing information, and they emphasize the content rather than the relationship (feeling) dimensions in an interaction. Establishing a good relationship is important in this type of an interview, but it is not the distinguishing characteristic. In health care settings, some of the many examples of this type of interview include admission interviews, history-taking interviews, selection interviews, performance appraisals, and research interviews.

Admissions interviews or intake interviews are used in health care agencies to acquire general demographic, biographical, and financial information about the client who has just entered the health care system. In some agencies, this information will be collected by clerical staff in an admissions office, while in other agencies this information may be gathered by the health professional. With shorter hospital stays and same-day admissions for surgical procedures, many admission interviews are now taking place by phone, prior to entering the hospital. Admission interviews are often used to obtain information (e.g., age, address, insurance) about a client.

History-taking interviews are used by some health professionals to gather information about the client's health history. They include obtaining information about the client's hereditary and family background (e.g., allergies, cancer, heart disease, epilepsy), past health problems (e.g., operations, trauma, psychological disorders), and present health status (e.g., respiratory system, neuromuscular system, medications). This information provides the basis upon which subsequent diagnoses and treatment plans are formulated.

Selection interviews are used in a health care organization to obtain information about individuals who are applying for a job, a transfer, or a promotion within the organization. In this type of interview, information about the individual is used to determine whether he or she is "the right person" for a new position. Information that is shared in this type of interview usually benefits both the interviewer and the interviewee.

Performance appraisals are interviews used by supervisory staff to provide a formal review and evaluation of an employee's past contributions to an organization and to provide a description of the expectations regarding the employee's future job performance. Information shared in this type of interview is usually evaluative in nature, and often serves as a basis for salary increases, promotions, and planning for the employee's future development.

Survey interviews are used by researchers to gather information systematically from a group (or sample) of individuals. Survey interviews are usually designed so that data, such as the beliefs, attitudes, or values of a group of people, can be analyzed using standard statistical procedures. The results of survey interviews in health care settings are often used to (1) assess a community's awareness of services offered by a health care organization, (2) evaluate the effectiveness of a recently created health care program, (3) assess the communication climate within an organization, or (4) determine areas of need for new health care services.

These are only a few of many types of information-sharing interviews used in health care. The common goals of each type of interview are to obtain information or share content within a specific area.

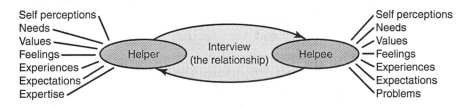

Figure 5–3. The helping relationship in the interview. (Reprinted from Brammer, L. M. [1979]. *The helping relationship: Process and skill* (2nd ed., p. 45). Englewood Cliffs, NJ: Prentice-Hall.)

Therapeutic Interviews

Whereas the primary emphasis in information-sharing interviews is placed on the acquisition of facts, ideas, and content, the primary emphasis in therapeutic interviews is placed on the development of a supportive relationship—the process dimension (Fig. 5–3). Therapeutic interviews are designed specifically to help clients identify and work through personal issues, concerns, and problems. Within the context of a therapeutic relationship, clients can feel free to express their personal thoughts and feelings; they gain new insights about past experiences, develop new problem-solving strategies, and find improved ways of coping with experiences.

Therapeutic interviews are conducted by health professionals in many different types of health care contexts. Social workers, nurses, physicians, chaplains, psychologists, and many others are required to do therapeutic interviews. The therapeutic interviews that we are referring to in this section are most commonly used by health professionals (e.g., clinical psychologists, social workers, or mental health nurse specialists) in settings where patients have personal problems that are primarily emotional or psychological.

There are two basic approaches to conducting therapeutic interviews: *directive* and *nondirective*. In the directive interview, the interviewer (therapist) guides, leads, or prescribes solutions for the interviewee (client). In the nondirective approach, the interviewer allows the interviewee to have control and to choose directions in solving his or her own problems. Both approaches can be placed on a single continuum (shown in Fig. 5–4) varying in degree of directiveness or nondirectiveness. Few therapeutic interviews fall at the extreme ends of the continuum because interviews are seldom entirely directive or entirely nondirective (Downs, Smeyak, & Martin, 1980).

Directive Interviewing

In the directive approach, the health professional often defines the nature of the client's problem and prescribes appropriate solutions for the problem. In this type of interview, the client looks to the professional for direction and guidance because the client perceives the professional as having special knowledge, experience, and expertise that can help the client cope with her or his circumstances. For example, in a directive interview with an over-

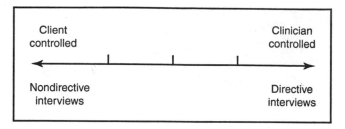

Figure 5–4. Continuum of approaches to therapeutic interviews. (From Patterson, L. E. & Eisenberg, S. [1983]. *The counseling process* (3rd ed., p. 192). Boston: Houghton Mifflin. Adapted by permission.)

weight client seeking help with weight control, the nutrition specialist would determine what type of diet plan the client needs to obtain a desired weight. The nutritionist would then provide the client with specific details about the diet. The directive approach is based on the assumption that the professional has more skills than the client in assessing health problems and choosing strategies to work through these problems (Downs, Smeyak, & Martin, 1980).

The directive approach has several advantages. First, this approach makes full use of the health professional's expertise. Clients receive help based on the professional's training and experience. Second, the directive approach provides specific, concrete information about the nature of a problem and possible solutions. For example, in a study of physicians, Woolliscroft and associates (1989) found that the use of narrowly focused questions was strongly related to obtaining critical data for clinical decision making. Third, the directive approach is much more efficient than the nondirective approach. Directive therapeutic interviews usually focus on the problem, and less time is spent exploring general areas of the client's concerns. In addition, the professional is given the responsibility to assess problems and prescribe solutions; thus, the interview seems to proceed more quickly because less negotiation and collaboration occur between client and professional.

Although there are advantages to the directive approach, there are also several disadvantages. First, the directive approach does not fully recognize the ability of the client to provide some useful assessment of his or her problem(s). This assumption that the professional is more competent than the client can belittle or downplay the importance of client observations and experiences. Second, the directive approach can be counterproductive to a client's well-being if the recommended advice from the health professional is the "wrong" advice or if it is not compatible with the way the client views the situation. Third, a directive approach that moves too quickly to formulate solutions without fully exploring the client's situation may lead to ineffective or misdirected solutions. In addition, the directive approach has the tendency to force the client into a submissive role while the professional plays the dominant role. When clients do not feel fully involved on an equal basis in an interview, they may not follow through on the solutions suggested.

Nondirective Interviewing

In the nondirective approach to therapeutic interviews, the client guides the interaction. Some research suggests that nondirective communication may be more important than directive communication for health professionals (Di Salvo, Larsen, & Backus, 1986). The nondirective approach originated in Roger's (1951, 1959) client-centered approach to psychotherapy. In this type of interview, the health professional serves as a facilitator who reacts supportively to the client's own explorations of a particular problem. Through empathic listening, the professional establishes a relationship in which the client is able to use his or her own resources to define, confront, and resolve problems. For example, if a client sought the help of a health professional for generalized feelings of anxiety, the therapist who uses a nondirective approach would provide a supportive atmosphere in which the client could verbalize feelings and develop his or her own understanding of the origins of the anxiety. The nondirective approach is based on the assumption that the client is the person best able to identify and resolve his or her problems.

The nondirective approach to therapeutic interviews has many positive features. It recognizes the innate potential of clients to identify and resolve their own problems. The nondirective approach encourages client involvement in the treatment process and recognizes that clients can affect and change their lives. In addition, this approach increases the chances that the client and the health professional will be addressing the "real" problem being experienced by the client: If the client identifies the problem, there is less chance that the problem will be defined incorrectly and less chance that the "wrong" problem will become the focus of the interview. Furthermore, the nondirective approach gives greater control to the client, who is treated as an equal partner in the interaction. Finally, when clients are active participants in the interview process, the probability increases that they will feel involved in the decision-making process and will follow through on necessary changes.

The nondirective approach to therapeutic interviews also has some unattractive features. A major criticism frequently leveled at the nondirective approach is that it usually requires large amounts of time, a scarce commodity in health care. Some health professionals believe that it is inefficient, costly, and unnecessary to allocate so much time to nondirective interviews. Also, some professionals may feel the nondirective approach does not make full use of their expertise. They may also feel that there are certain situations in which it is important and necessary to direct clients toward specific solutions that have been proven to be effective.

► PHASES IN THE INTERVIEW PROCESS

The interview process can be divided into four phases: (1) preparation, (2) initiation, (3) exploration, and (4) termination. For the purposes of our discussion, each phase will be analyzed separately; however, in actual interviews the phases blend into one another.

The length of time it takes to move through all four phases of the interview process depends on factors such as the goal of the interview, the severity of the client's problem, the skills of the clinician, and the number of problem areas that emerge (Wilson & Kneisl, 1996). In general, movement through all four phases will occur more rapidly (1) when the goal is information sharing rather than therapeutic change, (2) when the client's personality is well integrated as opposed to severely disorganized, and (3) when there is only a single problem rather than several problems.

In the following discussion of the phases of interviews, we will be using the term *interview* to refer to both single-session interviews, such as an admissions interview, as well as multiple-session interviews, similar to those used in therapeutic relationships. Strictly speaking, an interview occurs at one time and in one place; however, the concepts and theories that apply to specific interview relationships can also be applied to longer term therapeutic clinician–client relationships, which involve a series of interview sessions.

In this section, we will describe the characteristics and nature of each of the four interview phases. We will address the tasks that the health professional confronts in each phase, and we will also discuss some of the common problems that occur during each of the phases.

Preparation Phase

The preparation phase involves anticipating and planning for the actual interview. Sometimes the importance of this phase is minimized or even ignored. We have included it as one of the major phases because the planning or lack of planning has a significant impact on subsequent interview phases.

During the preparation phase, participants often develop preconceived ideas about each other and about how the interview will go. Clinicians seldom approach an interview without some notion about the clients with whom they will be meeting. At a walk-in clinic, for example, a clinician can learn the client's name, age, and ethnic background from the intake sheet. In emergency health care settings, information about a patient is often sent ahead of the patient's arrival. In a community health setting, a nurse who receives a referral from another agency may have considerable information about the client before their first interaction. In each of these examples, the health professional has acquired information that will affect his or her feelings about the interview process.

Clients, like clinicians, also actively anticipate their first meeting with the health professional. Some clients learn the professional's name, find out about his or her specialty, and obtain information on the professional's competence prior to their first meeting. Other clients may go through an extensive process of consulting friends, relatives, or other professionals in order to locate a professional with a certain expertise. Still others may spend time gathering information about a clinician's interpersonal style, therapeutic approach, or success in helping others. Based on the preinteraction information they obtain, clients form images and expectations about the clinician and about the first meeting.

Forchuk (1994) studied the preconceptions that nurses and psychiatric clients held for one another during the development of their therapeutic relationships. Preconceptions of both nurses and clients were evident very early in the relationship and underwent almost no change during the 6-month period of assessment. For example, psychiatric clients who held negative views of nurses as being controlling, unhelpful, and disinterested, tended to maintain these negative preconceptions throughout their relationship. Likewise, nurses who held very negative views of clients tended to maintain these views over time. Forchuk found that the type of preconception that clients and nurses held for one another was strongly related to the effectiveness of their interpersonal relationship—the more positive their preconceptions, the faster they were able to develop an effective working alliance with one another.

A major task for the health professional in the preparation phase is *to plan for the first meeting with the client* (Stuart & Sundeen, 1995). Interviews are more likely to be effective if the clinician is prepared and if the physical setting is also ready. Preparation can include studying about recent advances in treatments, getting assessment forms ready, having educational materials available, or locating an appropriate place to meet. In Chapter 4, we stressed the importance of the environment on the participants' communication. During the preparation phase the clinician can arrange for a comfortable setting that will make it easier to communicate effectively—for example, reserving a conference room, obtaining enough chairs to accommodate an entire family, or making sure that the interview will not be interrupted.

The second task of the preparation phase is *to assess one's own strengths and limitations* and to work through any personal anxieties (Stuart & Sundeen, 1995). Clients have many types of problems, and not all of them are easy for health professionals to handle. For example, some clinicians may find it hard to handle a client who has made repeated suicide attempts. Still other clinicians have problems helping a client whose alcohol intake has caused traumatic injuries to others. Health professionals need to be aware of which client problems are difficult for them to face or to deal with. Self-assessment in the preparation phase means that the clinician sorts through personal feelings, biases, and preconceptions, and if necessary, gets help in resolving personal anxieties related to problem areas.

If there is not enough preparation, difficulties are bound to occur in later phases. For example, if there is lack of adequate planning for room arrangements, the participants' interaction may be interrupted. Similarly, if a professional is unable to work through personal anxiety about a client's problem, considerable tension may pervade the initial meeting with the client and hinder the development of their therapeutic relationship (Forchuk, 1994). Thus, planning and self-assessment before the interview prepare the professional and the client for the first face-to-face encounter.

Initiation Phase

The initiation phase begins when the professional and client make their first contact with each other (e.g., a telephone conversation) or have their first meeting. Sundeen and her associates (1994) point out that the initiation phase is especially important because it sets the tone and creates the climate for the professional-client relationship. Forchuk (1988) found that the initiation phase was a significant factor in predicting how long psychiatric patients would be hospitalized. Patients in her study who moved more slowly through the initiation phase tended to be hospitalized for a longer period of time. Although the initiation phase is considered extremely important, surprisingly little research has been conducted in this area (Saltzman et al., 1976; Wilson & Kneisl, 1996).

During the initiation phase, the preconceived notions and expectations that clients and clinicians have developed in the preparation phase are either confirmed or revised. The following example illustrates how a client sometimes needs to change and revise preinteraction expectations about having an interview with a professional.

Joyce was a little apprehensive about her first meeting with a psychologist. A friend had given Joyce the psychologist's name and recommended him highly to her. Her friend had described the psychologist as a perceptive, understanding person in his mid-50s, with many years of clinical experience. Joyce formed a visual image of the psychologist as a rather gray-haired fatherly man, and she looked forward to her first meeting with him.

When Joyce arrived for her first session she was immediately taken aback by his appearance. He was dressed casually in a crewneck sweater and corduroy pants, and he appeared much younger and more attractive than Joyce had anticipated. Joyce felt disappointed and anxious during the first part of the session. She thought that her friend had misguided her and that she would not be able to relate to this young, attractive man, who was very different from the person she was expecting. As the interview continued, however, she found that in spite of his young appearance, the psychologist was understanding and empathic.

Although in this example it is the client who adjusted her expectations, it is equally important that professionals be able to adjust their own preconceptions of clients in the initiation phase.

After reconciling initial expectations, one of the first tasks for professionals in the initiation phase is *to establish a therapeutic climate that will foster trust and understanding.* A supportive atmosphere is particularly helpful at the beginning of the interview because it reduces the client's anxieties about new situations and relationships. A nonthreatening interview atmosphere makes it easier for clients to share their worries and concerns.

Communication plays an important role in creating a supportive interview climate. One type of communication that is often used to put participants at ease in the initial stage of an interview is phatic communication. Phatic communication refers to "small talk," such as the weather (e.g., "Did you have any trouble driving here through the snow?"), the parking (e.g., "Were you able to find a parking spot?"), or the setting (e.g., "Is that chair comfortable for you?"). A brief period of commonplace talk gives participants time to adjust to the setting and to each other before getting into a discussion of more personal information (Barnlund & Haiman, 1960). Phatic communication is used more often in professional–professional interviews (e.g., in selection interviews) and less often in therapeutic professional–client interviews. Too much of it can sidetrack an interview, make an interview seem phony, or produce an awkward atmosphere as the participants become unsure of how to move from superficial topics to more important issues.

Certain types of specific communication techniques such as open questions, reflection, restatement, and clarification also add to the development of a supportive atmosphere during the initial phase of an interview. These techniques are described and discussed at greater length in the last section of this chapter.

The second task of the initiation phase is *to clarify the purpose of the interview.* Benjamin (1981) encourages the interviewer to state clearly the purpose of the interview. He points out that ambiguous statements such as, "I think that we both already know why we are meeting today," can lead to second guessing or poor communication between participants. In a study of nurse–client interactions in community settings, Krisjanson and Chalmers (1990) found that in home visits the nurse was the one who usually stated the purpose of the visit, whereas if the client was interviewed in the clinic setting, the client usually explained the reason for the visit. The investigators found some instances in which the purpose of the interview was clearly stated and others in which it was only vaguely mentioned or not stated at all. In these latter situations, the interview took on a friendly rambling quality, but little exchange of health-related information occurred.

If the purpose of the interview is not stated, the participants may be unsure about their relationship (e.g., whether it is social or therapeutic) which ultimately hinders the focus of their interaction. Although stating the purpose of the interview is important, researchers found that few young physicians explained the purpose of the interview (Maguire, Fairbairn, & Fletcher, 1989). In an information-sharing interview, a statement such as, "I am a discharge planning nurse, and I would like to talk with you about what kind of care you are going to need at home," immediately lets the client know the clinician's expectations for the session. In a therapeutic interview, a statement such as, "Perhaps you could share some of the concerns that brought you here today and then we can decide which area would be most helpful for us to pursue," helps to identify the purpose of the interview. In both types of interviews, clarifying the purpose gives a structure to the relationship and gives a sense of direction for the interaction that is to follow.

The third task for professionals in the initiation phase is *to formulate a contract with the client.* A contract is a mutually agreed upon statement that provides specific guidelines about the nature of the interview. Essentially, a contract lets both participants know what to expect from one another during the relationship (Loomis, 1985). The contract often includes specific information such as the time and place of meetings, the length of each session, the number of sessions, the confidentiality of issues discussed, and plans for termination (Sundeen, Stuart, Rankin, & Cohen, 1994).

Contracts can be either spoken or written. Most contracts are established through verbal interaction, although the participants may never use the word *contract* in their conversations (Sundeen, Stuart, Rankin, & Cohen, 1994). Some clinicians prefer written contracts to verbal contracts. Steckel (1982), for example, believes that written contracts provide an observable, tangible mechanism to establish accountability between the clinician and client. Whether contracts are verbal or written, they clarify the details and structure of the interview process.

The fourth task of the initiation phase is *to establish mutual goals.* Mutual goal setting fosters collaboration between the client and the professional, and prevents either individual from imposing goals on the other. There is some indication, however, that goals are not always clearly established in therapeutic relationships. Farran, Carr, and Maxson (1988) studied goal setting between professionals and patients in a short-term psychiatric setting and found that nurses and physicians seldom communicated their goals to clients, nor did they elicit goals from clients. Patients and family members said they often did not know what to expect from the hospital nor from their relationships with professionals. The goals that are established during the orientation phase provide a sense of direction and readiness for the exploration phase that follows.

During the initiation phase, several communication problems may arise that will hinder the development of the interview process. Sayre (1978, pp. 176–177) identified several common errors that nursing students often make during the initiation phase of a nurse-patient interaction. The following examples illustrate these errors:

- Clinician uses vague introductions to explain the purpose of the interview.
- Clinician moves too quickly to get the patient to disclose uncomfortable information.
- Clinician has difficulty dealing with the client's request for personal information about the professional.
- Clinician is unsure of how to proceed with an interview after the initial introductions and moves instead into social conversation.

Potential problems in the initiation phase are more likely to occur when the clinician does not create a supportive climate or clarify the purpose of the relationship. The four tasks of the initiation phase are crucial because they provide a structure and direction for moving into the exploration phase.

Exploration Phase

After the structure and direction of the interview are established, the participants are ready to enter the exploration phase. This is often called the *working phase* because it is the part of the interview in which the client and the clinician try to confront, analyze, and work on the client's problems. During this working phase, the health professional tries to assist clients to master their anxieties, increase their sense of independence and responsibility, and acquire new coping abilities (Stuart & Sundeen, 1995).

A major task for professionals in this phase is *to help clients explore their personal problems*. During this phase, the clinician and the client can begin discussing emotionally charged topics. Benjamin (1981) contends that in the exploration phase a client's initial concern is often replaced by a different, more central concern. For example, a client may send out a trial balloon (a minor concern) in the initiation phase to see how the clinician responds to it. If the clinician seems to handle the first concern with sensitivity, the client then proceeds to share a more pressing concern. In addition, the goals formulated during the earlier phase are often modified as new information surfaces in the exploration phase. The following example illustrates this process.

A nursing student sought counseling to work through the tensions that she was experiencing at school. During the first session, the student said that she was having problems with low motivation, inability to concentrate, and difficulty meeting classroom deadlines.

At a later session, however, when the student was feeling more comfortable with the counselor, the student said that her real worry was her father's alcoholism and abuse of the younger children in her family. She said that these home problems were interfering with her ability to study. Based on this new information, she and the counselor agreed on different goals and discussed new ways of coping with the family stresses.

The task of exploration does not necessarily proceed at a smooth, consistent pace. As a rule, though, general themes and patterns emerge in the exploration phase that provide the basis for growth and positive change for the client.

A second task of the exploration phase is *to help clients manage feelings* generated by the discussion of stressful issues. The disclosure of personal and private information by clients during an interview session can generate anxiety. Clients may wonder if they have said too much, if the clinician will accept them, or if their feelings are typical of others who have experienced the same problems. In addition, for clients, the discussion of personal information may also bring out a wide range of feelings such as fear, anger, sadness, or hopelessness. In an atmosphere of acceptance and support, the clinician can help clients to manage and express these feelings.

The third task for health professionals in the exploration phase is to help clients *develop new coping skills*. Through the process of exploration, clients may question their previous behaviors, their usual ways of responding, and their rigid patterns of thinking. Even in short interviews (such as an intake interview), clients can become aware of their strong values or beliefs. The underlying goal of exploration is to help clients build their skills in coping with problems and stress.

The exploration phase is not easy for clients or professionals. Clients may be hesitant to discuss personal feelings, and clinicians may be uncertain about how to explore clients' feelings. Several common communication errors that can occur during this phase have been identified by Sayre (1978, pp. 178–180). They are listed below.

- Clinician is unable to maintain a sustained focus on an important issue. He or she prematurely changes topics or gives clients insufficient feedback to continue on a topic.
- Clinician frequently offers inappropriate advice, approval, or reassurances.
- Clinician responds in stereotyped ways to clients. He or she overuses the same communication techniques (e.g., reflective statements).

The errors cited by Sayre are just a few of many of the communication errors that can be made in the exploration phase.

There are no perfect guidelines for the exploration phase. The direction and flow of the conversation will vary considerably depending on the participants and the topics being discussed. Through the ongoing interaction the exploration process unfolds, goals are accomplished, and the termination phase begins.

Termination Phase

It is the termination phase that has been written about the most often, especially as it applied to therapeutic interviews (Lego, 1980). Perhaps so much has been written about this phase because termination evokes so many mixed feelings in people. Sundeen and her associates (1994) point out that at the close of a successful relationship, the satisfaction experienced by both participants at having met their mutually agreed upon goals must be balanced against the realization that they have to end a meaningful relationship. Termination is seldom easy for participants because it can evoke feelings of sadness, fear, or uncertainty at saying "goodbye."

Although it is sometimes difficult, termination is an essential phase of effective interviews. In this phase, the professional assists the client in finding closure to problems and concerns that have been discussed in the interview. Termination signals to the client that the purpose of the interview has been accomplished, the goals have been reached, and the end of the interview relationship is near.

The major task of this phase is *to plan for closure of the interview.* Ideally, the planning for termination begins in the initiation phase when the clinician and the client establish a contract. The fact that the interview is moving toward a conclusion is reinforced at various times throughout the other phases. At the very least, in interviews that continue for several sessions, termination issues should be considered in one or two sessions before the final meeting. In single-session interviews, termination issues should be discussed before the last few minutes of the interview. In either situation, the reminder that the interview is coming to an end enables the participants to reorient themselves and to tie up unfinished areas in the time that remains.

Planning for termination also involves making arrangements for needed follow-up resources. In a single-session interview, the participants may not have enough time to address some of the specific concerns that have been raised, and the clinician may need to refer the person elsewhere. For example, a school nurse who has the opportunity to meet only once with a troubled parent of a student who uses drugs may find it essential to refer the parent to another community resource for further help. In therapeutic interviews that have a number of sessions, the clinician may identify a follow-up resource person and link the client with the new resource person before the final meeting. For example, a student who is working with a client in a community mental health agency may plan one or two joint meetings between the client and the new resource person before the actual termination of the student–client relationship.

A few other factors should be included in plans for termination. At times it is helpful to decrease the frequency of the sessions or the length of each session as termination approaches. For instance, participants may decide to meet every other week rather than every week, or for 1/2 hour rather than 1 hour. Also, as termination approaches it is helpful for clinicians to direct clients toward discussion of topics that are less emotionally charged. Emotionally laden topics create anxieties in participants that can impede the closure process.

The second task of the termination phase is *to summarize issues and accomplishments.* The summary can be made by either the clinician or the client, but it is best when both people share in the process. It is helpful to clients to summarize areas that have been fully or partially resolved, as well as to summarize and repeat any "homework" assignments. Summaries are more beneficial if they are brief and specific, and if they underscore the movement in a relationship and in an interview.

The final task of the termination phase is *to assist clients to express their feelings about termination.* We mentioned earlier that termination often causes mixed feelings. Even if the termination is desired and the goals have been reached, it is fairly common to find feelings such as sadness, anger, abandonment, guilt, and helplessness during the termination process (Nehren & Gilliam, 1965; Sundeen, Stuart, Rankin, & Cohen, 1994). Perhaps it is not surprising that at times participants choose to extend the time set for termination, or skip the termination session altogether. However, by creating a climate and opportunity to work through these feelings, the clinician can bring the interview to a satisfying closure.

Several communication errors that can lead to ineffective movement through termination have been identified by Sayre (1978, pp. 182–183). She points out that students frequently make the following errors:

- Clinician prematurely terminates the interaction because the client is not responding in the expected way.
- Clinician does not allow enough time for termination and therefore deals with termination issues only superficially.
- Clinician brings up emotionally charged issues that should have been dealt with in an earlier phase.
- Clinician avoids dealing with termination issues because the clinician thinks he or she has not been helpful to the client.

These brief examples highlight some of the difficulties that can occur during termination. These errors are evident not only in students' interactions but also in the interviews conducted by practicing clinicians. Krisjanson and Chalmers (1990) found that some experienced nurses discussed termination, but others ended their meetings with clients very abruptly and without ever discussing plans for future follow-up. Many of the errors that occur during this phase can be eliminated by attending to the tasks of termination.

In general, it is best when termination can be planned and carried out after all the other phases have been completed. In reality, however, termination is not always neatly planned or perfectly timed. Terminations often occur unexpectedly when clinicians change jobs, students leave their clinical rotations, emergencies arise on a unit, or clients are transferred to another health care setting. In each of these cases, a departure terminates the participants' interaction.

Obviously, unexpected terminations or terminations with nebulous timelines are difficult to plan. For example, sometimes the actual termination date may be in limbo for a day or two, as in the case of a patient in an acute care hospital who has to wait for an available room in a rehabilitation center. In a situation such as this, it is not unusual for the patient to be transferred suddenly, with little or no time to terminate relationships with the hospital staff. Furthermore, if the patient's primary nurse or social worker is off work on the departure day, termination with these health professionals may be missed altogether. In situations such as these, where sudden and unplanned departures are a real possibility, it is important for health professionals to discuss aspects (e.g., resource planning or expression of feelings) of the termination process early.

All four phases of the interviewing process and the specific tasks associated with each phase are listed in Table 5–1. Like other developmental processes, the development of the interview relationship takes time. Each

TABLE 5–1. PHASES AND TASKS OF THE INTERVIEW PROCESS

Phases	Tasks
Preparation	Plan for first meeting
	Assess strengths and limitations
Initiation	Establish therapeutic climate
	Clarify purpose
	Formulate contract
	Establish mutual goals
Exploration	Explore problems
	Manage feelings
	Develop coping skills
Termination	Plan for closure
	Summarize issues
	Express feelings

Adapted from Stuart, G. W. & Sundeen, S. J. (1995) Principles and practice of psychiatric nursing (5th ed.). St. Louis: C. V. Mosby.

interview situation is different and each interview develops over time in unique ways. For example, Forchuk (1995) examined the development of the nurse–client relationship and found that the same individual, whether nurse or client, developed very different relationships with different people. However, nearly all interviews proceed either directly or indirectly through the four phases. By attending to the tasks of each phase, health professionals can reduce the possibility of problems occurring during the interview and also improve the quality of the health care interview.

Our discussion of phases may have implied that these interviews typically occur in a face-to-face interviewing context. While this may be the case for the majority of interviews, there is a growing use of telephone-based interviews. Same-day admissions for tests and procedures have necessitated the use of telephone interviews to obtain demographic, insurance, and medical history information prior to admission. Likewise, shorter hospital stays have necessitated the use of follow-up phone calls to verbally assess patients' health status, rate of recovery, and incidence of complications. For example, Keeling and Dennison (1995) used telephone interviews with myocardial infarction patients and/or their wives at 5, 14, and 21 days following discharge from the hospital to determine how the patient's recovery was progressing. Patients and their spouses expressed a great deal of appreciation and satisfaction with the follow-up phone interviews.

The same issues that are relevant for face-to-face interviews discussed earlier (e.g., clarifying a purpose, exploring problems, or planning for closure) are also relevant for telephone-based interviews. However, missing from the telephone interview are many of the dimensions of nonverbal communication. Without these nonverbal cues, participants need to rely more heavily on verbal communication to clarify and facilitate their communication.

► COMMUNICATION TECHNIQUES IN INTERVIEWS

Earlier in the chapter, we pointed out that interviewing is a special type of interpersonal communication that uses questions and answers and that is intended to acquire information or facilitate therapeutic outcomes. In this section of the chapter, we will describe specific communication techniques that are used by health professionals to conduct interviews. The techniques we will discuss are closed and open questions, silence, restatement, reflection, clarification, and interpretation. These are *only* techniques and their use does not guarantee that the interview will always fulfill its purpose. However, if these techniques are used together with the communication variables discussed in Chapter 2—trust, shared control, empathy, and confirmation—it is more likely that the interview will be effective.

Questions

The interviewer's ability to ask appropriate questions is the technique that is most important in effective interviews. Asking questions is the principal mode of carrying out interviews or, as Benjamin (1981) suggests, it is "the basic tool of the interviewer . . ." (p. 71). Although asking questions is the mainstay in health care interviews, health professionals should be cautious so as not to control interviews through the use of questions. For example, West (1983) studied a sample of 21 interactions between physicians and patients in a family practice center and found that physicians asked 773 questions compared to patients who asked 68. Furthermore, while patients responded to 98 percent of the questions, physicians responded to only 87 percent of the questions. Similarly, a study by Arntson, Droge, and Fassl (1978) found that pediatricians asked twice as many questions as parents. In another study of medical interviewing, Putnam and associates (1988) reported that medical residents had a difficult time listening to patients without asking questions. When they only listened, residents reported discomfort in allowing patients to talk about their illnesses in their own words. In health care interviews, it is important that both participants have equal opportunity to request information, and equal responsibility to receive and disclose information.

In general, there are two types of questions that can be used in interviews: closed questions and open questions. Each type is used for different purposes. A closer examination of each type of question will clarify how each can contribute to or detract from effective interviews.

Closed Questions

Questions that limit and restrict clients' responses to specific information are called *closed questions*. Closed questions have been likened to true-or-false and multiple-choice examination questions, because the respondent can only give specific or limited responses. Probably the most common type of closed question is one to which the client is asked to answer yes or no. In health care, closed questions are often used to gather demographic data, medical histories, or diagnostic information. Closed questions are used more frequently in information-sharing interviews than in therapeutic interviews.

The following examples are illustrations of closed questions:

- Do you think your breathing is better, worse, or about the same as yesterday?
- Are you feeling anxious about what the laboratory reports reveal about your condition?
- Do you have a history of heart problems in your family?

Clients could respond quickly to each of the preceding closed questions with straightforward and specific answers.

The main advantage of closed questions is that they can be used by professionals to get quick answers. They are efficient. In addition, this type of question does not demand deep introspection on the part of the client, while at the same time it provides the health professional with valuable information. However, there are also disadvantages to closed questions. Closed questions do not allow the client to explain feelings or emotions or give additional information. Thus, closed questions inhibit client communication and may lessen the client's sense of control.

Open Questions

Open questions do not restrict clients' responses; they allow clients to give extended and unlimited answers. As Benjamin (1981) points out, "The open question is broad; . . . allows the interviewee full scope; . . . invites him to widen his perceptual field; . . . ; [and] solicits his views, opinions, thoughts, and feelings" (p. 73).

Open questions are often used in therapeutic interviews as the primary means of encouraging clients to explore their personal thoughts and feelings. In an analysis of the communication used by expert nurses, Brown (1994) found that expert nurses frequently used open-ended questions in their interactions with clients. Open-ended questions were used by expert nurses at the beginning of interviews to elicit clients' concerns and again later in the interview to follow up on more personal issues, after rapport had been established between the client and nurse. Open questions draw clients out, allow for catharsis, and assist clients to express pent-up emotions. For medical patients, open questions are a means of getting patients to tell their story of what is wrong with them and to freely disclose about their situation (Sharf, 1984).

Open questions are illustrated in the following examples:

- You seem upset. What are you feeling right now?
- Describe what you think is going to happen.
- How did you feel when you first learned of your diagnosis?
- I think you've made considerable progress. What are your thoughts and feelings about how you're doing?

In each of the preceding examples, the questions are phrased so as to encourage the interviewee to talk and to describe his or her own frame of reference on a topic.

Open questions are advantageous and essential in health care interviews. Clients have a sense of control because they have the freedom to answer in whatever way they choose. In other words, clients can select what they want to say, how much they want to say, and how they want to say it. Open questions are also valuable because the interviewer obtains more information and description from the client. According to Roter and Hall (1987), who studied the interviewing styles of 43 primary care physicians, open questions are more strongly related to patient disclosure of medical in-

TABLE 5–2. CLASSIFICATION OF THE ADVANTAGES AND DISADVANTAGES OF OPEN VERSUS CLOSED QUESTIONS

	Efficiency	Emotionality	Depth	Control
Open questions	−	+	+	+
Closed questions	+	−	−	−

formation than are closed questions. With the added information, the interviewer can gain a better understanding of how the client thinks and feels. The only disadvantage of open questions is that they often require more interview time, which is at a premium in health care.

From the preceding discussion of open and closed questions, it is apparent that there are advantages and disadvantages of both types of questions. Table 5–2, summarized from the work of Berelson and Steiner (1964), compares the advantages and disadvantages of closed and open questions. In general, open questions give clients more control and encourage responses that have more breadth and more feelings; closed questions are more time efficient.

Silence

We have all heard the phrase, "Silence is golden." Silence can play a very valuable role and have very positive effects in the interview process, but it is not *always* positive. Sometimes silence is negative and counterproductive to effective communication. The major questions that confront interviewers are *when* to use silence and *how* to use silence most effectively.

In a classic article, Baker (1955) proposed a model of silence that illustrates two kinds of silences: positive silence and negative silence (Fig. 5–5). In Baker's model, silence that is negative (indicated by the notation S−) occurs when the participants in an interaction (person A and person B) feel uncomfortable, and when tension is high in their relationship. In addition, silence is also regarded as negative when no reciprocal identification (e.g., no empathy) is experienced by the participants for one another during the silence. As we move from left to right on the model, silence becomes more positive (indicated by S+), when tensions are reduced and the reciprocal identification between the participants increases. Baker suggests that positive silence is silence "in which arguments and contentions, whether expressed or not, have vanished, to be replaced by understanding acceptance on the part of the hearer (or hearers) and satisfied contentment on the part of the speaker" (p. 161).

Generally, silence is used less frequently in the initiation and termination phases of interviews and more often in the exploration phase. During the initiation phase, the clinician and client are trying to establish a relationship through conversation, and excessive use of silence detracts from this

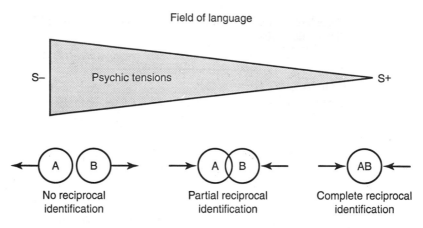

Field of language

Figure 5–5. The Baker model of silence. (Reprinted from Baker, S. J. [1955]. The theory of silences. *Journal of General Psychology, 53,* 159.)

process. At the end of an interview, silence may imply that the work of the interview has halted prematurely, which could work against a sense of planned closure. During the exploration phase, the use of silence by clinicians is more common because it provides a time for both the client and the clinician to think about the issues that they are actively exploring.

In an interview, silence can be used appropriately by a clinician to give a client the message, "Carry on and continue talking." The following example

---

Client: I'm really not sure I've done the right thing by deciding to put Mom in the nursing home. I feel like I should be taking care of her myself—at home. *(Client has wrinkled forehead.)*

Clinician: Mm'hm. *(Clinician nods.)*

Client: You know . . . going to a rest home is the last thing she would have chosen. She was normally so interested in everything we were doing. Our family is so close. It seems like we're just dropping her off and getting rid of her. *(Sighs.)*

Clinician: So you wish you could care for her yourself?

Client: Yes. But, I just can't do it. I should, but I don't think I can with all the problems she has. She can't walk by herself, she needs to be fed, she can't go to the bathroom alone, and she is confused most of the time. I don't know what to do. If only. . . . *(Pauses.)*

Clinician: *(Remains silent. Continues to look at client.)*

Client: . . . If only she hadn't had this stroke. I feel so guilty about not spending more time with her. But I guess I don't have any other good alternative at this point.

---

illustrates how silence can be used to stimulate the client to elaborate and expand upon a topic.

In the preceding example, the clinician's silence allows the client time to collect her thoughts and to think through the feelings that she has about placing her mother in a nursing home. In effect, the silence of the clinician is saying to the client, "Carry on. I'm with you on this. Do you have more you'd like to say? I'll listen." Silence is a useful technique that allows both the clinician and the client to collect their thoughts and ideas. Although long pauses for this purpose can be uncomfortable, shorter silences are an important element in effective interviews.

Although silence has several positive purposes, silence also has some drawbacks—it is *not* always golden. As is indicated in the Baker model, silence will create tension in situations where the interviewer and the client do not strongly identify with each other. For example, when two people are uncertain about what the other person is thinking during a silence, the silence may increase their discomfort and anxiety. Overuse of silence can also create a sense of directionlessness in interviews. Too many pauses or silent periods can result in participants feeling that the purpose of their conversation is unclear and unfocused. Finally, excessive use of silence may make clients feel that they are getting insufficient feedback on a topic.

Overall, it is important to be aware of both the positive and the negative effects that silence can produce in interviews. Effective interviewing requires clinicians to be sensitive to clients' needs and to use silence in situations where it will lead to positive outcomes.

Restatement

In Chapter 1, we discussed communication as a process in which there is feedback between the source and the receiver. In interviewing contexts, restatement acts as a feedback mechanism between the clinician and the client. Through restatement the clinician can communicate to the client that the clinician is listening and that the clinician understands what the client has said. Restatement is a technique that provides confirmation to clients because it directly acknowledges their point of view. Restatement gives clients a sense of validation—a feeling that they have been heard by another human being. The underlying assumption of restatement is that as clients feel validated or understood, they will also feel encouraged to continue speaking and examining their concerns.

As a communication technique, restatement involves paraphrasing or repeating the client's message. Although technically the clinician may restate the exact words of a client, it often seems more empathic and less mechanical to restate the message in slightly different words. In general, the clinician using restatement acts like a sounding board for the client. The following example illustrates how a clinician might use restatement:

....

Client: It is very hard for me to think about how my epilepsy is going to affect my wife and kids. I really wish they would carry on as if these seizures had never happened, but I'm concerned that my condition will upset them.

Clinician: It is difficult for you to think about the fact that your epilepsy will influence your family situation. You wish they could act as if everything was normal but you are worried that your potential to have more seizures will bother them and make things unnatural.

Client: Yes. I care an awful lot about them and I don't want to worry them.

Clinician: You really love your family and want the best for them.

Client: I sure do. They mean everything to me. That's why I'm feeling so down about this sickness. I just don't want it to affect them in any way.

....

In the preceding example, the clinician is paraphrasing or restating what the client has verbalized without adding any of his or her own personal feelings or thoughts.

In using restatement, health professionals often preface their responses to clients with phrases such as, "I hear you saying . . . ," or, "It sounds as if you feel . . . ," or, "Let me see if I understand you; you're saying. . . ." Prefaces such as these are useful in restatement because they help the clinician move into an other-directed frame of mind, and they help clients by expressing the intentions of the clinician to restate what the client has verbalized.

Reflection

As a communication technique, reflection is very similar to restatement. Both techniques aim to help clients to understand their thoughts and feelings, and both techniques also require the interviewer to act as an echo or sounding board for the client's expressions. In neither technique does the interviewer express her or his own perspectives. However, reflection is different from restatement and it does require a different approach on the part of the interviewer.

In reflection, the interviewer acts as a mirror for the expressed and sometimes unexpressed emotions and attitudes of the client. Unlike restatement, which centers on *what* the client has said (the content), the focus in reflection is on *how* something has been expressed, or the feeling dimension. "Reflection consists of bringing to the surface and expressing in words those feelings and attitudes that lie behind the interviewee's words" (Benjamin, 1981, p. 123). Reflection helps clients get in touch with their feelings and assists them in identifying and describing them.

Reflection is more difficult than restatement because it requires listening empathically for emotions and feelings. Clients are not always able to identify specifically their own emotional states. Reflection is a means of helping them in this process. To accurately understand clients, health professionals need to be attuned to the general emotion the client is expressing and the intensity of that emotion. In addition, health professionals need to be able to accurately communicate back to the client the precise feeling that has been expressed.

The following example of a professional-client interview illustrates how reflection can be used to help the client get in touch with feelings that are present:

Client: This hospital really makes me mad. One person tells me one thing and the next person tells me exactly the opposite. I wonder what's going on around here. *(Shakes head, throws hands up in the air.)*

Clinician: You are feeling pretty confused and angry by it all.

Client: Boy, am I! All my reports seem mixed up and everyone tells me something different. I just can't believe it has to be this way. *(Looks down.)*

Clinician: It seems that all the uncertainty over your reports is upsetting to you and that you feel helpless about how to respond.

Client: I guess so. I know they're doing everything they can—I just feel out of control and that worries me.

As the preceding example shows, in essence, reflection is a technique that helps clients to identify feelings that are enmeshed in the descriptions of their experiences. In short, reflection is a technique that helps clients get a handle on their feelings.

To use reflection effectively, health professionals themselves must have a broad vocabulary of feelings. In Table 5–3 we present a vocabulary of feelings developed by Hammond, Hepworth, and Smith (1977) that may be useful as a resource in identifying feelings. The vocabulary provides a list of feeling words that are strong, moderate, and mild variations of ten basic feeling categories (e.g., happy, depressed, lonely). Sometimes it is less threatening for clients to acknowledge mild feelings and more threatening for them to acknowledge strong feelings. For example, a client who is hesitant to discuss feelings may respond more readily to a clinician's reflection that the client is feeling "worried" (a mild feeling) than that he or she is "terrified" (a strong feeling) about a situation. As their relationship develops and the client experiences more trust in the clinician, the client may be comfortable enough to acknowledge stronger feelings. Being aware of the diversity of feeling words and the various levels of intensity of these words can enhance one's ability to accurately reflect the feelings that a client is experiencing.

TABLE 5–3. VOCABULARY OF FEELINGS

Levels of Intensity	Happy	Caring	Depressed	Inadequate	Fearful
Strong	Thrilled	Affection for	Dejected	Worthless	Terrified
	Ecstatic	Attached to	Hopeless	Powerless	Frightened
	Overjoyed	Devoted to	Bleak	Helpless	Intimidated
	Excited	Adoration	In despair	Impotent	Horrified
	Elated	Loving	Empty	Useless	Desperate
Moderate	Cheerful	Caring	Downcast	Inadequate	Afraid
	Lighthearted	Fond of	Sorrowful	Imcompetent	Scared
	Happy	Admiration	Demoralized	Inept	Fearful
	Serene	Concern for	Discouraged	Deficient	Apprehensive
	Aglow	Close	Pessimistic	Insignificant	Threatened
Mild	Glad	Warm toward	Unhappy	Lacking confidence	Nervous
	Contented	Friendly	Down	Unsure of yourself	Anxious
	Satisified	Like	Low	Uncertain	Unsure
	Pleasant	Positive	Sad	Weak	Hesitant
	Pleased	toward	Glum	Inefficient	Worried

Levels of Intensity	Confused	Hurt	Angry	Lonely	Guilt–Shame
Strong	Bewildered	Crushed	Furious	Isolated	Sick at heart
	Puzzled	Destroyed	Enraged	Abandoned	Humiliated
	Perplexed	Devastated	Seething	All alone	Disgraced
	Confounded	Disgraced	Infuriated	Forsaken	Degraded
	Befuddled	Humiliated	Violent	Cut off	Exposed
Moderate	Mixed-up	Hurt	Resentful	Lonely	Ashamed
	Foggy	Belittled	Hostile	Alienated	Guilty
	Adrift	Overlooked	Annoyed	Estranged	Remorseful
	Lost	Abused	Agitated	Remote	Demeaned
	Disconcerted	Depreciated	Mad	Alone	To blame
Mild	Uncertain	Put down	Uptight	Left out	Regretful
	Unsure	Neglected	Disgusted	Excluded	Wrong
	Bothered	Overlooked	Perturbed	Lonesome	Embarrassed
	Uncomfortable	Minimized	Chagrined	Distant	At fault
	Undecided	Unappreciated	Dismayed	Aloof	In error

Adapted from Hammond, D. C., Hepworth, D. H., & Smith, V. G. (1977). Improving therapeutic communication (pp. 86–87). San Francisco: Jossey-Bass.

Clarification

Clarification is a technique that can be used by clinicians to assist clients in moving from broad, elusive areas of discussion to narrower, more pinpointed areas of concern. Clarification serves as the vehicle that gets participants on the same wavelength and helps them find a common frame of reference about a particular set of events. In health care interviews, clarification helps the clinician to understand the client more clearly and helps the client to understand his or her own thoughts and feelings better.

The process of clarifying can take many different forms. It may involve eliciting more specific descriptions from a client who is talking in generalizations. For example, the clinician may ask the client to describe exactly *who* was involved, *what* was involved, *where* it occurred, or *when* it occurred (Peplau, 1960). Clarification can also involve asking the client who is vaguely describing a concern to give an *example* of the situation so that both the clinician and the client can share the same point of reference in their subsequent discussion. Clarification is also useful when the client raises several concerns at one time and the clinician is not certain which issue is most relevant or which problem the client feels is most pressing. In this situation, the clinician can ask the client which topic is of most concern to him or her so they can spend their time discussing it first.

Examples of clarification are illustrated in the following interaction:

Client: I can't ever get along with him. *(Shakes head.)*

Clinician: Who do you have trouble getting along with? *(Looking at client.)*

Client: My boss. I've tried all sorts of ways to get along with him and to try to get him to like me, but I still feel like he is putting me down all the time. *(Frowns.)*

Clinician: You sound frustrated about your relationship with your boss. What situation, recently, has been especially difficult for you?

Client: *(Pauses and thinks a moment.)* I guess . . . the time when I returned from my vacation. While I was gone all sorts of work had piled up and. . . .

In the preceding example, the clarifying techniques enable the clinician to get a better understanding of what exactly is bothering the client. Clarification also gives the client a chance to sort through general feelings of frustration and discomfort and attach these feelings to specific events. In general, clarification is a helpful technique for pinpointing an area of concern and for increasing the accuracy of communication between the participants in the interview.

Interpretation

Unlike the preceding communication techniques, all of which keep the focus of the interview on the client, interpretation is a technique in which the focus of the interaction shifts temporarily back to the interviewer. Interpretation is a process in which the clinician offers an explanation about the expressed concerns of the client. The goal or intention of interpretation is to offer the client a new frame of reference or a new way of looking at her or his experience, which will help the client to understand that experience better.

When interpretation is used, it is important that the client be given the opportunity to accept or reject the perspective offered by the clinician. Sometimes it is helpful if the interpretation is offered as the clinician's hypothesis or "hunch" about what is happening to the client. This tentativeness gives the client the chance to react to the validity of the interpretation. In the end, the interpretation needs to make sense to the client if it is going to be useful.

Although it is difficult to illustrate interpretation without an elaborate case description of a client's history and circumstances, the following example provides a sense of how a clinician uses interpretation.

....

Client: You know . . . before I retired . . . I used to be very busy. I'd see people in my office as late as 8:00 p.m. every night. But what was it all for? What difference does it make? Now I sit here, read a little, eat a bit, and that's it.

Clinician: I understand you to say that you devoted your whole life to helping people and now because you've retired it is difficult to find things to do that are meaningful. Is it possible that you are feeling the emptiness and loneliness of not being able to help or affect others' lives anymore?

Client: You could be right. The difference between my life now . . . and then . . . is like night and day. You know, my practice used to be one of the largest in the area. Now, I just sit, think, and reflect on how things used to be. It is nice not having the pressure that comes with knowing you always have to go to the office the next day. But I do miss it. . . .

....

As the example indicates, interpretation can be a useful tool in helping the client gain a different insight into his or her circumstances.

If interpretation is used appropriately, it can have a strong and positive impact on the client. To use interpretation appropriately, the following guidelines have been suggested by Brammer (1973):

1. Look for the *basic message* of the interviewee.
2. *Paraphrase* these to him or her.
3. Add *your understanding* of what his or her message means in terms of your theory or your general explanation of motives, defenses, needs, styles, and so on.
4. Keep the *language simple* and the *level close to his or her message.* Avoid wild speculation and statements in esoteric words.

5. *Introduce* your ideas with some kind of statement indicating that you are offering *your ideas tentatively* on what his or her words or behavior means. Examples are, "Is this a fair statement . . . ?" "The way I see it is. . . ." "I wonder if. . . ." "Try this one on for size. . . ."
6. Solicit the (interviewee's) *reactions* to your interpretations.
7. Your main goal is to *teach the interviewee* to do his or her own interpreting. Remember, you cannot give insight to others (p. 106).

With these guidelines in mind, interpretation can be a useful communication technique that will clarify and amplify clients' understanding of their situations.

In this section, we have discussed the major communication techniques that can assist the clinician in the interview process. Our intention has been to focus on communication techniques that facilitate effective interviews. In Table 5–4, we also present some common responses, such as putting clients on the defensive, glossing over their concerns, or making evaluative judgments about them, that can block effective interviewing (Bernstein & Bernstein, 1985; Peplau, 1960). Communication techniques that focus on the client, that demonstrate understanding of the client's perspective, and that facilitate the client's ability to understand and work through areas of concern will enhance the professional–client relationship and promote an effective interview process.

TABLE 5–4. COMMUNICATION TECHNIQUES THAT BLOCK EFFECTIVE INTERVIEWING

Response	Example	Outcome
Probing	"Why are you feeling so depressed about your son's situation?"	Puts client on the defensive and asks for information that the client may not have.
Giving advice	"If I were in your situation, I would call him back and try to convince him that. . . ."	Centers the interaction on the professional's needs and perspective rather than on the client's needs and perspective.
False reassurance	"Everything will work out eventually—I know it will."	Smooths over client's concerns and does not help the client to solve a particular problem.
Moralizing	"You acted too hastily; you should have thought through the consequences before you got involved."	Does not move interaction forward. Blames client and stagnates interaction.
Belittling	"I think that you're overreacting. Things aren't as bad as you make them seem."	Makes evaluative judgment about the client and restricts further discussion of client's concerns.

► SUMMARY

Overall, conducting interviews plays a prominent role in the communication of health professionals. *Interviewing* is defined as a special type of interpersonal communication that is purposeful and serious, usually involving questions and answers, with the goal of sharing information or facilitating therapeutic outcomes.

In health care settings there are two general types of interviews: information-sharing interviews and therapeutic interviews. Information-sharing interviews involve requesting or providing information. In this type of interview, the focus of the interaction is on purposeful content in a specific area of interest. Therapeutic interviews are concerned with helping clients identify and work through personal issues and concerns. More emphasis is placed on building a supportive relationship in this type of interview. Therapeutic interviews can be conducted by health professionals using directive as well as nondirective approaches.

The four phases of the interview process are preparation, initiation, exploration, and termination. The preparation phase occurs prior to the actual interview dialogue, and it involves anticipating and planning for the interview. During this phase, the major tasks of the health professional are to engage in self-assessment and to plan for the first meeting with the client. In the second phase, initiation, the stage is set for the rest of the interview. During this phase, the clinician's responsibilities focus on establishing a therapeutic climate, clarifying the purpose of the interview, formulating a contract with the client, and establishing mutual goals. The third phase, exploration, is often called the working phase. During this phase, the clinician and client confront, analyze, and struggle with the client's concerns. The clinician tries to assist the client in analyzing problems, managing feelings, and in developing coping skills. The termination phase signals to the client that the end of the interview relationship is near. During this phase, the clinician's responsibilities include planning for closure, summarizing major issues, and assisting the client in expressing feelings about termination.

Special communication techniques that are directly related to interviewing include closed and open questions, silence, restatement, reflection, clarification, and interpretation. Closed questions are questions that elicit yes or no answers. They take less time but only provide a restricted amount of information. Open questions elicit in-depth answers from clients and require more time. Silence may be used to encourage further response from the client. It can be positive or negative depending on how much empathy or tension exists between the participants. Restatement is used to repeat or paraphrase the content of a client's message, whereas reflection is used to focus on the feelings that the client is expressing beneath the words. Clarification moves the interaction from generalities to specifics, and interpretation offers the client a tentative new way of looking at his or her situation.

Practicing the appropriate use of each of these techniques can make health care interviews more effective.

▶ REFERENCES

Arntson, P., Droge, D., & Fassl, H. E. (1978). Pediatrician–patient communication: Final report. In B. D. Ruben (Ed.), *Communication yearbook 2* (pp. 505–522). New Brunswick, NJ: Transaction.

Baker, S. J. (1955). The theory of silences. *Journal of General Psychology, 53,* 145–167.

Barnlund, D. C., & Haiman, F. S. (1960). *The dynamics of discussion.* Boston: Houghton Mifflin.

Benjamin, A. (1981). *The helping interview* (3rd ed.). Boston: Houghton Mifflin.

Berelson, B., & Steiner, G. A. (1964). *Human behavior: An inventory of scientific findings.* New York: Harcourt, Brace & World.

Bernstein, L., & Bernstein, R. (1985). *Interviewing: A guide for health professionals* (4th ed.). Norwalk, CT: Appleton-Century-Crofts.

Brammer, L. M. (1973). *The helping relationship: Process and skills.* Englewood Cliffs, NJ: Prentice-Hall.

Brammer, L. M. (1979). *The helping relationship: Process and skill* (2nd ed.). Englewood Cliffs, NJ: Prentice-Hall.

Brown, S. J. (1994). Communication strategies used by an expert nurse. *Clinical Nursing Research, 3*(1), 43–56.

Di Salvo, V. S., Larsen, J. K., & Backus, D. K. (1986). The health care communicator: An identification of skills and problems. *Communication Education, 35,* 231–242.

Downs, C. W., Smeyak, G. P., & Martin, E. (1980). *Professional interviewing.* New York: Harper & Row.

Farran, C., Carr, V., & Maxson, E. (1988). Goal-related behaviors in short-term psychiatric hospitalization. *Archives of Psychiatric Nursing, 2*(3), 159–164.

Forchuk, C. (1992). The orientation phase of the nurse–client relationship: How long does it take? *Perspectives in Psychiatric Care, 28*(4), 7–10.

Forchuk, C. (1994). The orientation phase of the nurse–client relationship: testing Peplau's theory. *Journal of Advanced Nursing, 20,* 532–537.

Forchuk, C. (1995). Uniqueness within the nurse–client relationship. *Archives of Psychiatric Nursing, 9*(1), 34–39.

Hammond, D. C., Hepworth, D. H., & Smith, V. G. (1977). *Improving therapeutic communication.* San Francisco: Jossey-Bass.

Kahn, R. L., & Cannell, C. F. (1957). *The dynamics of interviewing: Theory, technique, and cases.* New York: Wiley.

Keeling, A. W., & Dennison, P. D. (1995). Nurse initiated telephone follow-up after acute myocardial infarction: A pilot study. *Heart & Lung, 24*(1), 45–49.

Kristjanson, L., & Chalmers, K. (1990). Nurse–client interactions in community-based practice: Creating common ground. *Public Health Nursing. 7*(4), 215–233.

Lego, S. (1980). The one-to-one nurse–patient relationship. *Perspectives in Psychiatric Care, 18*(2), 67–89.

Loomis, M. E. (1985). Levels of contracting. *Journal of Psychosocial Nursing, 23*(3), 9–14.

Maguire, P., Fairbairn, S., & Fletcher, C. (1989). Consultation skills of young doctors—Benefits of undergraduate feedback training in interviewing. In M. Stewart & D. Roter (Eds.), *Communicating with medical patients*. Newbury Park, CA: Sage.

Nehren, J., & Gilliam, N. R. (1965). Separation anxiety. *American Journal of Nursing, 65*(1), 109–112.

Patterson, L. E., & Eisenberg, S. (1983). *The counseling process* (3rd ed.). Boston: Houghton Mifflin.

Peplau, H. (1960). Talking with patients. *American Journal of Nursing, 60*(7), 964–966.

Putnam, S. M., Stiles, W. B., Jacob, M. C., & James, S. A. (1988). Teaching the medical interview: An intervention study. *Journal of General Internal Medicine, 3*, 36–47.

Rogers, C. R. (1951). *Client-centered therapy*. Boston: Houghton Mifflin.

Rogers, C. R. (1959). A theory of therapy, personality, and interpersonal relationships, as developed in the client-centered framework. In S. Koch (Ed.), *Psychology: A study of science, Vol. III. Formulations of the person and the social context* (pp. 184–256). New York: McGraw-Hill.

Roter, D. L., & Hall, J. A. (1987). Physicians' interviewing styles and medical information obtained from patients. *Journal of General Internal Medicine, 2*, 325–329.

Saltzman, C., Leutgert, M. J., Roth, C. H., Creaser, J., & Howard, L. (1976). Formation of a therapeutic relationship: Experiences during the initial phase of psychotherapy as predictors of treatment duration and outcome. *Journal of Consulting and Clinical Psychology, 44*(4), 546–555.

Sayre, J. (1978). Common errors in communication made by students in psychiatric nursing. *Perspectives in Psychiatric Care, 16*(4), 175–183.

Sharf, B. F. (1984). *The physician's guide to better communication*. Glenview, IL: Scott, Foresman.

Steckel, S. B. (1982). *Patient contracting*. Norwalk, CT: Appleton-Century-Crofts.

Stoeckle, J. D., & Billings, J. A. (1987). A history of history-taking: The medical interview. *Journal of General Internal Medicine, 2*, 119–127.

Stuart, G. W., & Sundeen, S. J. (1995). *Principles and practice of psychiatric nursing* (3rd ed.). St. Louis: Mosby.

Sundeen, S. J., Stuart, G. W., Rankin, E. D., & Cohen, S. A. (1994). *Nurse–client interaction: Implementing the nursing process*. St. Louis: Mosby.

West, C. (1983). "Ask me no questions . . ." An analysis of queries and replies in physician–patient dialogues. In S. Fisher & A. D. Todd (Eds.), *The social organization of doctor–patient communication* (pp. 75–106). Washington, DC: Center for Applied Linguistics.

Wilson, H. S., & Kneisl, C. R. (1996). *Psychiatric nursing* (5th ed.). Menlo Park, CA: Addison-Wesley.

Woolliscroft, J. O., Calhoun, J. G., Billiu, G. A., Stross, J. K., MacDonald, M., & Templeton, B. (1989). House officer interviewing techniques: Impact on data elicitation and patient perceptions. *Journal of General Internal Medicine, 4*, 108–114.

Small Group Communication 6
in Health Care

During the last decade, the health care field has seen groups take over functions that once were performed on an individual basis, or not at all. The number of self-help groups, for example, has increased dramatically in recent years. Many other types of groups are also being used to teach clients how to maintain health or overcome illness. Groups for people with eating disorders, for people with acquired immunodeficiency syndrome (AIDS), for adult children of alcoholics, and for parents of children who have suffered sexual abuse, are just a few of the many client-oriented groups that are part of health care today (Yalom, 1995). There is some evidence that such groups not only help people cope with illness but may also extend their survival. In a much-publicized study, investigators found that women with advanced breast cancer who participated in a weekly support group survived up to twice as long as women who received only standard medical care (Spiegel, Bloom, Kramer, & Gottheil, 1989). There is a growing awareness that groups may exert a powerful impact on the health and well-being of clients and at the same time help contain health care costs.

Groups are also being used more and more among health professionals in acute care and community-based settings. Interdisciplinary groups, advisory groups, task forces, management groups, stress reduction groups, and care-for-the-caregiver groups are some of the growing number of these professional-oriented groups. During a typical week, it is not uncommon for a health professional to be involved in several planned group meetings plus other informal groups.

With the increased use of groups in health care, it has become increasingly important for health professionals to understand how groups work and how members communicate within groups. In self-help, task, and therapy groups, effective communication is essential. In essence, when the communication in a group works well, the group has a good chance of working well. Communication is the process that connects members to one another and enables them to work interdependently.

The purpose of this chapter is to present, explain, and discuss communication concepts and theories that apply to small groups in health care. We begin by providing a definition of small group communication and then present a discussion of the central components that are common to most groups. The chapter concludes with a description of the four major phases that occur during the development of groups.

► DEFINITION OF SMALL GROUP COMMUNICATION

Before defining small group communication, it is useful to consider the question, What is a small group? Generally speaking, a small group refers to a set of three or more individuals whose relationships make them in some way *interdependent*. In their classic work on groups, Cartwright and Zander (1968) indicate that individuals usually exhibit one or more of the following characteristics in groups:

- They engage in frequent interaction.
- They define themselves as members.
- They are defined by others as belonging to the group.
- They share norms concerning matters of common interest.
- They participate in a system of interlocking roles.
- They identify with one another as a result of having set up the same model-object or ideals in their super-ego.
- They find the group to be rewarding.
- They pursue promotively interdependent goals.
- They have a collective perception of their unity.
- They tend to act in a unitary manner toward the environment (p. 48).

As indicated above, there are many qualities that can be used to characterize small groups.

Small group communication refers to the verbal and nonverbal communication that occurs among a collection of individuals whose relationships make them, to some degree, interdependent. Stated in another way, it refers to how a group of individuals who are dependent on each other share information and meanings through a common set of rules. The focus in studying group communication is on communication phenomena in small groups (Goldberg & Larson, 1975). This includes developing a better understanding of the communication process in small groups, being able to predict what communication outcomes will occur in small groups, and then learning to improve the communication among group members. Throughout this chapter we will discuss the transactions that occur in small groups and the factors that influence these transactions.

► TYPES OF HEALTH CARE GROUPS

The communication focus is different in different types of groups. By distinguishing among various types of groups, the communication implications for different groups in health care can be better understood (Cline, 1990).

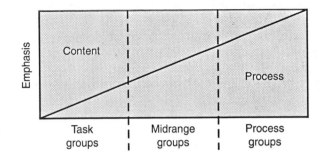

Figure 6–1. The emphasis on content and process in different types of groups. (Adapted from Loomis, M. E. [1979]. *Group process for nurses* (p. 102). St. Louis: Mosby.)

A general way of viewing the numerous groups in health care settings is according to whether they are process oriented or content oriented. Throughout this book the terms *process* and *content* have been used frequently to describe the components of a communication message. In group activity, the time spent discussing tasks and goals is referred to as the *content focus* of the group and the time spent relating and getting along with people is referred to as the *process focus* of the group (Loomis, 1979). Although *all* groups have both content and process elements, groups vary in the degree to which one or the other of these elements is emphasized.

Figure 6–1 illustrates types of groups along a content–process continuum. *Task groups*, which appear on the left end of the continuum, focus nearly all of their efforts on substantive issues such as the goal of the group, the activities that the group needs to accomplish, or the procedures the group will follow. A committee that is formed to revise staff policies is typical of a task group that is mainly concerned with content issues. *Process groups*, which appear at the right end of the continuum, focus on group members, how they are related, and how they communicate with each other. A therapy group in an inpatient psychiatric unit would be a familiar example of a process group. In a therapy group, most of the time is spent discussing how members feel about themselves, about other members of the group, and the group as a whole. Many groups fall midway between the two extremes of the task and process groups. These groups, referred to as *midrange groups*, have a blend of task and process (Loomis, 1979). For example, groups set up for ostomy patients generally emphasize content (e.g., physical care of the ostomy) as well as processing feelings among members (e.g., concerns about self-disclosure).

The content-process continuum provides a general way of differentiating groups into those that are more content oriented and those that are more process oriented.

► COMPONENTS OF SMALL GROUPS

In addition to being characterized as task oriented or process oriented, groups can also be described in terms of their components. Some of the major components include: goals, norms, cohesiveness, leader behavior, member behavior, and therapeutic factors that influence group functioning.

Goals

Every group needs a reason for its existence or else there would be no need for individuals to come together. Goals provide the rationale and motivation for people to form a group. For example, in a broad analysis of 75 teams that were selected from such diverse organizations as major corporations, hospitals, and sports teams, Larson and LaFasto (1989) found that without exception the teams that functioned most effectively had a very clear understanding of their objectives.

Typically, two types of goals operate in groups: individual goals and group goals. *Individual goals* are based on the particular needs and desires of each group member and may or may not be related to the goals of the group. *Group goals,* on the other hand, are shared (to some extent) by group members and involve some element of interdependence among the members. Both individual and group goals often operate simultaneously within a group. For example, a new employee may join a task force to study the parking problem at an agency as a way to get to know some other employees (individual goal) and also because of an interest in improving parking at the agency (group goal). Similarly, a nursing student may offer to co-lead a preoperative class for patients because the student is interested in helping the patients prepare for surgery (group goal) but also because the student wants to develop his or her own leadership skills (individual goal).

Problems can occur, however, when the individual goals held by one member are not *compatible* with the goals held by another member. This situation often leads to competition among group members especially when goal achievement by one member blocks the goal achievement of another member. In addition, members' incompatible goals can disrupt the flow of communication and reduce the degree of collaboration and the amount of friendliness among group members. In contrast, mutually shared goals lead to greater cooperation among the participants in a group.

Group goals also need to be *realistic*. When goals are set unreasonably high, members often feel overwhelmed by trying to reach the goal or frustrated when their attempts are unsuccessful. Yalom (1983) contends that therapists who set overly ambitious goals in groups can create anti-therapeutic effects: Members are set up for a situation in which they are likely to fail. On the other hand, goals that are too simplistic also present problems. Members of a task group, for example, may have difficulty getting interested or motivated in working in a group whose goals offer little interest or challenge (Zander, 1994). Group goals need to be realistically attainable within the time available to the group.

Another important issue to be considered regarding group goals is their degree of *clarity.* Clarity refers to the amount of certainty that members have about the nature of group goals and about how they should go about meeting those goals. In order for people to work together, they need to have a common understanding about the mission of the group. Ambiguous or vague goals can lead to uncertainty and annoyance among group members. For example, Klein (1981) reported that the lack of clear goals can be especially problematic in patient–staff community meetings in a psychiatric unit. He observed that an inability to specify clear goals for the group leaves members wondering how long the meeting should last, what topics are appropriate for discussion, and what type of participation is desired from patients and staff. In addition, he observed that when goals and task boundaries are not clearly established, topics in the meeting shifted rapidly and unpredictably, the level of disclosure varied, the meetings lacked continuity, and the anxiety of group members increased.

Goal clarity can be enhanced if the leader helps members to identify group goals and removes the obstacles to meeting these goals (House, 1971). For example, in a health education group for diabetics, the leader can outline the general goals of the group before the meeting so that clients can determine if the proposed group will meet their needs. When the goals of a group are clear, realistic, and shared by group members, the group will function more effectively.

Norms

Norms are the rules of behavior that are established and shared by group members to ensure consistency in the behavior of group members. Norms often suggest what type of behavior is appropriate or *should* be exhibited by group members, thus adding to the predictability within a group. Norms do not emerge on their own—they are the outcome of people interacting together (Stech & Ratliffe, 1976). However, a group does not develop norms for every single behavior within a group, only for those behaviors that are important to the group.

Norms can be overt or covert. *Overt norms* are usually verbally agreed-upon rules that are generally known to all members. For example, a group of health professionals may agree to show up on time for their weekly treatment planning meetings rather than straggle in 5 to 10 minutes late for each meeting. In this group, punctuality becomes the norm and new members who enter the meetings are quickly reminded of this rule of behavior. *Covert norms* are not usually verbally acknowledged by group members. For example, a communication norm that often operates in groups is that when one person talks, all others should listen. Group members who violate this norm often receive disapproving glances or other nonverbal messages from group members. Another example of a covert norm could be the seating arrangement in a group. If everyone knows where he or she is "supposed" to sit without its being discussed, a covert norm is operating within the group.

Norms can also be enabling or restrictive (Loomis, 1979). *Enabling norms* assist the group in meeting its goals. For example, in a task group, the norm that "all members do their homework and come to the meeting prepared" enables the group to make decisions more efficiently. In a process group, such as a parent effectiveness group, the norm that "members share experiences and offer constructive feedback to one another" enables members to learn more about parenting from one another. *Restrictive norms* hinder the group's movement toward goals. When norms develop in a group that allow members to attack one another verbally or to be chronically tardy, the group is restricted from accomplishing its goal. In health care settings, some professionals are paged during meetings, or leave before meetings are concluded, creating restrictive norms. The following example illustrates how the restrictive norms in a group can hinder group development.

Two students were asked to assume a leadership role in an ongoing group in a community mental health center. The group consisted of clients from the state psychiatric hospital who were presently living in the community. The group was called a "relating" group and was designed to improve the members' interpersonal skills. Before taking over as leaders of the group, the students observed several sessions of the group and became aware of norms operating in the group. They observed that several members frequently arrived 15 to 30 minutes late for the meeting. Other members made frequent trips to the bathroom or to the coffee machine during the meeting.

Due to the constant movement of members in and out of the group, members who left the group were unsure about what topic was being discussed when they returned. Members who remained in the meeting were constantly interrupted by members who were returning. Although "relating" was the title of the group, little interpersonal relating went on in the group.

Over a period of time the new student leaders, with the help of a few influential group members, tried to change the norms in the group. They limited the entry of late members to the group, encouraged members to take bathroom and beverage breaks before the meeting, and also complimented members on their increased attentiveness to one another. Under the new leadership, norms gradually changed in the group.

In the above situation the norms operating in the group were restrictive; they interfered with the group goal that members learn how to relate to one another. New norms gradually developed that enabled the group to meet its goals.

Generally, there is some latitude in the amount of conformity demanded by group members of other group members. Groups seldom demand 100 percent conformity. Although groups may tolerate more deviance from some norms (e.g., punctuality) than from others (e.g., no smoking), individuals who deviate considerably from important or highly valued norms will receive reprimands from other group members.

Norms are an important component of group functioning. Norms develop very early in the life of a group and once developed are very difficult to change (Yalom, 1995). Group leaders and members need to attend closely to early norm development and try to shape norms that will maximize group effectiveness.

Cohesiveness

Cohesiveness is often considered an elusive but essential component of groups. Group members frequently have an intuitive sense of when there is a high degree of cohesion in their group, but they have difficulty describing what cohesiveness is or how it developed. Cohesiveness is often described as a sense of "we-ness," the cement that holds groups together, or as the *esprit de corps* that exists within a group. It should be pointed out that groups are neither cohesive nor uncohesive in an absolute sense, but rather have varying degrees of cohesion (Jones, Barnlund, & Haiman, 1980). Groups without any cohesion would most likely cease to exist.

Cohesion has been associated with a number of positive outcomes for group members (Cartwright, 1968; Shaw, 1976). First, high cohesiveness is frequently associated with increased participation and better interaction among members. People tend to talk more readily and to listen more carefully in very cohesive groups. Second, in highly cohesive groups, group membership tends to be more consistent. Members are attracted toward one another and will want to attend group meetings. Third, highly cohesive groups are able to exert a strong influence on group members. Members conform more closely to group norms and engage in more goal-directed behavior for the group. Fourth, member satisfaction is high in cohesive groups; members tend to feel more secure and find enjoyment in participating in the group. Last, members of a cohesive group usually are more productive than are members of a less cohesive group. Members of groups with greater cohesion can direct their energies toward group goals without spending extensive time working out interpersonal issues and conflicts.

Recognizing the importance of cohesiveness, what factors influence the development of cohesiveness in a group? Cartwright (1968) identified several factors that affect group cohesiveness: clarity of the group's goals, similarity among group members, a sense of interdependence within the group, a democratic style of leadership, decentralized communication patterns (i.e., increased member–member interactions), and a group size that is appropriate to the nature of the task being undertaken. Although some of these factors may be more influential in one type of group than another, attention to these factors and the way in which they are helping or hindering cohesiveness increases group effectiveness.

In addition to factors that foster the development of group cohesiveness, there are also factors that threaten cohesion. Loomis (1979) has identified four *threats to cohesiveness* that she encountered in health care groups: (1) unstable membership, (2) group deviants, (3) subgrouping, and (4) leadership problems. According to Loomis, cohesiveness is threatened in groups with *unstable membership* because members are uncertain about the goals and the norms of the group. For example, a hospital operations committee, which has different individuals attending it each month, would be less cohesive than a committee that has a stable membership. Similarly, a drop-in group at a center for senior citizens may lack cohesiveness because of unstable membership. *Group deviants,* the second threat identified by Loomis, hinder group cohesiveness because they vary so much from the group norms and group goals. Other members often have to expend considerable time and energy to get the deviant to conform to the group. *Subgrouping* also threatens cohesiveness because members can become more committed to the needs of the subgroup rather than those of the whole group. Subgroups or cliques often form within a large group when the needs of many members cannot be adequately addressed and satisfied. The last threat identified by Loomis is *leadership problems.* She contends that if the leader lacks the ability to develop the group's cohesiveness, it is likely to diminish.

Cohesiveness, like norms and goals, is an important component in effective group functioning. Cohesion does not develop instantaneously but is created gradually as members communicate with one another. Group effectiveness is enhanced when health professionals focus on helping groups to build cohesiveness.

Leader Behavior

Leader behavior is a fourth component that influences group functioning. The leader plays a pivotal role in guiding the group to meet its goals, in developing group norms, and in facilitating communication among group members.

Communication is necessary for effective leadership. Leadership does not take place within a vacuum or in isolation from followers; it exists within a group or organization. *Leadership* refers to the process in which one person attempts to influence others in order to attain some mutually agreed-upon goal. It is not a linear, or one-way event, but occurs through the ongoing *transactions* between the individual who is designated as the leader and those who are the followers. *Communication* becomes the means or vehicle that the leader uses to bring about change in others. For example, Hawks (1987) found that leaders' interactions had a strong effect on members' interactions. When leaders were facilitative and communicated directly to group members, the members were significantly more effective in their own communication with others. An effective leader selects methods of communicating that are likely to have a positive impact on followers and that will result in progress toward the desired goal (Graen & Uhl-Bien, 1995).

Fisher (1974) has identified the positive communication behaviors that account for successful leader emergence. Foremost, emergent leaders are verbally active, fluent, and express their thoughts articulately in group interaction. They initiate new ideas in conferences, seek opinions from others, and express their own opinions with firmness but not rigidity. Although this list is not exhaustive, these are the kinds of communicative behaviors that emergent leaders exhibit.

On the negative side, Geier (1967) has identified the behaviors that eliminate individuals from emerging as successful leaders. These negative communicative behaviors included low participation, uninformed contributions, rigid argumentation, overly directive comments, stilted language, and incessant talking. Individuals who engage in these types of communication are less likely to emerge as leaders in health care organizations.

Lieberman, Yalom, and Miles (1973) studied the behaviors of encounter group leaders and identified four dimensions that they believed explained leader behavior in therapy or personal growth groups. The four behaviors were (1) emotional stimulation, (2) caring, (3) meaning-attribution, and (4) executive function.

Emotional stimulation is characteristic of a leader who assumes an active role in encouraging members to express feelings, assists members in confronting their ideas and values, and models ways to share concerns in the group. *Caring* includes those behaviors in which the leader demonstrates kindness, warmth, openness, and sincerity with group members. *Meaning-attribution* involves cognitive activities in which the leader provides explanations or helps members to understand why they are acting or feeling a certain way. Meaning-attribution also involves assisting group members to look at either the meaning of the group's behavior as a whole or at the meaning of the behavior of individual members within the group. *Executive functioning* describes the managerial aspects of a group in which the leader sets limits, monitors rules, and attends to various procedures in the group.

It is important to realize that different leader behaviors are called for by different types of groups. Effective leaders attempt to match their styles to the needs of the group (Carew, Parisi-Carew, & Blanchard, 1990; Hersey & Blanchard, 1993). Certain groups need leaders to be very directive and task focused, whereas other groups demand a relationship approach from leaders. For example, the leader of a community task force to improve interagency communication would be concerned with structuring the meeting so that members could discuss problems and formulate solutions within a given period of time. If, however, the same leader were leading a group with dialysis patients, the leader would be more concerned with establishing a group climate that would foster sharing and support interactions among group members. In other words, the leader would use different behavior in different types of groups. Similarly, different leader behavior is needed for different types of clients. For example, Burnside (1994) contends that group work with older adults is different from group work with younger adults. With older adults, the leader needs to pay closer attention to sensory losses experienced by group members; move the group at a slower pace, since older clients dislike feeling rushed; and plan group meetings during the day, since older clients tire more readily by the evening hours. For successful group outcomes, the leader needs to attend to the specific goals of the group and the specific needs of group members.

Member Behavior

Member behavior is just as important to effective group functioning as is leader behavior. Too often, however, the responses of group members toward one another are often overlooked or considered of only minor importance to group functioning. It is not uncommon, for example, to hear students blame a boring seminar entirely on a student leader. While blaming only the leader, students overlook the way in which their behavior (e.g., failing to participate) contributed to the ineffective and boring group. Similarly, health professionals sometimes complain about a leader who allows a group to get sidetracked on an irrelevant issue that consumes much of the committee's allotted time. Like the students, these individuals have minimized their role in group functioning and have placed responsibility solely on the leader. Effective group functioning is influenced by *both* leader and member behavior; it is a shared responsibility.

Member behavior in small groups has been assessed in a number of ways. In this section, member behavior will be examined by looking at the roles and interaction patterns among group members.

Member Roles

Early work on *member roles* in small groups was conducted by Benne and Sheats (1948), who classified the roles of group members into three broad categories: (1) group task roles, (2) group-building and maintenance roles, and (3) individual roles. Although Benne and Sheats's work was reported a number of years ago, their role categories are still recognized as useful in understanding group functioning, especially in task groups. Benne and Sheats believed that group members often fulfill more than one role in a particular group and that the various roles can be played by either the leader or individual group members.

The first category, *group task roles*, includes members' roles that contribute to the group's ability to perform its task. These roles are concerned primarily with members obtaining and sharing information so that they can solve particular problems. The names of the group task roles and a brief description of each role are listed below:

1. *Initiator-contributor:* Suggests new ideas or a new way of viewing the group task.
2. *Information seeker:* Asks for clarification or for additional information about the problem being discussed.
3. *Opinion seeker:* Asks for clarification of values that may be involved in the goal or task that the group is discussing.
4. *Information giver:* Offers facts or personal experiences that are related to problems being discussed in the group.
5. *Opinion giver:* States his or her personal beliefs that are pertinent to the group's discussion.
6. *Elaborator:* Expands on ideas being discussed by offering an example or the rationale for a suggestion.
7. *Coordinator:* Pulls together various ideas and suggestions made by group members or tries to coordinate group activities.
8. *Orientor:* Defines the present position of the group in relation to its goals or raises questions about the direction in which the discussion is moving.
9. *Evaluator–critic:* Considers the practicality or logic of suggestions offered in the group.
10. *Energizer:* Stimulates the group toward an action or decision.
11. *Procedural technician:* Assists group movement by carrying out routine tasks for the group.
12. *Recorder:* Writes down suggestions or activities decided on by the group.

As the names of these various group task roles indicate, these members' roles assist the group in meeting its task or goal obligations.

The second category, *group-building and maintenance roles*, includes roles that promote cohesiveness among group members and enhance members' ability to work together as a group. These roles focus more on developing good working relations among the members rather than on the particular task of the group. The specific roles in this category are as follows:

1. *Encourager:* Provides praise and acceptance of other members' contributions.
2. *Harmonizer:* Mediates the differences among various group members.
3. *Compromiser:* Offers to modify his or her position to maintain group harmony.
4. *Gatekeeper:* Regulates the flow of communication, facilitates quiet

members' contributions, and limits the comments from members who are dominating the discussion.

5. *Standard setter:* Reminds group members of the standards they are trying to achieve.
6. *Group observer:* Comments on the various aspects of group process that are operating within the group and, in doing so, enables members to be more aware of how well they are functioning as a group.
7. *Follower:* Goes along with the movement of the group.

The final category of group roles described by Benne and Sheats includes *individual roles.* Unlike the previous two categories of roles that facilitate the effective functioning of groups, these roles are nonfunctional and unhelpful to the group. *Individual roles* are used by group members to satisfy their own particular needs. These roles do not help the group to accomplish its task (group task roles) or to facilitate good member relationships (group-building roles). The roles in this category are listed below:

1. *Aggressor:* Attacks or disapproves of others' suggestions, feelings, or values.
2. *Blocker:* Resists, without good reason, or becomes extremely negative to others' suggestions.
3. *Recognition seeker:* Calls attention repeatedly to own accomplishments and diverts the group's attention.
4. *Self-confessor:* Uses the group's time to express personal, non-group-oriented feelings or comments.
5. *Playboy–playgirl:* Plays around and displays other behavior that indicates he or she is not involved in the group process.
6. *Dominator:* Tries repeatedly to assert own authority and often interrupts other group members.
7. *Help seeker:* Tries to elicit sympathy from other group members.
8. *Special interest pleader:* Speaks for a particular group or person (e.g., "the union," "the unemployed") but is really using the group to meet personal needs and to cloak personal biases and prejudices.

According to Benne and Sheats, it is helpful when group members are able to fulfill a variety of roles so that they can meet the group's needs at various points in time. They also believe that some roles will be more helpful to a particular group at one time and less useful at another. For example, a newly formed task group may have a higher need for an initiator–contributor than for an evaluator–critic. The evaluator–critic role may be more helpful later when members start to weigh the pros and cons of various alternatives.

How, then, can these three categories of group member roles be helpful to health professionals interested in group process? First, these categories remind health professionals that as members of various groups, they can influence group functioning by the type of role that they assume. Sec-

ROLE ASSESSMENT CHECKLIST		
Roles	Roles I usually play in groups	Roles I need to practice in groups
Group Task Roles		
1. Initiator-contributor		
2. Information seeker		
3. Opinion seeker		
4. Information giver		
5. Opinion giver		
6. Elaborator		
7. Coordinator		
8. Orienter		
9. Evaluator-critic		
10. Energizer		
11. Procedural technician		
12. Recorder		
Group Maintenance Roles		
1. Encourager		
2. Harmonizer		
3. Compromiser		
4. Gatekeeper		
5. Standard setter		
6. Group observer		
7. Follower		
Individual Roles		
1. Aggressor		
2. Blocker		
3. Recognition seeker		
4. Self-confessor		
5. Playboy/playgirl		
6. Dominator		
7. Help seeker		
8. Special interest pleader		

Figure 6–2. Checklist of role behaviors. (Adapted from the role categories described by Benne, K. D. & Sheats, P. [1948]. Functional roles of group members. *Journal of Social Issues, 4*(2), 41–49.)

ond, these categories can serve as a useful assessment tool to help professionals identify the roles that they tend to assume in groups or the roles that they *need* to use more in groups (Fig. 6–2). Third, these categories can help leaders and members to diagnose group problems. For example, if a curriculum committee is repeatedly unable to get at its task of resolving curriculum problems, the members (either alone or as a group) can analyze roles that are counterproductive in the group and concentrate on developing new roles that will increase group productivity. These role categories do not prescribe or offer a formula for determining which roles at which time will assure optimal group functioning. They do, however, provide a way of looking at how various roles assumed by group members can influence group process.

Communication Networks

Member behavior in small groups can also be understood by analyzing interaction patterns or the *communication networks* that exist among group members. Communication networks indicate whether communication is centralized (all messages flow to one person) or decentralized, and whether channels are open or closed between participants. Communication networks do not describe who sits next to whom in a group but rather the lines of communication between members.

Several common communication networks are portrayed in Figure 6–3. The symbol "o" represents a person and the line(s) connecting the "o's" represents channels of communication between participants. Individuals may not always be able to change a particular communication network, but by being aware of existing channels they can work toward opening new channels and closing others. In addition, health professionals may find that

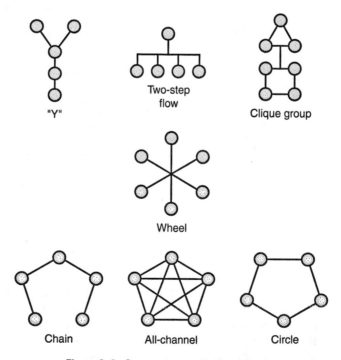

Figure 6–3. Common communication networks.

one type of communication network is more effective with a specific type of group than is another. For example, the all-channel network, with high interaction among members, is often considered more effective in a therapy group than is a wheel pattern, in which all communication is directed through the leader. On the other hand, a wheel or Y pattern may be the most useful network for transmitting information in certain health care situations where time is limited and the issue is not complex. Not all groups will fit into the patterns that have been identified. Only a few of the many patterns that have been described by communication specialists have been presented in this chapter.

Another way of looking at the interaction patterns of group members is to draw a *sociogram*. A sociogram provides a means of charting "who is talking to whom" and "how often" in a small group setting. Figure 6–4 is a sociogram depicting the interaction patterns of a group of health care members during one treatment planning session. Each line indicates that a verbal interaction has taken place between group members. Arrows indicate who sent the message. In this sociogram, the physician and psychologist direct most of their communication toward one another. Only occasionally do they direct communication toward the group as a whole or to other team members. The diagram also illustrates that the student and dietitian are

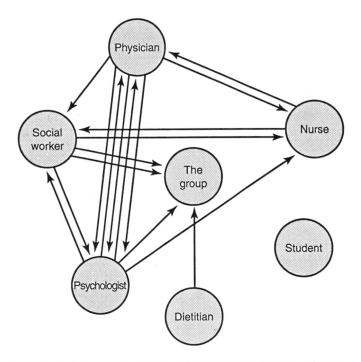

Figure 6–4. Sociogram of an interdisciplinary treatment planning conference.

quiet members; the dietitian directed only one comment to the group and the student did not send or receive any comments. In addition, the sociogram shows that most of the communication occurs between physician, nurse, social worker, and psychologist. For the most part, members direct their comments to specific members; little communication is directed to the group as a whole. Assuming that the goal of this particular group is to resolve a unit problem that requires input from all group members, this sociogram suggests that the dietitian and student need to be drawn into the discussion, the physician and psychologist need to direct less communication toward each other, and all members need to direct more communication to the group as a whole.

Figure 6–5 illustrates a sociogram of a group of clients in a newly formed group for adolescent single parents. In this group, the leader occupies the central position where he or she receives the majority of member interaction. Very little communication is occurring between group members. If the goal of this group is to have members share experiences and concerns about single parenting, then the leader needs to move out of the central "switchboard position" and encourage more member–member or member–group interaction.

Diagrams illustrating interaction patterns among group members, whether in the form of *common communication network* diagrams or *group-specific sociograms,* help to illustrate the flow of communication in small groups. These diagrams help members to understand another important aspect of member behavior that ultimately influences how well the group functions.

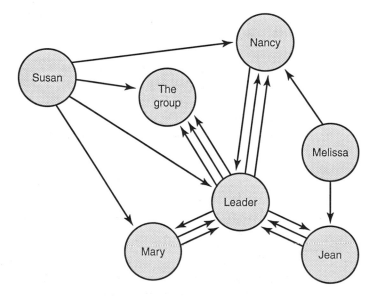

Figure 6–5. Sociogram of a client group.

Therapeutic Factors

How do groups help people change? What interpersonal processes in groups are beneficial to members? Are there specific factors in groups that can be called "therapeutic"? Questions such as these have motivated researchers to study various groups in an effort to identify those factors that have a positive influence on group members. These studies have identified a series of positive forces, often referred to as therapeutic factors, that operate in groups. Yalom (1995) has written most extensively about these curative factors, and his writing will be used as the primary source for the following discussion.

Based on his research and clinical experience, Yalom (1983) identified 11 therapeutic factors that are crucial to the process of change. Yalom states that some of these factors are actually mechanisms of change, whereas others exist more as conditions for change. The therapeutic factors can be viewed as a cluster of factors that, taken together in varying combinations, exert a positive influence on group members. Any one factor by itself is not sufficient to create change. These therapeutic factors are generally thought of as forces operating within therapy groups, but some of these factors can operate in other groups as well.

The first therapeutic factor is called *instillation of hope*. This factor is essential in groups, especially during the initial phase of the group when members are not sure if the group will be able to help them. Members often become hopeful as they meet others in a group who have been in a similar situation (or worse) and who have been able to overcome their difficulties. For example, new hemodialysis patients often feel more hopeful about their ability to adjust to hemodialysis after talking with "veteran" dialysis patients (Steinglass, Gonzalez, Dosovitz, & Reiss, 1982). From the realization that others have succeeded, or from the encouragement received from other group members, the individual gains optimism that he or she will also be able to overcome similar hurdles. Self-help groups such as Recovery Incorporated and Alcoholics Anonymous rely heavily on providing hope. In these groups, seasoned members give testimonies to new members about how they were able to stop drinking or to cope with mental stress in spite of numerous difficulties.

Universality, the second therapeutic factor, occurs as group members realize that they are not alone—that their circumstances are shared by others. Universality is similar to instillation of hope but places more emphasis on the fact that, although each individual is unique, human problems are universal or shared to some extent by other people. This curative factor helps to break down the isolation that people often experience as a result of their problems. A person with cancer, for example, may frequently feel that he or she is the only person struggling with a life-threatening illness. However, when this person joins an "I Can Cope" group, the person realizes that he or she is not alone; others are also struggling with a serious illness.

Examining the benefits of a support group for people with brain tumors, Leavitt, Lamb, and Voss (1996) found that the group provided a safe haven for patients and their family members, where participants found acceptance, understanding, and a shared experience. Some patients removed their hats and wigs, as feelings of isolation and stigma were counteracted by feelings of safety within the group. Participants also validated the "reasonableness" of one another's responses or feelings, because they too, had experienced the difficulties associated with brain tumors.

In multicultural groups, special attention needs to be directed to promoting universality. Yalom (1995) has noted that in some groups, the minority group members may feel excluded because they have different beliefs about disclosure or expression of feelings. In these settings, group leaders need to help members move beyond their cultural differences and focus on their transcultural, shared human experience.

Imparting information includes the advice, suggestions, educational information, and other ideas that the leader(s) and members give to one another. In health care groups, this therapeutic factor is frequently evident when clients are offered health teaching or practical suggestions from others. For example, a nurse may provide information on infant care to a group of new parents, or a person who has already had cardiac bypass surgery may tell patients being oriented to a cardiac surgery unit what to expect. Information becomes curative when it gives people a greater sense of control and knowledge of what to expect in their experiences or circumstances.

Altruism occurs when one group member assists another and feels good about having helped. According to Yalom, this therapeutic factor is often minimized by group members who frequently wonder how they can possibly help others when they are so absorbed and overwhelmed by their own problems. Altruistic behavior helps the giving individuals to realize that in spite of their own difficulties or concerns they still have the strength and capability to help others. Altruism reinforces the positive resources that people retain even in times of stress.

The *corrective recapitulation of the primary family group* also serves as an important therapeutic factor in groups. During group experiences, some members often respond to other group members or to the group leaders in ways that are similar to how they responded to parents or other family members. For example, in an inpatient therapy group, a young male adolescent may play the male co-therapist against the female co-therapist in much the same way that he pitted his father against his mother. The adolescent also uses the same tactics to create tension in the group as he did to create tension in his family. As these parallels surface, group members can gain awareness of how they respond to family members outside the group, and they can use the group to practice new ways of behaving.

The *development of socializing techniques* also can occur within the group setting. In some groups (e.g, "relating" groups or "social awareness" groups), the development of social skills will be the primary focus of the group. In other groups, such as problem-solving groups, the development of socializing skills will not be the main focus, but it will still occur as members continually interact with one another about how to make decisions and learn to solve problems. For instance, the development of socializing techniques was evident in one group in which a young woman initially was very withdrawn and never contributed to the group. During the course of the group, other group members frequently drew the woman into the group discussion and complimented her on her insightful observations. Through the assistance of group members, this woman was encouraged to participate more, and in so doing she gained more confidence and skill in socializing with others.

Imitative behavior occurs in groups when group members start to model their behavior, appearance, or language after the leader or other group members. For example, the behaviors of the therapist of a battered women's group were often imitated by members of the group. The therapist, who was also battered at one time in her life, spoke assertively in the group and demonstrated respect for herself as well as for others. Members frequently would adopt this woman's mannerisms and dress. One explanation that Yalom (1995) offers for the curative effect of imitative behavior is that it enables members to break out of old patterns and try on new behaviors so that they can determine if the new behaviors will also work for them.

Interpersonal learning occurs as members provide one another with feedback about their interpersonal behavior. Some members may seldom have received constructive feedback from others. With this new information, members can alter their behavior or learn more effective ways of interacting with others. To illustrate, a student was referred to the counseling center at the university because of the trouble she was having communicating with clients during her clinical rotation. The student set high standards for herself as well as for others, and she frequently treated clients in a condescending manner. During the group experience, the student received feedback that she frequently displayed disgust (nonverbally) toward group members when they did not behave or respond in exactly the way that she desired. From this feedback and from the other things she learned in the group, the student became more aware of how she often gave negative interpersonal cues to others and how this behavior could interfere with her communication with clients. In another study, Gordon and associates (1988) found that women who participated in a therapy group reported significantly less depression and more self-esteem following group meetings, and the change lasted 3 years longer than for women in a no-treatment control group. According to the investigators, women in the therapy group learned and tried new communication skills that endured long after the group was discontinued.

Cohesiveness another therapeutic factor identified by Yalom, was also discussed earlier in this chapter. Yalom states that group cohesion facilitates the development of many positive outcomes in group members, such as acceptance, belonging, and feeling valued as a human being. According to

Yalom (1995), group cohesiveness is not merely a therapeutic factor but a necessary precondition for effective therapy. In a study that utilized group therapy with elderly clients, Young and Reed (1995) found that bonding or developing a sense of connectedness to one another was one of the strongest therapeutic factors operating in the group.

Catharsis, as a therapeutic factor, means more than just the expression of pent-up feelings. Catharsis becomes an important therapeutic factor when the ventilation of feelings is coupled with interpersonal learning. Yalom believes that "learning how to express feelings" or acquiring the skill of expressing feelings is more important than the mere act of getting them out. For example, Mr. B., a first-time criminal offender, was attending weekly group sessions at a rehabilitation center. At one meeting, Mr. B. started to cry and told the group about some of his traumatic childhood experiences that he had never told anyone before. Mr. B. received a great deal of support from other members, and he learned that it was important and acceptable for him—a man—to cry and to express feelings.

In the group setting, participants are given the opportunity to share feelings and fears that they might have withheld from family members or others outside of the group (Cella & Yellen, 1993). This was evident in a support group for health professionals who worked with persons with AIDS. Within the security of the group, members felt comfortable discussing their fear of contracting the disease or their fear that they might already test positive for the human immunodeficiency virus (HIV)—feelings that they were not comfortable discussing with family and friends (Lego, 1994). Members were grateful for a secure place where they could discuss their fears and anxieties, without a need to defend their positions.

Existential factors are the last of the therapeutic factors identified by Yalom. Group members realize that life is sometimes not fair, that pain cannot always be escaped, and people need to take responsibility for the way that they live their lives. Part of this curative factor is the need for people to grapple with issues of responsibility, choice, and meaning in life. Existential factors can play an important role in groups where members have terminal or progressive illness. Existential factors become curative to the extent that members are supported as they struggle with existential concerns, find their own answers to difficult questions, and find meaning in their circumstances.

For health professionals working in groups, it is important to assess which therapeutic factors are operating and which factors can be fostered to increase the benefit of the group for clients. Yalom (1995) states that some factors will be more important in one phase of the group than others. For example, instillation of hope and universality are especially important during the early phase. In addition, some curative factors will be more useful to some members than others (Yalom, 1983). For example, certain members may benefit a great deal from socializing techniques while other members may benefit more from imparting information. All in all, the therapeutic process of groups is strongly influenced by these 11 factors, which often operate in a group setting.

In this section, we have discussed the various components that influence how various groups function. In general, groups will function more effectively with clear group goals, facilitative norms, a leader who is attuned to the needs of group members, and members who occupy roles and use interaction patterns that assist the group to complete its goal. In addition, effective groups will try to build group cohesiveness and will use some of the therapeutic factors that can have a positive influence on group members.

▶ PHASES OF SMALL GROUPS

In the previous section, we described the makeup or components of small groups. Now we will shift our discussion to an explanation of how groups develop and proceed over time—the phases of small groups.

Several models have been proposed to explain the phases that occur in small groups (Bales & Strodtbeck, 1951; Bennis & Shepard, 1956; Fisher, 1974; Schutz, 1958; Tuckman, 1965). Some of these models have been constructed by assessing the various stages in task groups, while other models have been constructed through observations of different phases in therapy (process) groups. Considered together, this research provides a basis for suggesting that most groups go through a consistent sequence of identifiable phases. As Shaw (1976) points out, "It is probable that the kind and sequences of phases in group development are similar for all groups, although the content and duration of phases vary with the kind of group and with the group task" (p. 97).

Generally, small groups proceed through five phases: (1) orientation, (2) conflict, (3) cohesion, (4) working, and (5) termination. The time it takes to complete a single phase may vary from group to group. For example, short-term ad hoc groups may proceed through all five phases in a single session, while long-term therapy groups may spend many weeks in a single phase. Movement from one phase to another usually occurs in sequence, even though the group may return to a previous phase at one time or another. Although each phase has identifiable characteristics and qualities that make it distinct from other phases, the phases often overlap and blur into each other (Yalom, 1995).

Orientation Phase

The beginning period in the small group process is called the orientation phase. During this phase, individuals spend time assessing their purpose for joining the group and also figuring out where they fit in the group. The focus of communication in the orientation phase is on questions of "in or out" (Schutz 1958). In other words, members are often trying to determine how included or excluded they are in the group. Yalom (1995) points out that during the orientation phase "members wonder what membership entails. What are the admission requirements? How much must one reveal himself or give of himself? What type of commitment must one make?" (p. 296). These concerns are illustrated by the comments made by one woman in a mastectomy support group.

When I first read about this group in the newspaper, I wasn't sure that the group was for someone like me. I felt that I had adjusted well to my mastectomy and I wondered if the group was more for women who were having a hard time accepting their mastectomies. I also was unsure what happens in a "support" group. I had never been to one before and didn't know what to expect.

At the first session I still felt uncertain about why I was there, how I would fit in with the rest of the group, and what we were going to do.

After the meeting, I felt more comfortable. The leader helped to make me feel at ease. It helped to meet the other women and talk to them. Each of us had a different story to tell. I still felt unsure of myself, but I knew I was going to continue on in the group.

Schutz (1958) suggests that in the orientation phase members want to become included in the group as unique individuals; they want to belong and be related to the group but they do not want to lose a sense of who they are. Members need to feel that they can retain their unique identity even though they are joining in a group experience with others.

Tuckman (1965), whose perspective is derived from a synthesis of 50 articles on the sequential phases of groups, has labeled the orientation stage of groups the *forming phase.* He suggests that during the forming phase, members engage in testing the other members and the leader to determine what is appropriate and acceptable behavior within the group. Tuckman points out that members often express a strong sense of dependence on the leader or some other important group member for guidance regarding appropriate boundaries in a new situation. In a task group, for example, members spend time at this point trying to identify the nature of the task and the ground rules operating within the group. They frequently ask and give information about the group goal and also look to the leader for direction.

Communication during the orientation phase is often stereotypical and restricted (Yalom, 1995). Group members, who are unsure about their position in the group or the norms of the group, do not want to "rock the boat" at the beginning. As a result, members frequently introduce safe topics of conversation. For example, Schutz (1958) says it is common for new groups to engage in conversations about "goblet issues" during this early phase. The term *goblet issues* originates from a description of cocktail party conversations when people (with goblets in hand) talk about seemingly unimportant, ritualistic subjects such as the weather or common acquaintances (e.g., "Do you know so and so?"). Goblet issues serve a valuable function; they allow individuals to size up others and to determine how others will respond to them. Goblet issues give members the chance to communicate in ways that have little risk, while they simultaneously determine where they fit in the group. In general, communication during the orientation phase remains at a superficial level and there is little self-disclosure until members gain more trust in one another and feel more secure in the group setting.

For example, in a group established for women who were survivors of childhood incest, Carlson and Harrigan (1995) found considerable distrust during the orientation phase among group members. Not only were women hesitant to share their incest secret, but they were also reluctant to share their last names or to exchange their telephone numbers. Although it took several weeks for members to get to know one another and develop trust, a caring bond eventually developed as members realized they shared a similar inner pain.

Leadership in the orientation phase is directed toward helping group members satisfy their needs for belonging. It requires helping members to feel a part of the group but also to feel a sense of privacy, trust, and independence. In addition, an effective leader provides a degree of structure for the group, establishes group guidelines, shapes group norms, and assists group members in understanding the role they play in the overall purpose of the group. If the leader can help members through some of the discomfort in the orientation phase, the work of group members in subsequent phases becomes easier.

Conflict Phase

The second phase in the developmental sequence of group process is called the *conflict phase*. During this phase, members become less interested in orientation issues, such as how they are fitting into the group, and become more interested in control issues, such as how they are influencing the group. Each member wants to be perceived by others as a competent group member with something to offer others. During this time, members are concerned with the relative amount of control and authority they have, compared to other members and the leader, on group decisions. Communication in this phase focuses on issues of "top or bottom," that is, who will have more influence in the group (top position) and who will have less influence in the group (bottom position) (Schutz, 1958). According to Schutz, during this stage there are often leadership struggles and increased competition among members. In addition, frequent discussions typically occur about what task needs to be completed, which rules of procedure will be followed, and how decisions will be made in the group.

Conflicts resulting from struggles for control are common as a group develops. As Yalom (1995) states, "The struggle for control is part of the infrastructure of every group: it is always present, sometimes quiescent, sometimes smoldering, sometimes in full conflagration" (p. 298). In psychotherapy groups, conflicts between group members and the therapist are inevitable during this phase (Yalom, 1995). In addition to leader–member conflicts, struggles for control can also cause the development of coalitions or subgroups (Bennis & Shepard, 1956). Coalitions represent members' needs to express their own power within a subframework of the group.

The following example illustrates a task group in the conflict phase of group process.

A task group was meeting for the second time to discuss the implementation of primary care nursing on a unit that had previously used functional nursing assignments (e.g., medication nurse, treatment nurse). Although in the first meeting there seemed to be agreement and excitement among members about implementing the primary care system, in this second meeting there was considerable conflict among members. Disagreements arose over how the new system should be implemented and even if the new system should be implemented.

As the meeting progressed, one subgroup formed among staff from the day shift, who argued for implementation of the proposed plans as soon as possible. Another subgroup formed among the evening shift who argued that implementation be delayed. The evening staff contended that the recent reduction in evening personnel would make implementation of primary care impossible on their shift. The full group was unable to reach a consensus during this meeting; they had reached an impasse. Additional meetings were needed to resolve their conflicts and to reach agreement on the primary care plan.

In the Tuckman (1965) schema, the conflict phase is called *storming*, which refers to the stormy intragroup conflicts that typically occur during this phase. Tuckman suggests that members' hostility during this phase is an indication of their resistance to forming a new group structure. Members want to maintain their individuality while they struggle with the unknown of a new set of interpersonal relationships. In regard to task issues, members during this phase exhibit a greater degree of emotional response to what the group task demands of them as individuals. Specifically, members weigh options more carefully and consider how changes will affect them personally. The members of the task group mentioned in the case study, for example, started expressing concern about how the new primary care system would affect them on their particular shift.

Leadership in this phase is directed toward helping the group members accept and work through group conflicts. Group members often fear that conflict and criticism will harm cohesiveness. Members also worry that group debates and indecision are symptomatic of poor group functioning. Leaders can help members realize that increased emotional expression or conflict is normal during this phase (see Chap. 7). Leaders can also help members understand that group decisions take time and that a "mulling-over time" helps groups to make high-quality decisions (Fisher, 1974).

Furthermore, leaders can assist group members to satisfy their needs for control or influence within the group during the conflict phase. Some members may want a lot of responsibility and influence, while others may prefer less (Schutz, 1958). Leaders can help both types of group members. For example, a leader could give a special assignment to a member who wants more influence and have that member report back to the group in the following session. Leaders can also allow other members with lower desires for control to maintain lower profiles in the group during this time. As members satisfy their needs for control, conflicts eventually lessen and the group moves to the third phase.

Cohesion Phase

The third phase in the development of groups, the *cohesion phase*, usually follows on the heels of the control struggles and conflicts. This phase can emerge for a variety of reasons. For example, members of a task group may become aware of time pressures and realize that they need to start moving toward consensus in order to meet their objectives. Members of a therapy group may become more understanding of one another's differences and more able to accept these differences in the group. Still others may observe the splits and factions of the previous stage and feel the need to move closer rather than farther away from others. Essentially, members want to develop unity during this phase.

Communication in this phase often focuses on issues of "near or far" (Schutz, 1958). Group members want to maintain close positive relationships with each other but they also do not want to become too intimate. As group members start feeling more positive about each other and the group, they also feel more secure expressing their opinions; members now think that others will listen and be supportive of them. Yalom (1995) points out that during this phase there is an increase of morale among members; their trust in one another builds and they dare to tell others more about themselves. In addition, during this phase it is not unusual for group members to suppress negative comments and feelings for the sake of group unity.

The cohesion phase is similar to the *norming phase* in Tuckman's model. Tuckman (1965) points out that during the norming phase, group members accept the idiosyncrasies of fellow group members and they try to maintain and perpetuate the group and its norms. For example, a group member may shrug off a bizarre comment or an eccentric behavior by another group member and say, "Oh, that's just the way he acts when he's nervous." Members also attempt to protect the uniqueness of the group and to ensure harmony within the group. During this phase there is greater expression of ideas, opinions, and observations on task issues.

Leadership during this phase poses fewer problems than during other phases because of the positive feelings and the unified sense of direction in the group at this time. The leader can put the group on "automatic pilot" during this phase as members work in harmony on group objectives. The leader provides guidance and direction only as needed and essentially assumes a nondominant role during this phase.

Working Phase

The fourth phase in group development is called the *working phase*. This phase is similar to the cohesion phase but it involves more time, greater depth, and increased disclosure among group members. There can be considerable variability in this stage from one type of group to another. In long-term therapy groups, this phase can take a couple of months to develop. In some short-term task groups, a distinct working phase may never be clearly observable; the work of this phase may actually be carried out in the conflict and cohesion phases.

Tuckman (1965) calls this phase the *performing phase,* because members now perform the work they have set out to do. At this point, members feel secure to express both positive and negative emotions in task groups, yet communication usually remains positive, even to the point of members joking and praising each other (Fisher, 1974). The group spirit and the feeling of unity among members are often high during the working phase.

Little directive leader behavior is needed in task groups during this phase, since members are actively solving problems and working with one another in goal-directed activity. In therapy groups, leader behavior will vary according to the various issues in the group. (See Yalom, 1995, for a more extensive discussion of the therapist's responsibilities during the working phase.) Some groups will require more intervention by the therapist than others.

Termination Phase

The last phase is called the *termination phase.* This phase usually occurs when the goals of a group have been fulfilled or when the allotted time has run out and the members begin to consider the implications of ending the group. Yalom (1995) points out that "the end of the group is a real loss. It can never really be reconvened, and even if relationships are continued in pairs or small fragments of the group, the entire group, as members then know it—will be gone forever" (p. 367). As we discussed in Chapter 5, termination is a time when individuals experience a whole range of emotions, from guilt to fear, depending on their own unique previous experiences with the termination process. For example, survivors of incest have reported that feelings of loss were a critical issue as they faced termination (Carlson & Harrigan, 1995). Some members felt they were being abandoned after they had finally learned to trust group members. Others were anxious and worried that the group was ending and they were not fully "healed."

Schutz (1958) contends that groups often go through a cycle during termination that is the reverse of what they experience during the formative phases. He suggests, for example, that during this disintegration phase, group members deal first with their *affectional* ties; they express positive and negative feelings about the group. Next they focus on *control* issues; they consider their relationships to the leader. Lastly, they discuss issues related to *inclusion* as a group member; they discuss their commitment to group members and contemplate what it will be like to no longer be in the group (Schutz, 1958, p. 174).

During the termination phase, leaders need to summarize the work of the group, emphasize the goals that have been achieved, and help group members find a sense of closure as they confront their feelings about the approaching end of group meetings and the members' relationships. Each group member will confront termination in a unique way and the leader can help the group by being sensitive to these differences. Finally, leaders also need to express their own feelings about the group's coming to an end.

In summary, most groups progress through five phases: orientation, conflict, cohesion, working, and termination. Table 6–1 summarizes the communication that often occurs during each phase, although at times there is overlap between the phases. By being aware of these phases and the issues that often surface in each phase, health professionals can increase their capacity to work effectively in groups.

TABLE 6–1. TYPICAL KINDS OF COMMUNICATION IN DIFFERENT PHASES OF GROUPS

Orientation	Conflict	Cohesion	Working	Termination
Safe topics	Disagreements and debates	Supportive comments	Positive comments	Summary of discussions
Goblet issues	Discussions about rules and procedures	Greater self-disclosure	Consensus statements	Expression of feelings
Little self-disclosure	"Top or bottom" discussions	Suppression of negative feelings	Problem-solving comments	Closure statements
"In or out" discussions		"Close or far" discussions	In-depth self-disclosure	

► SUMMARY

Small group communication refers to the verbal and nonverbal communication that occurs among a collection of individuals whose relationships make them to some degree interdependent.

Many different types of small groups exist in health care settings. The various types of health care groups can be distinguished in a general way according to the degree to which they are content oriented or process oriented.

There are several components of small groups that can affect the groups' functioning. First of all, goals provide the reason and motivation for people to form a group. It is important that goals be clear, realistic, and shared to a considerable extent among group members. Norms are the rules established by group members that indicate what types of behaviors are appropriate within the group. Norms can be overt or covert, and they can facilitate or restrict the group's activity. Cohesiveness is the sense of "we-ness" shared by group members that stimulates members to stay in a group. Leader behavior plays an important role in guiding the group, developing norms, and facilitating communication. Specific leader behaviors such as emotional stimulation, caring, meaning–attribution, and executive functioning are linked to effective group functioning. Member behavior, often overlooked, is also an important component. Member behavior can be described in terms of the roles occupied by group members (task roles, group-building and maintenance roles, and individual roles) or in terms of the interaction patterns used by group members. Therapeutic factors, often referred to as curative factors, are also an important component in group functioning. Eleven therapeutic factors that can have a positive influence on group members have been identified as operating in groups at one time or another.

Groups commonly progress through five phases: orientation, conflict, cohesion, working, and termination. The orientation phase occurs at the beginning as members try to determine how they are related to each other and to the group goal. Communication usually stays on safe topics with limited amounts of self-disclosure during this phase. The conflict phase centers around issues of authority and control as members try to determine how much influence they have in the group. In this phase, communication is frequently marked by disagreements and dissent. During the cohesion phase, group members draw closer together and develop a greater sense of unity. Members often suppress negative communication and become more supportive of one another during this time. The working phase is marked by greater disclosure and more profound discussion of group issues. The termination phase occurs at the end of the process as the group completes its tasks or goals. During this time, issues are summarized and members' feelings toward one another and the group are expressed.

▶ REFERENCES

Bales, R. F., & Strodtbeck, F. L. (1951). Phases in group problem-solving. *Journal of Abnormal and Social Psychology, 46*, 485–495.

Benne, K. D., & Sheats, P. (1948). Functional roles of group members. *Journal of Social Issues, 4*(2), 41–49.

Bennis, W. G., & Shepard, H. A. (1956). A theory of group development. *Human Relations, 9*, 415–437.

Burnside, I. (1994). Group work with older persons. *Journal of Gerontological Nursing, 20*(1), 43.

Carew, D., Parisi-Carew, E., & Blanchard, K. (1990). *Group development and situational leadership II.* Escondido, CA: Blanchard Training & Development.

Carlson, R. R., & Harrigan, A. K. (1995). Group intervention: The healing journey of incest. *Journal of Holistic Nursing, 13*(1), 19–29.

Cartwright, D. (1968). The nature of group cohesiveness. In D. Cartwright & A. Zander (Eds.), *Group dynamics: Research and theory* (3rd ed.). New York: Harper & Row.

Cartwright, D., & Zander, A. (Eds.) (1968). *Group dynamics: Research and theory* (3rd ed.). New York: Harper & Row.

Cella, D. F., Yellen, S. B. (1993). Cancer support groups: The state of the art. *Cancer Practice, 1*(1), 56–61.

Cline, R. J. W. (1990). Small group communication in health care. In E. B. Ray & L. Donohew (Eds.), *Communication and health: Systems and applications* (pp. 69–92). Hillsdale, NJ: Erlbaum.

Fisher, B. A. (1974). *Small group decision making: Communication and the group process.* New York: McGraw-Hill.

Geier, J. G. (1967). A trait approach to the study of leadership in small groups. *Journal of Communication, 11*, 316–323.

Goldberg, A. A., & Larson, C. E. (1975). *Group communication: Discussion processes and applications.* Englewood Cliffs, NJ: Prentice-Hall.

Gordon, V. C., Matwychuk, A. K., Sachs, E. G., & Canedy, B. H. (1988). A three-year follow-up of a cognitive–behavioral therapy intervention. *Archives of Psychiatric Nursing, 2*(4), 218–226.

Graen, G.B., & Uhl-Bien, M. (1995). Relationship-based approach to leadership: Development of leader–member exchange (LMX) theory of leadership over 25 years: Applying a multi-level multi-domain perspective. *Leadership Quarterly, 6*(2), 219–247.

Hawks, I. K. (1987). Facilitativeness in small groups: A process-oriented study using lag sequential analysis. *Psychological Reports, 61*, 955–962.

Hersey, P., & Blanchard, K. H. (1993). *Management of organizational behavior: Utilizing human resources* (6th ed.). Englewood Cliffs, NJ: Prentice-Hall.

House, R. J. (1971). A path-goal theory of leader effectiveness. *Administration Science Quarterly, 16*, 321–338.

Jones, S. E., Barnlund, D. C., & Haiman, F. S. (1980). *The dynamics of discussion: Communication groups* (2nd ed.). New York: Harper & Row.

Klein, R. H. (1981). The patient-staff community meeting: A tea party with the mad hatter. *International Journal of Group Psychotherapy, 31*(2), 205–222.

Larson, C. E., & LaFasto, F. M. J. (1989). *Teamwork: What must go right, what can go wrong.* Newbury Park, CA: Sage.

Leavitt, M. B., Lamb, S. A., & Voss, B. S. (1996). Brain tumor support group: Content themes and mechanisms of support. *Oncology Nursing Forum, 23*(8), 1247–1256.

Lego, S. (1994). AIDS-related anxiety and coping methods in a support group for caregivers. *Archives of Psychiatric Nursing, 8*(3), 200–207.

Lieberman, M. A., Yalom, I. D., & Miles, M. B. (1973). *Encounter groups: First facts.* New York: Basic Books.

Loomis, M. E. (1979). *Group process for nurses.* St. Louis: C. V. Mosby.

Schutz, W. C. (1958). *FIRO: A three dimensional theory of interpersonal behavior.* New York: Holt, Rinehart & Winston.

Shaw, M. E. (1976). *Group dynamics: The psychology of small group behavior* (2nd ed.). New York: McGraw-Hill.

Spiegel, D., Bloom, J. R., Kraemer, H. D., & Gottheil, E. (1989). Effect of psychosocial treatment on survival of patients with metastatic breast cancer. *Lancet, 2*(8668), 888–891.

Stech, E., & Ratliffe, S. A. (1976). *Working in groups: A communication manual for leaders and participants in task-oriented groups.* Skokie, IL: National Textbook Company.

Steinglass, P., Gonzalez, S., Dosovitz, I., & Reiss, D. (1982). Discussion groups for chronic hemodialysis patients and their families. *General Hospital Psychiatry, 4*(1), 7–13.

Tuckman, B. W. (1965). Developmental sequences in small groups. *Psychological Bulletin, 63*(6), 384–399.

Yalom, I. D. (1983). *Inpatient group psychotherapy.* New York: Basic Books.

Yalom, I. D. (1995). *The theory and practice of group psychotherapy* (4th ed.). New York: Basic Books.

Young, C. A., & Reed, P. G. (1995). Elders' perceptions of the role of group psychotherapy in fostering self-transcendence. *Archives of Psychiatric Nursing, 9*(6), 338–347.

Zander, A. F. (1994). *Making groups effective* (2nd ed.). San Francisco: Jossey-Bass.

Conflict and Communication in Health Care Settings 7

Conflict is inevitable in human organizations. In health care organizations, the potential for conflict is heightened because within these settings individuals must address life and death issues. They have to function both independently and interdependently within a system containing considerable role ambiguity and complex lines of authority. Health professionals need to be highly skilled both in technical areas and in human relationships. Other organizations may demand similar qualities from individuals, but seldom to the same extent that they are required of professionals in health care. These demands on health professionals make conflict unavoidable.

Conflict creates the need *for* change and it occurs as the result *of* change. When confronted with conflict, we often feel uncomfortable because of the strain, controversy, and stress that accompany conflict. To manage conflict, we have to change our own behavior or we have to change the situation around us. Conversely, change itself can create conflict. Most of us like a degree of consistency in our work and in our relationships; thus, when rules or procedures change or when people change, we are thrown off balance and we feel somewhat disoriented. These dissonant feelings that accompany change can in turn lead to conflict.

Although conflict is uncomfortable, it is not unhealthy nor is it necessarily bad. Conflict will always be present in health care organizations and it will usually produce change. The important question for us to address is not, How can we *avoid* conflict and *eliminate* change? but rather, How can we *manage* conflict effectively and produce *positive* change? If conflict is managed in effective and productive ways, the result is a reduction of stress, an increase in creative problem solving, and the strengthening of interpersonal relationships.

In this chapter, we will approach conflict from a communication perspective. Conflict can be placed at the center of the health communication model presented in Chapter 1. Conflict occurs in the *transactions* between people in professional–professional, professional–client, professional–family, and family–client *relationships* in various health care *contexts*. Throughout the book, we have tried to emphasize that health communication is multidimensional, and we have stressed the importance of viewing communication in health care relationships as a transactional process. Similarly, conflict is not a static or unidirectional event but a process that is transactional.

When conflict exists in human relationships it is recognized and expressed through communication (Folger, Poole, & Stutman, 1993; Hocker & Wilmot, 1995, Lulofs, 1994). Communication becomes the means that people use to express their disagreements or differences. It also provides the avenue by which conflicts can be successfully resolved, or by which conflicts can be escalated to produce negative results.

This chapter will emphasize ways to manage conflict. First, we will present selected definitions of conflict. Next, we will discuss two basic kinds of conflict (content and relational), and two theoretical approaches that have been taken in the study of conflict. The chapter will conclude with an examination of specific conflict management styles and communication approaches for dealing with conflict.

► CONFLICT DEFINED

When we think of conflict in simple terms, we think of a struggle between people, groups, organizations, cultures, or nations. Conflict involves confrontation—two opposing forces brought face to face. When conflict occurs it is usually painful or at least causes stress.

Generally, conflict has been investigated from three perspectives: personal conflict, interpersonal conflict, and social conflict. Personal conflict research has focused on the conflict that occurs *within* individuals, the dynamics of personality that predispose individuals to experience conflict within the self. Psychoanalytical theorists as well as other personality theorists discuss personal conflict at great length. Interpersonal conflict refers to conflict *between* individuals, especially between people who are different. Social conflict refers to clashes between societies and nations. Studies in this field include research on the causes of international conflicts, war, and peace. Our discussion in this chapter will focus on the communication that occurs between individuals who are in conflict—the interpersonal conflict perspective.

A review of the definitions employed in the research literature on conflict provides us with a more explicit meaning for the term *conflict*. Sociologist Coser (1967) provides a frequently cited definition of conflict:

a struggle over values and claims to scarce status, power, and resources in which the aims of the opponents are to neutralize, injure, or eliminate the rivals. (p. 8)

Deutsch (1973) suggests that conflict exists whenever there are incompatible activities between people, groups, or nations. An incompatible activity is one that obstructs, interferes with, or prevents another activity. Both Coser and Deutsch emphasize that conflict need not be destructive but that it can be turned to constructive ends.

Hocker and Wilmot (1995) also emphasize the positive aspects of conflict. They define conflict from a communication perspective as

---

an expressed struggle between at least two interdependent parties who perceive incompatible goals, scarce resources, and interference from others in achieving their goals. (p. 21)

They suggest that conflict should not be viewed as abnormal or undesirable but rather as constructive and growth producing.

The approach we will take in this chapter incorporates several dimensions of conflict suggested by Hocher and Wilmot. First, conflict is a *struggle;* it is the result of opposing forces coming together. For example, conflict exists between a physician and a nurse when they oppose each other on whether or not a patient is ready to be discharged from the hospital. A conflict exists between two community health professionals when they oppose each other on the type of sex education program that could be adopted in a school system. Similarly, conflict occurs when two individuals are arguing opposite positions on an issue such as abortion. Conflict involves a clash between individuals.

Second, there needs to be an element of *interdependence* between individuals for conflict to take place. If health professionals could function entirely independently of each other, there would be no reason for conflict. Everyone could do his or her own work and there would be no area of contention. However, personnel in health care organizations do not work in isolation from one another. In fact, health care personnel often need to function with a high degree of interdependence. Clients depend on nurses, nurses depend on social workers, physicians depend on nurses, administrators depend on staff, and so on. This interdependence sets up an environment in which conflict is very likely.

When two parties are interdependent, each is forced to deal with questions such as: How are we related to each other? How much influence do I want in this relationship? How much influence am I willing to accept from the other party? Because of our interdependence, questions such as these cannot be avoided. In fact, Hocker and Wilmot (1995) contend that these questions permeate most conflicts. In highly important relationships, Hocker and Wilmot suggest that these questions can be addressed openly and directly and in transient relationships they often need to be addressed on a more tacit level.

Third, conflict always contains an *affective* element. Conflict involves the arousal of feelings (Brown & Keller, 1979). When our beliefs or values on a highly charged issue (e.g., the right to strike or autonomy over professional practice) are challenged or blocked, we become upset and usually feel it is important to defend them or fight for our position.

The primary emotion connected with conflict is not necessarily anger or hostility. An array of emotions can accompany conflict. Hocker & Wilmot (1995) found that many people report feeling lonely, sad, or disconnected during conflict. For some, interpersonal conflict creates feelings of abandonment—that their human bond to others has been broken. As we mentioned earlier, it is the feelings aroused in these situations that produce the discomfort that surrounds conflict.

Fourth, conflict involves *differences* between individuals that they perceive to be incompatible. Conflict can result from differences in individuals' beliefs, values, and goals (content issues); or from differences in individuals' desires for control, status, and affiliation (relational issues). The opportunities for conflict are almost endless because each of us is unique and each of us has developed a particular set of beliefs, needs, and behaviors. These differences are a constant breeding ground for conflict.

Based on these four elements, we will be using the following definition of conflict: *Conflict is a felt struggle between two or more interdependent individuals over perceived incompatible differences in beliefs, values, and goals, or over differences in desires for control, status, and affection.* This definition of conflict will be the base from which we discuss conflict in this chapter.

► KINDS OF CONFLICT

There are two major kinds of conflict: conflict over content issues and conflict over relationship issues (Fig. 7–1). Both kinds are present in health care settings. These two kinds of conflict parallel the communication perspective, which states that all interpersonal messages contain a content and a relational component (see Chap. 1). Conflict over content issues involves struggles between health professionals who differ on issues such as policies or procedures. Conflict over relationship issues involves struggles between

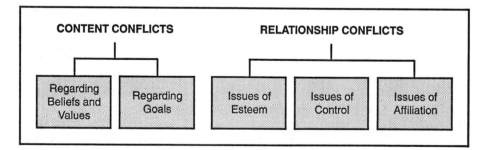

Figure 7–1. Different kinds of content and relational conflicts.

health professionals about how they are related to each other. Although both kinds of conflict are distinct, they do have an impact on each other. A closer examination of each kind of conflict will provide us with a clearer picture of each and also give us a basis from which we can discuss theories of conflict and styles of effective conflict management.

Conflict on the Content Level

Debating with someone about the advantages or disadvantages of a particular organizational change is something that is familiar to all of us. In fact, a large portion of the time we spend in discussions with other health professionals is spent talking about the pros and cons of health care issues such as managed care, allocation of resources, staffing needs, and related topics. Strong disagreements on these topics are not uncommon. These disagreements are considered conflicts on the content level when they center on differences in (1) beliefs and values or (2) goals and ways to reach those goals.

Content conflicts are quite prevalent in interpersonal relationships. In fact, there may be a tendency for individuals to emphasize content and ignore relationship issues during conflict (Wilmot, 1987). For example, Carrocci (1985) found that although individuals in conflict situations could in fact identify both the content issues (e.g., statements about goals) and the relationship issues (e.g., statements about one another or their relationship), they usually generated content- rather than relationship-type responses when they responded to these conflict situations. Perhaps content issues are the primary battleground for our interpersonal conflicts.

Conflict Regarding Beliefs and Values

Each of us has a unique system of beliefs and values that constitutes a basic philosophy of life. We each have had different and unique parents, educational experiences, and work experiences. When we communicate with others, we become aware that others' orientations are often very different from our own. If we perceive what another person communicates as incompatible with our own viewpoint, a conflict in beliefs or values occurs.

In health care, conflict arising from differences in beliefs and values can be illustrated in several ways. For example, patients from certain religious faiths who do not believe it is right to have blood transfusions may be in conflict with health professionals who believe blood transfusions are an appropriate way to maintain a patient's life. Another example of conflict of beliefs can occur when some health professionals believe they should have the right to strike while others feel that health care professionals should not be allowed to withhold services. Still another example would be the conflict that takes place in a discussion when one professional favors national health care while another is vehemently opposed to it. In each of these examples, conflict occurs because one individual feels that his or her *beliefs* are incompatible with the position taken by another individual on the issue.

Conflicts over differences in beliefs and values are often manifested in the conversations, debates, or arguments that occur between individuals.

In his play *Whose Life It Is Anyway?*, Brian Clark (1978) vividly illustrated a conflict in values between a health professional and a client. Clark's play provides a moving account of the experiences of a young sculptor who becomes a quadraplegic as a result of an accident. In the play, the sculptor (Ken) is in conflict with his physician (Dr. Emerson) over who is to control Ken's destiny. Ken wants to leave the hospital, which means he will die because he cannot care for himself without the help of others. Even though he would die, Ken prefers to leave the hospital because he thinks existing in the hospital would be meaningless. Dr. Emerson wants Ken to remain in the hospital where he can receive continuing care that would sustain his life. The following interaction begins with a nurse (Sister) preparing medication for Dr. Emerson to give to Ken.

Dr. Emerson: Have you the Valium ready, Sister?

Sister: Yes, sir. *(She hands him the kidney dish. Dr. Emerson takes it. Sister makes to follow him).*

Dr. Emerson: It's all right, Sister. You've plenty of work, I expect.

Sister: There's always plenty of that. *(Dr. Emerson goes into Ken's room.)*

Ken: Hello, hello, they've brought up the heavy brigade. *(Dr. Emerson pulls back the bed clothes and reaches for Ken's arm.)* Dr. Emerson, I am afraid I must insist that you do not stick that needle in me.

Dr. Emerson: It is important that I do.

Ken: Who for?

Dr. Emerson: You.

Ken: I'm the best judge of that.

Dr. Emerson: I think not. You don't even know what's in this syringe.

Ken: I take it that the injection is one of a series of measures to keep me alive.

Dr. Emerson: You could say that.

Ken: Then it is not important. I've decided not to stay alive.

Dr. Emerson: But you can't decide that.

Ken: Why not?

Dr. Emerson: You're very depressed.

Ken: Does that surprise you?

Dr. Emerson: Of course not; it's perfectly natural. Your body received massive injuries; it takes time to come to any acceptance of the new situation. Now I shan't be a minute. . . .

Ken: Don't stick that - - - - - - - thing in me!

Dr. Emerson:	There. . . . It's over now.
Ken:	Doctor, I didn't give you permission to stick that needle in me. Why did you do it?
Dr. Emerson:	It was necessary. Now try to sleep. . . . You will find that as you gain acceptance of the situation you will be able to find a new way of living.
Ken:	Please let me make myself clear. I specifically refused permission to stick that needle in me and you didn't listen. You took no notice.
Dr. Emerson:	You must rely on us, old chap. Of course you're depressed. I'll send someone along to have a chat with you. Now I really must go and get on with my rounds.[1]

Some health professionals place a high value on the patient's right to make choices and exert personal control. Other health professionals, like Dr. Emerson, place a greater value on sustaining and preserving human life by using all the available medical technologies. The value conflict between Dr. Emerson and Ken is acute. At the same time, both individuals are highly interdependent on one another: To carry out his decision to leave the hospital, Ken needs Dr. Emerson's agreement; to give medical care, Dr. Emerson needs cooperation from Ken. Both individuals perceive the other's values as incompatible and this makes conflict inevitable. The communication between Dr. Emerson and Ken illustrates conflict over a particular content area—values.

Conflict Regarding Goals

A second common type of content-related conflict occurs in situations where individuals have different goals. In a study of the dimensions of interpersonal conflict in small group contexts, Knutson, Lashbrook, and Heemer (1976) identified two types of conflict that occur regarding group goals: (1) procedural conflict and (2) substantive conflict.

Procedural conflict refers to differences between individuals with regard to the approach they wish to take in attempting to reach a goal. In essence it is conflict over the best means to an agreed-upon end. The struggle in procedural conflict is over the *method* that will be used to achieve the goal, not over *what* goal to achieve. In health care, conflicts can be observed in many situations—from the best technique for giving an intramuscular injection to the optimal method for intubating a patient, and from the most effective way to approach a depressed patient to the best approach for teaching a woman how to breast-feed her baby. In each instance, conflict can

---

[1]Reprinted by permission of Dodd, Mead & Company, Inc., from *Whose Life Is It Anyway?* by Brian Clark. Copyright 1978 by Brian Clark.

occur when individuals do not agree with each other on what is the best way to achieve a goal.

Substantive conflict occurs when individuals differ with regard to the substance of the goal or what the goal should be. For example, a health maintenance organization (HMO) administrator whose goal is to decrease the length of hospital stays for patients may have a conflict with a doctor whose goal is to optimize patients' recovery times. Two public health professionals may have different viewpoints on whether the goals of a public health agency should be directed to developing more treatment services or to preventing disease. In health care agencies in general, substantive conflicts often occur between administrators whose goals for more accurate record keeping conflict with staff goals to spend more time providing direct services to clients. These illustrations by no means exhaust all the possible examples of substantive conflict; however, they point out that conflict can occur as a result of two or more individuals disagreeing on what the goal or goals are to be in a health care agency.

Conflict on the Relational Level

Have you ever heard someone say, "I don't seem to get along with her (or him); we have a personality clash"? The words *personality clash* are another way of describing a conflict on the relational level. Sometimes we do not get along with another person, not because of *what* we are talking about (conflict over content issues) but because of *how* we are talking about it. *Relational conflict* refers to the differences we feel between ourself and others concerning how we are relating to each other. It is typically caused neither by one person nor the other, but arises in their relationship. Relational conflict is usually related to incompatible differences between individuals over issues of (1) self-esteem, (2) control, and (3) affiliation (see Fig. 7–1).

Relational Conflict and Issues of Esteem

The need for esteem and recognition has been identified by Maslow (1970) as one of the major needs in an individual's hierarchy of human needs. Each of us has needs for esteem—we want to feel significant, useful, and worthwhile. We desire to have an effect on our surroundings and to be perceived by others as worthy of their respect. We attempt to satisfy our esteem needs through what we do and how we act, particularly in how we act in our relationships with clients and other health professionals.

When our needs for esteem are not being fulfilled in our relationships, we experience relational conflict because others do not see us in the way we wish to be seen. For example, a nursing technician may have repeated conflicts with a head nurse if the head nurse fails to recognize the unique contributions the technician can make to the overall health care process. Similarly, older staff members may feel hostile and upset when they do not receive the respect they feel they deserve because of their experience. So, too, younger nurses may want recognition for their innovative approaches to problems but older staff may fail to give it.

At the same time that we want our own esteem needs satisfied, other persons want their esteem needs satisfied as well. If the supply of respect we can give each other *seems* limited (or scarce), then our needs for esteem will clash. We will see the other person's needs for esteem as competing with our own or draining the limited resource away from us. To illustrate, consider a situation in which an occupational therapist and a physical therapist are both working with a person who has had a stroke, and both staff members feel they have contributed to the progress that the patient has made in her or his rehabilitation. In this instance, if one or both of the staff members believe that they are not receiving sufficient credit for their contribution to the patient's recovery, conflict may result. As their conflict escalates, the effectiveness of their working relationship and the quality of their communication may diminish. When the amount of available esteem (validation from others) seems scarce, a clash develops regarding who is to receive credit for the work that has been done.

Health professionals want to receive respect for their competence from other health professionals as well as from clients. When others interact with health professionals in ways that do not give them the recognition they believe they deserve, the result is often conflict.

Relational Conflict and Issues of Control

As we discussed in Chapter 2, effective communication in health care relationships is strongly related to how individuals share control in their relationships. Because many jobs and roles in a health care setting are not always clearly defined, the control or power inherent in any one role is also seldom explicit. Furthermore, the power structures in health care units today are also changing, leading to greater uncertainty about who has how much power over whom. It is no longer true that the lines of authority are simple and straightforward, (e.g., physician–nurse–patient). In recent years, power has become more widely distributed among many roles (Heineken & Wozniak, 1988).

Relational conflict also occurs when individuals in health care roles (e.g., patient, medical social worker, nurse) perceive that the actual control that they have in their relationships is incompatible with the amount of control that they would ideally like to have. Each of us has different needs for control. Some people like to have a great deal, while others are satisfied (and sometimes even more content) with only a little. In addition, our needs for control may also vary from one time to another. For example, there are times when a person's need to control others or events is very high; at other times, this same person may prefer that others take charge. Relational conflict over control issues develops when there is a clash between the needs for control that one person has at a given time (high or low) and the needs for control that others have at that same time (high or low). If, for example, my need to direct events is compatible with yours, no conflict will take place; however, if I perceive your needs for control to be getting in the way of my control needs, then we will soon find ourselves in conflict. As struggles for control ensue, the communication among the participants may include negative, challenging remarks as each person tries to gain control over the other or undermine the other's control.

A graphic example of a conflict over relational control is provided in the exerpt from *Whose Life Is It Anyway?*, which we discussed in the previous section. The patient (Ken) and the health professional (Dr. Emerson) are engaged in a major conflict over who will control Ken's present care and future plans. When Dr. Emerson gives the Valium against Ken's will, he is exerting control over Ken. This behavior of the physician clashes dramatically with Ken's desire to exert control over the process by refusing treatment. Ken and Dr. Emerson both want control, and this struggle brings out many strong negative feelings and challenging comments toward one another.

Relationships between participants in health care contexts are replete with struggles for control. They are frequent occurrences between health professionals and other health professionals, and between health professionals and clients (see Chap. 3). In the final section of this chapter, we will present some conflict management strategies that are particularly helpful in coping with relational conflict that arises from issues of control.

Relational Conflict and Issues of Affiliation

In addition to the need for control, Schutz (1966) has suggested that individuals also have a need to be included and loved by others. Each of us has a need to be involved in our relationships, to be liked, and to receive affection. If our needs for closeness are not satisfied in our relationships, we feel frustrated and experience feelings of conflict. Of course, some people like to be very involved and very close in their relationships, while others prefer less involvement and more distance. In any case, when others behave in ways that are incompatible with our own desires for warmth and affection, feelings of conflict emerge.

Relational conflict over these affiliation issues is illustrated in the following two examples. While working together on a hospital ethics review board, a nurse and physician, both of whom are married, develop a strong platonic relationship which they both find rewarding. They enjoy their committee work together and find their consultations regarding patients positive. As time goes by, the physician begins contacting the nurse more frequently and the nurse begins feeling uncomfortable with the relationship. In this situation, interpersonal conflict may occur between the physician and the nurse over their different needs for affiliation. The physician wants to increase his closeness with the nurse. The nurse, who has strong affiliations outside the job, feels flattered but is unable to fulfill the affiliation needs of the physician. Their incompatible desires concerning affiliation create conflict.

Conflict over needs for affiliation is also evident in rehabilitation centers. In this type of setting, patients often develop strong relationships with staff members. For example, a patient who gradually makes big strides in physical therapy may become attached to the physical therapist who is responsible for directing the treatment. As the physical therapist attempts to withdraw from this intense relationship and to shift the primary responsibility for the therapy back to the patient, the patient may feel a loss of warmth and closeness. In this situation the patient's feeling of loss of affection or of rejection can create conflict.

Relational conflicts—whether they are over affiliation, esteem, or control—are seldom overt. Due to the subtle nature of these conflicts, they are often not easy to recognize. Even when they are recognized, relational conflicts are often ignored (Carrocci, 1985). In addition, because it is difficult for many individuals to openly communicate that they want more recognition, control, or affection, these relational conflicts are difficult to resolve.

According to communication theorists, relational issues are inextricably bound to content issues, as discussed in Chapter 1. This means that relational conflicts will often surface during the discussion of content issues. For example, what may at first appear to be a conflict between two professionals regarding the *content* of a community-based stop-smoking program may really be a struggle over which of the persons will ultimately have *control* of the program. As we mentioned, relational conflicts are complex and not easily resolved.

Communication remains central to managing different kinds of conflict in health care settings. Health professionals who are able to keep channels of communication open with others will have a greater chance of understanding others' beliefs, values, and needs for esteem, control, and affiliation. With increased understanding, many of these common kinds of conflict will seem less difficult to resolve and more open to negotiation. In the next section, we will discuss theories that have been advanced to explain content conflicts as well as conflicts on the relational level. In addition, we will discuss how both kinds of conflict can be resolved.

▶ THEORETICAL APPROACHES TO CONFLICT

Many theories have been advanced by researchers to explain human conflict. Game theory and conflict resolution theory are the two major theoretical perspectives that have emerged in the research on conflicts between individuals and between groups. A brief examination of each of these approaches will help to clarify the nature of interpersonal conflict. At the beginning of this chapter, we mentioned that human conflict was inevitable and that it need not be considered bad. As Deutsch (1973) has suggested, "The point is not how to eliminate or prevent conflict but rather how to make it productive" (p. 17). Each of the following theoretical approaches emphasizes the ways in which conflict can be used to produce constructive outcomes.

Game Theory

An abundance of research on conflict uses game theory as its basis (Deutsch, 1973; Rapoport, 1960; Von Neumann & Morganstern, 1944; and others). Game theory focuses on the logical aspects of conflict and various strategies that can be employed to win a game. The players use a series of moves during the game that maximizes their likelihood of gain and minimizes their chance of loss. Game theory assumes that individuals will select strategies and make choices that are beneficial to their own self-interest. Because game players' choices are usually interdependent, their self-interests often collide—which produces conflict.

Game theory is a useful approach for studying conflict. It allows researchers to control some of the situational factors surrounding conflict by establishing predetermined payoffs and losses. In the laboratory, researchers can directly observe how specific conditions foster competition or cooperation, how communication influences the outcomes, and how other variables affect interpersonal conflict. However, as we mentioned in Chapter 2 in our discussion of the Prisoner's Dilemma Game, results based on "laboratory" games cannot always be generalized or applied to real world settings. In real-life situations, the complexities of interpersonal conflict are seldom as clear-cut as in the laboratory setting.

Conflict Resolution Theory

A second theoretical approach to conflict—conflict resolution theory—encompasses a large body of research literature. Deutsch's book, *The Resolution of Conflict* (1973), and Jandt's work, *Conflict Resolution Through Communication* (1973), provide substantive overviews of this theoretical approach. Given the definition of conflict discussed earlier, what is the best way to solve interpersonal conflicts? How can conflict be resolved so as to produce positive outcomes?

To answer these and similar questions, Filley (1975) proposed a model of conflict resolution represented in Figure 7–2 which was based on his own research and that of Pondy (1967) and others. Filley argues that the conflict resolution process moves through six steps: (1) antecedent conditions, (2) perceived conflict, (3) felt conflict, (4) manifest behavior, (5) conflict resolution or suppression, and (6) resolution aftermath (see Fig. 7–2 and Table 7–1). As Filley's model is frequently cited and often used in discussions of conflict, we will describe each of the six steps in more detail in the following sections.

Antecedent Conditions

Filley's model suggests that there are several antecedent conditions that set the stage for conflict. The potential for conflict is greater when

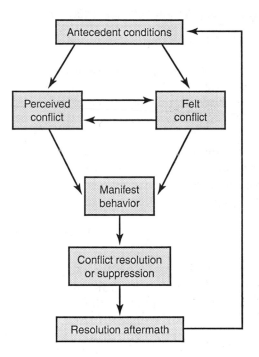

Figure 7–2. The conflict process. (From Filley, A.C. [1975]. *Interpersonal conflict resolution* (p. 8). Glenview, IL: Scott, Foresman. Reprinted by permission.)

- Individuals' responsibilities and roles are ambiguous.
- There is competition for resources.
- There are barriers to communication.
- Individuals are forced to depend on others.
- There is a high degree of differentiation in organizational levels and job specialties.
- Joint decision making and consensus are a necessity.
- There are many rules, procedures, and policies.
- There are unresolved prior conflicts (Filley, 1975).

Many of these conditions are present in health care settings. In hospitals, for example, nearly all the antecedent conditions mentioned above are frequently present. As we pointed out in Chapter 3, the roles of health professionals in the hospital are not always explicitly defined, and they often overlap with the responsibilities of other health professionals. For example, dietitians' responsibilities overlap those of nurses, nurses' duties intersect with those of physicians, physical therapists' responsibilities overlap those of occupational therapists, and social workers' responsibilities may coincide with those of nurses, to list a few. Also, in light of hospitals' emphasis on containing costs, the competition for resources between departments and

TABLE 7–1. STEPS IN THE CONFLICT RESOLUTION PROCESS

Antecedent conditions. Certain conditions exist which *can* lead to conflict, although they do not always do so.

Perceived conflict. Two or more individuals logically and objectively recognize that their aims are incompatible.

Felt conflict. Individuals experience feelings of threat, hostility, fear, or mistrust.

Manifest behavior. Overt action or behavior takes place—aggression, competition, debate, or problem solving.

Conflict resolution or suppression. The conflict is resolved—or suppressed—either by all parties' agreement or else by the defeat of one party.

Resolution aftermath. Individuals experience or live with the consequence of the resolution.

Adapted from Filley, A. C. (1975). Interpersonal conflict resolution (pp. 8–9). Glenview, IL: Scott, Foresman.

even between professional groups can be intense. Furthermore, barriers to communication in hospitals are created by having rotating shifts for personnel (day, evening, and night shifts) or by placing highly interdependent departments far apart from each other. Moreover, personnel are often required to engage in joint decision making while being governed by a multitude of rules, procedures, and policies. Finally, because hospitals are organizations with many levels of authority and numerous job specialties, the potential for communication difficulties and conflict is increased.

Perceived Conflict and Felt Conflict

Assuming that the conditions necessary for conflict are present, the next steps in the conflict process are *perceived conflict* and *felt conflict* (see Fig. 7–2). Conflict occurs more readily if the perceptions of the opposing parties are very far apart. When person A perceives a problem differently from person B, they are more likely to come into conflict. For example, physicians and nurses may have two very different perspectives on patient care. Physicians often highlight the importance of diagnostic procedures and the *cure* component of health care. Nurses and other health professionals, on the other hand, often highlight the importance of psychosocial interventions and the *care* component of health care. Their perceptual differences about what comprises good patient care can create a *perceived conflict* between professionals. On the other hand, if doctors view their duties as including considerable care and nurses share a concern for correct diagnosis, the perceived conflict is considerably reduced.

Felt conflict refers to the level of emotional involvement in a problem situation. Many times conflict between individuals is not based on rational elements but is the result of the emotional reactions of individuals. In fact, as we mentioned near the beginning of this chapter, it is this *affect* dimension that makes us uncomfortable with conflict, and may even make us try to avoid it at times. One mental health worker commented on the conflict she experienced with the director of her agency.

I was so angry with her [the director] that I felt like my blood was boiling. I was intensely frustrated at what I felt was a blocking move on her part. I tried to avoid her as much as I could. I was worried that if I saw her I would burst out in anger and put my job in jeopardy.

Clearly, if we can learn to cope with the intense emotions felt in conflict, our ability to resolve the conflict will be enhanced.

Manifest Behavior

Manifest behavior refers to the behavior and action of individuals in response to conflict. These are the signs of conflict that are observable to bystanders. Individuals manifest primarily two kinds of behaviors in response to perceived and felt conflict: (1) conflictive behaviors (negative) and (2) problem-solving behaviors (positive). *Conflictive behavior* is characterized by the conscious attempts of one person to compete, dominate, and win over a second person. For example, conflictive behavior would be manifested by a health professional in an interdisciplinary meeting who consciously tries to block the innovative program suggested by another health professional. The dominating professional may try tactics such as discrediting the proposed program or diverting the discussion to a completely different topic in order to prevent program adoption. *Problem-solving behaviors*, on the other hand, are conscious attempts to find mutually acceptable alternatives—to find approaches to problems that have positive outcomes for both parties.

Conflict Resolution or Suppression

The next step in the conflict model is conflict resolution or suppression. In conflict situations, individuals can either suppress conflict or engage in activity that will lead to its resolution. Behavior directed toward the resolution of conflict can be characterized by three different *strategies:* (1) win–lose, (2) lose–lose, or (3) win–win.

WIN–LOSE STRATEGIES. The win–lose strategy of conflict resolution is quite common, and most of us have used it at one time or another. Our culture and society, which are very competitive in nature, reinforce a win–lose approach toward conflict. However, it is not the optimal way to resolve conflict because one of the participants loses. This strategy is characterized by attempts of one individual to control or dominate another so as to obtain his or her own goal(s) even at the expense of another's goal(s). In this type of conflict, the parties (1) frequently see each other as adversaries; (2) define their goals individually rather than mutually; and (3) emphasize the problem rather than the long-term nature of the relationship (Filley, 1975, p. 25). The following case illustrates a win–lose strategy.

Financial reports indicated that revenues in a large metropolitan hospital were down 10 percent. In light of the reduced income, the vice-presidents of the various departments within the hospital were told to cut their departmental expenditures by 10 percent. (In this particular hospital 68 percent of the overall costs were for personnel.) One of the vice-presidents met with the director of social services and told her to make the necessary cuts within her department.

During their meeting, the social service director reminded the vice-president that the administration and medical staff had recently approved a new "open" referral policy to the social service department. Under the new policy, any staff member, patient, or family member could initiate a referral and no longer needed to go through a physician. The director showed the vice-president records that indicated the number of social service referrals had increased by 40 percent during the 6 months in which the policy had been in effect. The vice-president listened to the director's arguments but said that considering the total hospital situation, the social service department would just have to "make do" with the reduced budget.

The social service director left the meeting frustrated and decided to submit a proposal to the budget committee and get their decision on the matter. The director was well aware that the vice-president, who was on the budget committee, would argue against the proposal.

The conflict between the director and the vice-president evolved into a win–lose situation. If the budget committee approved the proposal, the director would win and the vice-president would lose. If the budget committee rejected the proposal, the opposite would occur. In either situation, there would be long-term implications for both the social service department and the vice-president's reputation, and also for the ongoing working relationship between the director and the vice-president.

LOSE–LOSE STRATEGIES. The lose–lose approach to conflict is obviously one we would all like to avoid when possible. Most people do not intentionally select a lose–lose strategy, but they end up with this outcome when other strategies, such as a win–lose strategy, fail. In lose–lose conflicts, both parties try to win over the other but both end up losing to each other. Neither person's goals are achieved and the relationship is weakened. The following case study illustrates a lose–lose form of conflict resolution.

A school of nursing was seeking a new director. Administrators at the college strongly desired to have an "in-house" person assume the position, since that person would already be familiar with the program and would have faculty support. Two faculty members said that they would like the position and both tried to line up faculty support. In their attempt to gather faculty support, strong disagreements developed between the two candidates and two distinct factions developed within the faculty. Both factions of faculty members threatened to quit if the person of their choice was not selected. In the end, neither in-house candidate was appointed director of the program; instead a person from the outside who was less qualified had to be hired for the position. The tension and conflict that were generated within the two faculty groups resulted in many long-term problems for the faculty. Their negative feelings toward each other were surpassed only by their overall dislike for the new director. It was a lose–lose situation.

WIN–WIN STRATEGIES. Individuals who employ win–win strategies approach conflict in ways that are significantly different from the strategies used by individuals who take win–lose or lose–lose approaches toward conflict. The win–win strategy is an approach that allows both individuals to feel they have attained all or part of their goals. This strategy tries to satisfy mutual needs, to solve problems creatively, and to develop relationships. There is no attempt by one party to win over or control another party in this approach.

Win–win strategies are not easy to use because they entail a great deal of time and energy. They also require effective interpersonal communication, because an individual must argue strongly for his or her own goal and at the same time listen closely to the thoughts and feelings of the other individual arguing for another goal. When using this approach, individuals have to be attuned to creative alternatives that allow both parties to obtain what they want. However, in the midst of interpersonal conflict, when we are absorbed by our own feelings and needs, it is often difficult to perceive or feel the other person's needs. Finding win–win solutions to conflict means suppressing but not sacrificing our own needs to listen to the needs of others. Whether it be a conflict over a policy or procedure or a conflict for control or esteem, win–win strategies mean both parties communicate in ways that allow each of them to satisfy at least some needs.

Win–win solutions strengthen relationships. They make individuals feel better about how they are related to others. Over time, the strengthening of relationships has the advantage of helping individuals in future conflict resolution. The following case study helps to illustrate a win–win strategy for conflict resolution.

The director of a nursing program at a liberal arts college in a small midwestern community was very concerned about the lack of available nurses with master's degrees to teach in the program. He also noticed that a number of the master's-prepared faculty that he did employ were leaving to work in a nearby service setting where the salaries were higher and where faculty could use their "rusty" clinical skills.

A director of a large hospital in the same community was concerned about the lack of strong role models for the young staff at her hospital. The director also experienced a constant need for highly educated nurses to offer inservice programs in the hospital. For a short period of time, both directors found themselves competing for the few highly educated nurses who lived in this community. The directors, becoming aware of their similar problems, started to work together to find ways of attracting more specialized professionals into their community and also to make better use of the persons that were already available. After numerous extended dialogues, they agreed to design and develop a joint-appointment program in which staff could spend part of their time working for the school of nursing and part of their time working for the hospital. They found that this type of program would benefit both institutions as well as the individual staff members. In the ensuing years, the directors not only developed the program, but they were also able to obtain a grant to fund their collaborative program.

Win–win solutions are facilitated if the individuals can engage in *creative problem solving*. This technique, which originated from Dewey's (1910) work on critical thinking, usually involves five steps:

1. Mutually define the problem(s).
2. Identify potential solutions to the problem(s).

3. Assess the advantages and disadvantages of each of the solutions.
4. Select the solution that represents the best alternative to solving the problem.
5. Discuss and evaluate the fit between the selected solution and the problem.

This problem-solving process is one format for arriving at win–win solutions and does not need to be followed exactly. The form of problem solving used should depend on the type of problem being addressed. For some conflicts, identifying the problem will be the most difficult part; in other conflicts, finding the best solution from a series of alternatives will be the primary concern. No matter which segment is highlighted, this process will aid conflict resolution. However, each step requires that participants communicate their ideas clearly to one another, listen thoughtfully to the suggestions of others, and evaluate the suggestions and the alternatives that are proposed in an objective, nonjudgmental manner.

Resolution Aftermath

The final aspect of conflict in the Filley conflict model is resolution aftermath (see Fig. 7–2). During this phase, participants experience feelings directly related to the outcome of the resolution process. If the conflict is resolved in a positive fashion, the participants will have good feelings about themselves, about each other, and the situation. This was the case in the example involving the director of the school of nursing and the director of the hospital. Participants using a win–win strategy will find that they are strongly committed to the agreed-upon solution and to maintaining a good relationship with other participants. On the other hand, if the conflict is resolved in an unproductive style, participants will have negative feelings about themselves, each other, and the relationship. This was evident in the case studies about the social service director and the hospital vice-president and the nursing school seeking a new administrator. In win–lose and lose–lose situations, participants may feel less cooperative, more distrustful, and prone to further conflicts (Filley, 1975, p. 18). Obviously, the preferred goal of conflict resolution is to arrive at solutions that result in positive feelings, productive interactions, and cooperative relationships among the participants.

▶ STYLES OF APPROACHING CONFLICT

We have discussed the nature of conflict, different kinds of conflict, theoretical perspectives on conflict, and strategies for resolving conflict. Now we will address the questions, Do individuals have different ways of handling conflict? and, How do the styles employed by individuals affect the outcomes of the conflicts?

Researchers have found that individuals approach interpersonal conflict using basically five styles: (1) avoidance, (2) competition, (3) accommodation, (4) compromise, and (5) collaboration. This five-category scheme for classifying conflict was developed by Kilmann and Thomas (1975, 1977) and is based on the work of Blake and Mouton (1964). Each of the styles in the category system is unique and can be applied to conflicts that are typical in health care settings. To measure conflict styles, Thomas and Kilmann (1974) have developed a conflict mode instrument that assesses individual behavior in conflict situations.

A model developed by Kilmann and Thomas (1975) illustrates the interrelationships between the conflict styles (Fig. 7–3). As you can observe, the model describes conflict styles along two dimensions: assertiveness and cooperativeness. Each conflict style is characterized by how much assertiveness and how much cooperativeness an individual shows when confronting conflict. *Assertiveness* refers to attempts to satisfy one's own concerns, while *cooperativeness* represents attempts to satisfy the concerns of others. In conflict situations, both sets of concerns are present. Effective conflict management is a mix of assertiveness and cooperativeness—it involves attending to concerns for self and others simultaneously.

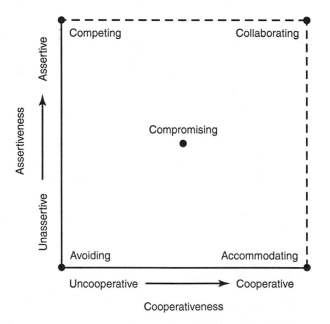

Figure 7–3. A diagram depicting the relationship between assertiveness, cooperativeness, and styles of approaching the personal conflict. (Adapted with permission of authors and publisher from Kilmann, R. H., & Thomas, K. W. [1975]. Interpersonal conflict-handling behavior as reflections of Jungian personality dimensions. *Psychological Reports, 37,* 972.)

In the model, five commonly observed styles of conflict are identified along the assertiveness and cooperativeness dimensions. In conflict situations, a person's individual style is usually a combination of these different styles. "Each of us is capable of using all five conflict-handling modes; none of us can be characterized as having a single, rigid style of dealing with conflict" (Thomas & Kilmann, 1974, p. 13). Nevertheless, because of past experiences or situational factors, some persons may have a tendency to rely more heavily on one conflict style than on others. *Successful conflict resolution occurs when individuals select the conflict style that most appropriately meets the demands of the situation.*

In the next section, each of the five conflict styles will be discussed in more detail. As you read the descriptions of these styles, perhaps you can identify which style of conflict management you most commonly use in your communication with others. Is that style productive or counterproductive? Of all the styles described, is there one or more that you could develop to enhance your conflict-handling skills?

Avoidance

Avoidance is both an unassertive and an uncooperative conflict style. As the word suggests, avoidance is a style characteristic of individuals who are passive and who do not want to recognize conflict. These persons generally prefer to ignore conflict situations rather than confront them directly. In conflict-producing circumstances, these individuals are not assertive about pursuing their own interests nor are they cooperative in assisting others to pursue their concerns.

Avoidance as a style for managing conflict is usually counterproductive and often leads to stress and further conflict. However, there are some situations in which avoidance may be useful—for example, when an issue is of trivial importance or when the potential damages from conflict would be too great. King (1982) points out that overemphasizing minor conflicts can be counterproductive, costly, and time consuming. Avoidance can also provide a cooling-off period (Thomas & Kilmann, 1974). Generally speaking, though, it is better if individuals confront conflict and attempt to resolve it, if at all possible.

In health care settings, avoidance is not an uncommon conflict style. In fact, there are times when avoidance may almost be necessary. For example, one department in a hospital may frequently be in conflict with another department that is always slow in responding to requests. If the request is directly related to the survival of a patient, the interdepartmental conflict becomes less important than just getting the service immediately—and avoiding conflict may be the best way. Health care practitioners are often dealing with life and death decisions for patients; consequently, they often need to suppress their own concerns or conflicts with other staff members in order to perform the necessary services. In these critical situations, avoiding conflict may facilitate the health care delivery process.

In general, however, avoidance is not a constructive style of confronting conflict. Health professionals who are continually required to avoid conflict experience a great deal of stress. They bottle up their feelings of irritation, frustration, anger, or rage inside themselves, creating more anxiety, instead of expressing them or resolving the situation. Furthermore, avoidance is essentially a static approach to conflict; it does nothing to solve problems or to make changes that could prevent conflicts. In health care organizations, the problems that exist will seldom be alleviated or resolved by avoidance.

Competition

Competition is a conflict style characteristic of individuals who are highly assertive about pursuing their own goals but uncooperative in assisting others to reach their goals. These individuals attempt to resolve a struggle by controlling or persuading others in order to achieve their own ends. A competitive style is based on a win–lose conflict strategy.

Competition is widespread in our culture and frequently turns up in health care. In a study of physician–nurse relationships, Prescott and Bowen (1985) found that competition was the predominant mode used by nurses and physicians to handle disagreements. In some situations, competition can produce short-term solutions to conflicts that are more productive than if competition were not present. For example, in a community in which hospitals are in conflict over who is to provide specific services, the quality of the services will be higher, and the cost to the public will usually be lower than if there were no conflict. In the area of cost containment, a competitive approach to conflict can generate innovative cost-saving solutions to complex problems. Similarly, on the interpersonal level, when two professionals compete to provide quality care, the outcomes can be very positive for clients. In effect, competitive approaches to conflict can challenge participants to make their best efforts, and this can have positive results.

Generally, though, competitive approaches to conflict are not the most advantageous because they are more often counterproductive than productive. They involve one party "beating" another, which means somebody will always come out the "loser." In failing to take others' concerns into account, we do others a disservice. When we attempt to solve conflict with dominance and control, communication can easily become hostile and destructive. Too much competition among health professionals can direct energy away from patient care and toward unnecessary interprofessional struggles. For example, Prescott and Bowen (1985) found that the competitive conflict-handling modes of nurses and physicians were inefficient and often resulted in unnecessary delays in patient care. Too much competition between health care facilities can lead to a duplication of services within communities (e.g., two magnetic resonance imaging machines (MRIs), two dialysis units) and duplication increases health care costs. Competitive approaches to conflict may create unstable situations as one party is constantly striving to attain or maintain dominance over the other party. Finally, competition is disconfirming; in competition, individuals fail to recognize the concerns and needs of others.

Accommodation

Accommodation is a conflict style that is unassertive but cooperative. It is an approach to conflict that is "other-directed." An accommodating individual attends very closely to the needs of others and ignores her or his own needs. Using this style, individuals confront problems by deferring to others.

In the beginning of this chapter, we defined conflict as a felt struggle between individuals over incompatible differences. Accommodation is one way for individuals to move away from the uncomfortable feelings of struggle that conflict inevitably produces. By yielding to others, individuals can lessen the frustrations that conflict creates. In accommodating, an individual essentially communicates to another, "You are right, I agree; let's forget about it." The felt struggle is reduced through acquiescence.

The problem with accommodation is that it is in effect a lose–win strategy. Individuals who accommodate may lose because they fail to take the opportunity to express their own opinions and feelings. Their contributions are not fully considered because they are not actively expressed or forcefully advocated. Prescott and Bowen (1985) contend that accommodation is wasteful and potentially hazardous to quality patient care. This style is primarily a submissive style that allows others to take charge. To illustrate accommodation, consider the following conflict between a nurse and a physician regarding the use of pain medication with a terminally ill cancer patient. The physician believes that pain medication should be given no sooner than every 4 hours. In contrast, the nurse believes that the patient should be allowed to request pain medication as necessary and should not have to adhere to a rigid 4-hour schedule. After only a brief discussion of their differences, the nurse decides to give in—to accept the physician's approach to the situation. The nurse in this situation suppresses his or her values regarding pain management in order to maintain an amicable nurse–physician relationship and prevent further conflict. Although the accommodating approach to conflict probably resolves conflict faster than some of the other approaches, the drawback of this approach is that the accommodator sacrifices his or her own values and possibly the quality of care in order to maintain smooth relationships with others.

From a positive perspective, accommodation can be useful in situations in which preserving harmony is necessary. Consider the example of two professionals who differ on an issue: One professional is deeply interested in the particular issue while his or her colleague is less involved in the issue. In this instance, it can be useful for the professional who finds the issue less important to go along with the concerned professional in order to maintain good personal relations. Accommodation can also be effective in conflict-arousing situations such as staff scheduling. If individuals accommodate others in schedule conflicts, it helps to reduce tension among staff members and it enhances the overall quality of their professional–professional relationships. In general, accommodation can at times be an effective means of eliminating conflict. As a rule, however, accommodation is not a preferred conflict style.

Compromise

As Figure 7–3 indicates, compromise occurs halfway between competition and accommodation, which means it includes both a degree of assertiveness and a degree of cooperativeness. In using compromise to approach conflict, an individual attends to the concerns of others as well as to her or his own concerns. On the diagonal axis of Figure 7–3, compromise occurs midway between avoidance and collaboration. This means that persons using this approach do not completely ignore confrontations but neither do they struggle with problems to the fullest degree. Thomas and Kilmann (1974) point out that this conflict style is often chosen because it is expedient and provides a quick means to find a middle ground. It partially satisfies the concerns of both parties.

While growing up, children are often taught that it is important to be able to compromise when a fight or conflict occurs with others. Although it was never easy to compromise, we were taught that we should strive for it. To a certain extent this is correct; compromise is a positive conflict style because it requires that individuals attend to others' goals as well as their own. Compromise reminds us of the golden rule: "Do unto others as you would have them do unto you." The problem with compromise is one of degree. It does not go far enough in resolving conflict. As two persons give in to one anothers' demands, both individuals also pull back from fully expressing their own demands. Both individuals suppress personal thoughts and feelings in order to reach solutions that are not completely satisfactory for either side.

In health care, the compromise strategy may sometimes be seen in the communication among health professionals in interdisciplinary team meetings. One person may soften his or her own position considerably in order to resolve a problem so that each of them can get back to other responsibilities. Although this may be efficient and conserve time, innovative solutions are sacrificed in favor of quick solutions. In compromising, individuals also make themselves submissive to others and squelch their uniqueness. The need for harmony supersedes the need for optimal solutions to conflict.

Collaboration

Collaboration, the most preferred of the conflict styles, requires both assertiveness and cooperation. It involves attending fully to others' concerns while not sacrificing or suppressing one's own concerns (see Fig. 7–3). Collaboration is the ideal conflict style because it recognizes the inevitability of human conflict. It confronts conflict, and then uses conflict to produce constructive outcomes.

Although collaboration is the most preferred style, it is the hardest to achieve. Collaboration requires energy and hard work among participants. To resolve incompatible differences through collaboration, individuals need to take enough time to explore their differences, to identify areas of agreement, and to select solutions that are mutually satisfying. This often involves extended conversation in which the participants search for entirely new alternatives to existing problems. In nurse–physician relationships, col laborating is difficult because nurses and physicians do not spend large amounts of time in face-to-face interaction (Katzman & Roberts, 1988; Lamb & Napodano, 1984) and because they lack a full understanding of the kinds of problems the other group faces (Mechanic & Aiken, 1982). Collaboration requires sharing control in an effort to obtain innovative solutions that are mutually acceptable. The results of collaboration are positive because both sides win, communication is satisfying, relationships are strengthened, and negotiated solutions are frequently more cost-effective in the long run.

The five styles of approaching conflict—avoidance, competition, accommodation, compromise, and collaboration—can be observed in various conflict situations. Although there are advantages and disadvantages to each style, the conflict-handling style that meets the needs of the participants while also fitting the demands of the situation will be most effective in resolving conflict. An effective style such as collaboration and a productive strategy such as the win–win approach both require that participants attend closely to one another's opinions and proposals, then interact in ways that result in solutions acceptable to all parties. Effective communication is the pivotal element that prevents differences among individuals from escalating and facilitates constructive resolution to conflict situations.

▶ COMMUNICATION APPROACHES FOR CONFLICT RESOLUTION

Throughout this chapter, we have emphasized the complexity of conflict and the difficulties that arise in addressing it. There are no panaceas or simple paths. In fact, except for a few newsstand-type books that claim to provide quick cures to conflict, only a few sources give practical techniques for resolution. In this section, we describe several practical communication approaches that play a major role in the conflict resolution process: these include differentiation, fractionation, and face-saving.

Differentiation

Differentiation describes a process that occurs in the early phase of conflict and that involves attempts by both parties to define and clarify their positions. It is very important to conflict resolution because it establishes the nature and parameters of the conflict. Differentiation requires that individuals explain and elaborate their own position, frequently focusing on their differences rather than their similarities. Differentiation represents a difficult time in the conflict process because it is more likely to involve a heating up or escalating of conflict rather than a cooling off. During this time, fears may arise that the conflict will not be successfully resolved (Folger, Poole, & Stutman, 1993). Differentiation is also difficult because it initially personalizes the conflict and brings out feelings and sentiments in people that they themselves are the cause of the conflict (Folger, Poole, & Stutman, 1993).

The value of differentiation is that it defines the conflict. It helps both parties realize how they differ in regard to the issue being considered. Being aware of these differences is useful for conflict resolution because it focuses the conflict, gives credence to both parties' interest in the conflict issue, and in essence depersonalizes the conflict.

The following example illustrates both the difficulties and advantages of differentiation.

Hospital X is a 500-bed urban hospital that employs 1,200 nurses on a full-time basis. In addition to nurses with bachelor's degrees, the hospital also employs 100 nurses aides, which the hospital calls patient care assistants (PCAs). To become more cost effective, the hospital developed a plan to increase the ratio of PCAs to nurses.

On many of the units in the hospital, there were reports of communication breakdowns between PCAs and nurses. In general, nurses complained that PCAs were not adequately carrying out their job responsibilities. PCAs complained that they were not getting respect and not being dealt with fairly.

To address these issues, the hospital brought together a series of working groups comprised of half PCAs and half nurses that met weekly for 2 months.

For the first several meetings, the participants in the groups spent a lot of time describing how they felt about their roles and responsibilities, especially compared to others'. These meetings were often heated and involved in a lot of gut-feeling talk as well as confrontive language. During the meetings, participants complained of "not getting anywhere," "feeling angrier than when they started," and "scared that the whole thing was an insurmountable problem."

On the positive side, the meetings resulted in both the nurses and PCAs learning new things about their work situation. Nurses were able to clarify their expectations of PCAs and to express frustrations about their work habits. PCAs were able to describe how nurses ignored them and often ineptly asked them to perform various tasks that fell outside the PCA's job description. Both the nurses and PCAs found out that the problems they experienced were common throughout the hospital and not unique to any individual.

In essence, the meetings helped the PCAs and nurses to view their conflicts less personally and to be less defensive about them. Both groups learned to talk about their concerns without losing control. They found out that their conflict could be viewed as an external problem that needed to be addressed mutually by both parties.

In subsequent sessions, the nurses and PCAs tried to use their new insights to resolve their communication breakdowns.

In the above example, differentiation occurred among group members as they attempted to lay out on the table their thoughts and feelings about PCA–nurse communication. It was a difficult process because it demanded that each participant talk about his or her feelings about why there were communication difficulties at the hospital, and exposing these feelings was threatening. The group meetings were beneficial because they helped the participants as well as other hospital personnel to clarify the underlying issues in PCA–nurse communication.

Fractionation

Fractionation is a strategy for resolving conflicts that involves breaking down large conflict circumstances into smaller, more manageable units (Fisher, 1971; Hocker & Wilmot, 1993). Like differentiation, fractionation usually occurs in the early stages of the resolution process. It is an intentional process that demands active choice on the part of the participants. In fractionation, the participants agree to "downsize" a large dispute into smaller disputes; they agree to confront a part of the larger conflict in which they are involved.

Fractionation is an important strategy in conflict resolution for several reasons. First, fractionation gives focus to conflict. By narrowing down large conflicts, individuals are able to give clarity and definition to their difficulties instead of trying to solve a whole host of problems at once. Second, fractionation reduces the conflict itself by sizing it down to smaller more manageable conflicts. It is helpful for individuals to know that the conflict they are confronting is not a huge amorphous mass of interpersonal difficulties, but rather a specific and delimited issue or issues. Third, fractionation facilitates a better working relationship between participants in the conflict. During fractionation, participants mutually redefine the large conflict into a smaller one. In agreeing to address a reduced version of a conflict, the participants confirm their relationship and validate with one another their desire and ability to work through problems.

The following case example, which is an extension of the case described in the previous section, illustrates how fractionation can be used to facilitate conflict resolution in a health care setting.

Hospital X wanted to confront the issues that existed between nurses and patient care assistants (PCAs). In the working groups that the hospital established to address these problems, the facilitators asked the nurses and the PCAs to describe at length the communication difficulties they were experiencing. The descriptions were lengthy, involved, and very personal.

The statements made by participants included a huge array of difficulties. PCAs made statements such as, "Nurses sit at their desks and ask me to do things they could do themselves," "Nurses don't let us go to report so we don't know a lot of important details on patients," and "Nurses don't value us as part of the health care team." Nurses, on the other hand, made statements like, "PCAs just can't be trusted to do what you ask them to do," "PCAs are slow; you ask them to do an accucheck and it's never done on time," and "PCAs don't care about the unit; you never see them stay overtime.

Given these descriptions and statements, the facilitator assisted the participants in choosing one issue to confront—how patient information was shared between nurses and PCAs. During these discussions, the participants agreed not to bring up other topics or concerns. Discussions about patient information included talking about what information PCAs needed, what information nurses could and could not share, when nurses were available to talk with PCAs, and the pros and cons of having PCAs sit in on the shift-to-shift report.

The outcome of these discussions was that nurses learned "what" and "how much" information PCAs actually wanted to know about patients. More importantly, perhaps, they learned that PCAs cared a great deal about the health status of patients. PCAs learned how important their duties (e.g., doing accuchecks on time) were to the overall care plan of patients. They also learned how much nurses depended on them to complete their job responsibilities.

A major change that occurred as a result of these discussions was that the nursing staff agreed to conduct a 15-minute daily meeting with PCAs to give them updates and status reports on each of the new and old patients. When the PCAs and nurses finished talking about the access to information issue, they expressed an interest in trying to resolve other problems, as well.

In the above example, fractionation was used to narrow down the nurse–PCA communication problems. In agreeing to focus their discussions on patient information, the participants began the conflict resolution process and were able to restrain themselves from the frustration and anxiety of confronting all of the PCA–nurse problems at one time. Instead of being frustrated by the magnitude of their problems, the participants gained a sense of accomplishment by successfully resolving the patient information issue, and they saw that they could work with each other in an effective relationship.

Face-Saving

A third strategy that assists in the process of resolving conflicts is face-saving. *Face-saving* refers to communicative attempts to establish or maintain one's self-image in response to a real or perceived threat (Folger, Poole, & Stutman, 1993; Goffman, 1967; Lulofs, 1994). Face-saving includes messages on the relational level of how individuals think others see them and how they want to be seen by others. The intent of face-saving messages is to obtain from others a validation of our perceptions of ourselves.

In conflict, which is often threatening, participants may become concerned about how others view them in regard to the position they have taken on issues. This concern for self can be counterproductive to conflict resolution because it shifts the focus of the conflict away from substantive issues and onto personal issues. Instead of confronting the central concerns of the conflict, face-saving messages force participants to deal with the self-images of the participants as they relate to the conflict. In essence, face-saving messages can inhibit the progressive process of conflict resolution.

Interpersonal conflicts can be made less threatening if individuals try to communicate so as to preserve the self-image of the other. Conflict issues should be discussed in ways that minimize threat to the participants. It is important to be aware of how people want to be seen by others, how conflict can threaten those desires, and how our communication can minimize those threats (Lulofs, 1994).

In trying to resolve conflicts, face-saving should be a concern to participants for two reasons. First, if possible, participants should try to avoid letting the discussions during conflict shift to face-saving issues. Although not easy, this can be done by staying focused on content issues and maintaining interactions that do not challenge the other person's self-image. Second, during the later stages of conflict, face-saving messages can actually be used to assist participants in giving each other validation and support for how they have come across during conflict. Face-saving messages can confirm for others that they have handled themselves appropriately during conflict and that their relationship is still healthy.

The following case example illustrates how face-saving can affect conflict resolution.

At a large university hospital, significant disruptions occurred when 1,000 nurses went on strike after contract negotiations failed. The issues in the conflict were salary, forced overtime, and mandatory coverage of short-staffed units.

The strike created a great deal of upheaval in the community. People took sides on whether it was appropriate for professionals to strike. There was much name-calling and many personal attacks between nurses and administrators. Many letters were written "to the editor" of the local newspaper regarding the inappropriate behaviors of the nurses and hospital administrators. The 12-week strike was finally settled when a mediator was brought into the negotiations.

During the negotiations, both the hospital administrators and the nurses released many statements to the media. The hospital stressed that its position was reasonable and that it was good for the community. The nurses stressed that they were only demanding fair wage increases and working conditions that would promote quality patient care.

At one point during the negotiations, the hospital ran a full-page advertisement in the paper titled "A message to striking nurses and their families. A misunderstanding?" In the ad, they described their proposal and why they thought their proposal was misunderstood. At the end of the ad, the hospital stated "We respect your right to strike. A strike is a peaceful and powerful means by which you communicate your concern or dissatisfaction."

In the final outcome on the strike, (1) the nurses received a substantial salary increase, (2) nurses were given the opportunity to have input into the process of how nurses were assigned to low-staffed units, and (3) administrators retained the control of the use of staff for overtime.

After the strike was over, both sides issued statements saying they wanted to get back to the business of delivering the best health care available in the state. Neither side stressed what they gained in the negotiations or what their opponents failed to receive. The messages emphasized pulling together for the good of the community.

This case shows how face-saving can function negatively and positively during conflict. Much of the early negotiations were inhibited by name-calling and the subsequent face-saving efforts of both sides to establish an image that what they were doing was appropriate given the circumstances. As a result, these images and issues of "right and wrong" became the focus of the conflict rather than the substantive issues of salary and overtime. If the parties had avoided these face-saving efforts, perhaps the conflict could have been settled sooner.

The case also illustrates how face-saving messages can advance the conflict resolution process. During the middle of the negotiations when the hospital ran the advertisement about clearing up misunderstandings, the administration was obviously trying to save face for itself but also it was trying to save face for nurses by expressing to them that being on strike was not illegal, and that the hospital was willing to accept the nurses' behavior and continue to have a working relationship. Similarly, the media messages that both parties released at the end of the strike included affirmation of the other party's self-image. The nurses did not try to claim victory nor point out what the hospital lost in the negotiations. In turn, the hospital did not emphasize what they had won or that the nurses were bad because they had gone out on strike. The point is that these gentle face-saving messages helped both sides to feel good about themselves—to re-establish their image as good health care providers.

In summary, resolving conflicts is not a simple process. By being aware of differentiation, fractionation, and face-saving, health professionals can enhance their abilities and skills in the conflict resolution process.

▶ SUMMARY

In human relationships, interpersonal conflict is inevitable. Conflict is defined as a struggle between two or more individuals over perceived incompatible differences in beliefs, values, and goals, or over differences in desires for control, status, and affection. If it is managed in appropriate ways, conflict need not be destructive but can be constructive and used to positive ends. Communication plays a central role in the conflict and in its resolution.

Conflict occurs between individuals on two levels: content and relationship. Conflict on the content level involves differences in beliefs, values, or goal orientation. Conflicts regarding goal orientation can be further divided into procedural and substantive conflicts. Procedural conflicts involve differences regarding the best way of approaching a goal, whereas substantive conflicts occur over struggles about the nature of the goal itself. Conflict on the relational level refers to differences between individuals with regard to their desires for esteem, control, and affiliation in their relationships. Relational conflicts are seldom overt, which makes them difficult for people to recognize and resolve.

The major theoretical approaches advanced by researchers to explain human conflict are game theory and conflict resolution theory. Game theory focuses on the payoffs and losses that people encounter in trying to resolve conflict in a game situation. Game theory is most useful in understanding conflict in laboratory settings. Conflict resolution theory, based on Filley's model, is helpful in describing conflict in real-life situations. This model identifies six steps that occur in conflict resolution: antecedent conditions, perceived conflict, felt conflict, manifest behavior, conflict resolution or suppression, and resolution aftermath.

To resolve interpersonal conflict, there are basically three strategies: win–lose, lose–lose, or win–win. Individuals attempt to dominate or control one another in the less effective win–lose and lose–lose conflict strategies. Win–win strategies are constructive because they emphasize mutual satisfaction of needs and relationship development, with no attempt by one party to control another. Win–win strategies are facilitated by the process of creative problem solving, which includes (1) mutually defining a problem, (2) identifying solutions, (3) assessing the merits of each solution, (4) selecting the best solution, and (5) evaluating the fit between the solution and the problem.

Five styles of approaching conflict are avoidance, competition, accommodation, compromise, and collaboration. Each of these styles characterizes individuals in terms of the degree of assertiveness and cooperativeness they show when confronting conflict. The most constructive approach to conflict is collaboration, which requires that individuals recognize, confront, and resolve conflict by attending fully to others' concerns without sacrificing their own. Managing conflicts effectively leads to stronger relationships among participants and more creative solutions to problems.

Three practical approaches to conflict resolution are differentiation, fractionation, and face-saving. Differentiation is a process that helps participants to define the nature of the conflict and to clarify their positions with one another. Fractionation refers to the technique of sizing down large conflicts into smaller, more manageable conflicts. Face-saving consists of relational messages that individuals express to each other in order to maintain their self-image during conflict. Together or singly, these approaches can assist health professionals in making the conflict resolution process more productive.

► REFERENCES

Blake, R. R., & Mouton, L. S. (1964). *The managerial grid.* Houston: Gulf Publishing.

Brown, C. T., & Keller, P. W. (1979). *Monologue to dialogue: An exploration of interpersonal communication.* Englewood Cliffs, NJ: Prentice-Hall.

Carrocci, N. M. (1985). Perceiving and responding to interpersonal conflict. *The Central States Speech Journal, 36*(4), 215–228.

Clark, B. (1978). *Whose life is it anyway?* New York: Avon Books.

Coser, L. A. (1967). *Continuities in study of social conflict.* New York: Free Press.

Deutsch, M. (1973). *The resolution of conflict.* New Haven and London: Yale University Press.

Dewey, J. (1910). *How we think.* Boston: Heath.

Filley, A. C. (1975). *Interpersonal conflict resolution.* Glenview, IL: Scott, Foresman.

Fisher, R. (1971). Fractionating conflict. In C. G. Smith (Ed.), *Conflict resolution: Contributions of the behavioral sciences.* South Bend, IN: University of Notre Dame Press.

Folger, J. P., Poole, M. S., & Stutman, R. K. (1993). *Working through conflict: Strategies for relationships, groups, and organizations* (2nd ed.). Glenview, IL: Scott, Foresman.

Goffman, E. (1967). *Interaction ritual: Essays on face-to-face behavior.* New York: Anchor Books.

Heineken, J., & Wozniak, D. A. (1988). Power perceptions of nurse managerial personnel. *Western Journal of Nursing Research, 10*(5), 591–599.

Hocker, J. L., & Wilmot, W. W. (1995). *Interpersonal conflict* (4th ed.). Dubuque, IO: Wm. C. Brown.

Jandt, F. E. (1973). *Conflict resolution through communication.* New York: Harper & Row.

Katzman, E. M., & Roberts, J. I. (1988). Nurse–physician conflicts as barriers to the enactment of nursing roles. *Western Journal of Nursing Research, 10*(5), 576–590.

Kilmann, R. H., & Thomas, K. W. (1975). Interpersonal conflict-handling behavior as reflections of Jungian personality dimensions. *Psychological Reports, 37,* 971–980.

Kilmann, R. H., & Thomas, K. W. (1977). Developing a forced-choice measure of conflict handling behavior: The "mode" instrument. *Educational and Psychology Measurement, 37,* 309–325.

King, B. W. (1982). Teamwork/personnel conflicts. *Journal of Emergency Nursing, 8*(1), 51–54.

Knutson, T., Lashbrook, V., & Heemer, A. (1976). *The Dimensions of Small Group Conflict: A Factor Analytic Study.* Paper presented to the annual meeting of the International Communication Association, Portland, OR.

Lamb, G. S., & Napodano, R. J. (1984). Physician–nurse practitioner interaction patterns in primary care practices. *American Journal of Public Health, 74*(1), 26–29.

Lulofs, R. S. (1994). *Conflict: From theory to action.* Scottsdale, AR: Gorsuch Scarisbrick.

Maslow, A. (1970). *Motivation and personality* (2nd ed.). New York: Harper & Row.

Mechanic, D., & Aiken, L. H. (1982). A cooperative agenda for medicine and nursing. *The New England Journal of Medicine, 307*(12), 747–750.

Pondy, L. R. (1967). Organizational conflict: Concepts and models. *Administration Science Quarterly, 12,* 296–320.

Prescott, P. A., & Bowen, S. (1985). Physician–nurse relationships. *Annals of Internal Medicine, 103,* 127–133.

Rapoport, A. (1960). *Fights, games, and debates.* Ann Arbor: University of Michigan Press.

Schutz, W. C. (1966). *The interpersonal underworld.* Palo Alto, CA: Science and Behavior Books.

Thomas, K. W., & Kilmann, R. H. (1974). *Thomas–Kilmann conflict mode instrument.* New York: XICOM.

Von Neumann, J., & Morganstern, O. (1944). *The theory of games and economic behavior.* Princeton, NJ: Princeton University Press.

Wilmot, W. W. (1987). *Dyadic communication* (3rd ed.). New York: Random House.

Ethics and 8
Health Communication

New technologies, changing health care delivery systems, and limited health resources have dramatically increased the number of ethical dilemmas confronting professionals in health care today. Special areas of concern for professionals include advanced directives, clinical trials, "Do Not Resuscitate" (DNR) orders, organ transplantation, assisted suicide, genetic advances, rationing health care, and access to services. Inherent in each of these areas are difficult ethical questions about what is right and who is going to decide for individuals and society.

Communication is an important aspect of biomedical ethics. In health care, communication functions as the medium for ethical decision making and it also affects the outcomes of biomedical choices. This chapter addresses several major ethical issues in health care from a communication perspective.

The chapter begins with a description of the nature of medical ethics and the basic principles that undergird ethical decision making in health care. The second section looks at the area of informed consent and how communication affects its use in health care settings. Section three addresses honesty and truth telling. The chapter concludes with a discussion of ethics committees and the process of ethical decision making. Throughout the chapter, a series of case studies illustrate the content discussed and raise questions for further consideration.

▶ DIMENSIONS OF BIOMEDICAL ETHICS

Before we discuss the interface between communication and ethics, it is important that we have a common understanding of what is meant by biomedical ethics. In this section, we define biomedical ethics and discuss the major tenets, including the Hippocratic tradition, beneficence, paternalism, autonomy, and justice. Much has been written in the area of biomedical ethics in the last 20 years because of significant advances in technology and profound changes in the health care delivery systems (Aroskar, 1994; Beauchamp & Childress, 1994; Caplan, 1983; Cranford & Doudera, 1984;

Katz, 1984; O'Connor, 1996; Veatch, 1989; Winters, Glass, & Sakurai, 1993). The field is constantly and rapidly developing.

Biomedical Ethics Defined

Ethical theory has a lengthy history dating back to Plato and Aristotle. The word *ethics* has its roots in the Greek word *ethos*, which means customs or character. Hence, the area of ethics deals with the kinds of conduct and human virtues that an individual or society finds desirable or appropriate. Specifically, *ethics* refers to a system of rules or principles that are used to guide human behavior. In addition, ethics is used to describe attributes such as "goodness" or "virtuousness" of individuals and their motives. *Biomedical ethics* is concerned with the application of ethical principles and theories to the problems that occur in the fields of health care and medicine (Beauchamp & Childress, 1994).

What is "right" and what is "wrong" or what is "good" and what is "bad" are the basic questions in ethical situations. In any given circumstance, ethical questions are either implicitly or explicitly involved when a decision has to be made by an individual or society about what is the appropriate thing to do. The choices that individuals make about how to respond to life events are informed and directed by their ethics.

Hippocratic Tradition and Beneficence

The Hippocratic oath that physicians take declares that physicians will dedicate themselves to helping the sick and to doing them no harm, and that they will do their best to act on the behalf of patients. Although this oath is taken only by physicians, there has been a tradition among health professionals in all areas to act in specific ways that will help patients. The Hippocratic tradition still influences biomedical ethics because it implies that health professionals "ought" to make choices that benefit patients. Furthermore, it promotes the underlying values and beliefs that it is good to be helpful and to take care of others.

The principle of beneficence is directly related to the Hippocratic tradition because it refers to the duty to help others achieve their interests and to protect others from harm (Beauchamp & Childress, 1994). It has been challenged in recent years because it is sometimes interpreted to mean that physicians or other health professionals have a duty to make choices *for* patients rather than *with* patients. In addition, the principle of beneficence can conflict with other principles, especially in situations where health professionals' actions are directly opposite to the wishes of patients or family members. For example, Sherry (1990) describes this dilemma in a home care situation in which an elderly man with an amputation who had developed decubiti on his back was lying in his own excrement but wanted to be "left alone." The ethical struggle facing the home care nurse is between wanting care for the patient's wounds (beneficence) and wanting to respect the patient's desire to be left alone (autonomy).

The following case study also illustrates the conflict that can occur between beneficence and other ethical principles. Although beneficence is being challenged more often, it is still an important ethical principle that guides the behavior and practice of health professionals.

Mr. D., a 61-year-old divorced man, was admitted to the hospital because of ongoing difficulty with controlling his epileptic seizures. Numerous medications were tried to control his seizure activity with virtually no success. Eventually, Mr. D. became comatose and a neurological consultation revealed evidence of bilateral frontal lobe bleeding. Over the past 2 days, there was minor improvement in his neurological status: he made some response to noise, blinked at visual stimuli, and grimaced in response to noxious stimuli in the left arm. His right arm remained paralyzed and he had "dense aphasia."

Mr. D.'s prognosis was listed as poor even though it was too early to determine what his ultimate level of functioning might be if the bleeding could be stopped and if the seizures could be controlled. It was clear, however, that Mr. D. would not be able to return to independent living nor be able to care for himself in any kind of independent manner.

Mr D.'s sister and his nephew said that he had been a very independent, hard-working salesman before his neurological problems started. After he began having seizures, he became very concerned about becoming a burden to his family. He stated adamantly on a number of occasions that if his condition deteriorated he did not want to be maintained on any type of machine or tubes.

The physician caring for Mr. D. felt a strong responsibility to act in what he considered was the patient's best interest. He had a reputation among his medical colleagues for doing all that he could do to help patients. The physician insisted that Mr. D. have a gastrostomy so that he could receive some nutrition in the hospital. The physician is reported to have said, "We can't starve him!"

Ethical Questions:

How are *beneficence* and respect for *autonomy* shown in this case? What role does family–physician communication play in the resolution of this conflict?

What role do other health professionals (e.g., nurses, chaplains, and social workers) play in this situation?

Paternalism

Rooted in the Hippocratic tradition is the notion of paternalism, which is the process of making choices on behalf of others without their consent (Childress, 1979; Thomasma, 1983). It implies that one individual believes he or she knows better than another what is good for the other person. As the term suggests, paternalism involves the fatherlike behavior of helping others even when they may not have asked for or selected the help that is being provided. When health professionals do things to help patients without first checking if patients want help, their actions are paternalistic.

A classic example of paternalism, discussed earlier in the book (see Chap. 7), is the physician's treatment of Ken in the play *Whose Life Is It Anyway?* The physician (Dr. Emerson) believed that it was best for Ken to be rehabilitated and he ordered an injection of Valium for Ken, even though Ken did not want rehabilitation nor help with his depression. Dr. Emerson faced an ethical dilemma. On the one hand, to "help" the patient meant to give Ken medication to relieve his depression; on the other hand, to "help" meant to comply with his wishes and not give him medication. Dr. Emerson resolved his dilemma by choosing to help Ken by giving him the injection. Although this example is extreme, it illustrates paternalism and the ethical dilemmas that health professionals often face when they try to act on patients' behalf.

The nature of our health care system places health professionals in a dominant position regarding patient information, and this position carries a special ethical burden. Because health professionals frequently have more knowledge, expertise, and access to information, they have more power in professional–patient and professional–family relationships. This power dramatically increases the professional's ability to act with beneficence, to promote patient autonomy, and to push for issues of social justice.

Autonomy

Since the early 1960s, we have seen a growing emphasis in our culture on individual rights and responsibilities. During the 1990s, there has been an increased emphasis on self, with a rapid growth of the number of self-help groups that are available to assist people with health problems. A growing consumer movement stressed that people should be involved in matters of their own health, while a growing health care movement stressed self-care (Orem, 1995) and the belief that patients should be taught how to care for themselves. These societal and health care trends emphasized the ethical position of autonomy because they placed the individual at the nexus of decision making.

Autonomy is a principle of biomedical ethics that suggests that the rights of the individual are paramount in making decisions about health-related issues. It emphasizes that individuals should be in charge of matters related to their own health; each person has the right to self-determination. The basic appeal of autonomy is that it helps to establish a person's moral independence and enables an individual to retain control over important health care decisions (see the following case study). Autonomy is not an "all or nothing" issue; instead, it is manifested in degrees. The critical question that needs to be answered is, "What is a sufficiently autonomous choice?" (Shatz, 1986).

Mrs. A. was a 49-year-old single woman who lived alone. She had two grown daughters and four grandchildren. Mrs. A. placed a high value on her independence. When not working in her job as a teacher's aide, she loved to spend time babysitting her grandchildren. Mrs. A. was very religious and relied heavily on her faith in making decisions about her life. Her church family was her primary support system.

Mrs. A. was a diabetic and had controlled her disease well for 15 years. Because of her diabetes, she developed end-stage renal disease, which made it necessary to start dialysis. Mrs. A. was quite hesitant to start dialysis because she was not sure it would allow her the control that she wanted to maintain her independent lifestyle. After 14 months of dialysis, Mrs. A. became very frustrated. She said she felt terrible. She required oxygen to breathe comfortably. It was very difficult to do anything. She could not shop or get to church without the help of someone else. She could no longer work at the school. Even going to the park with her grandchildren was a major task.

In spite of the fact that Mrs. A.'s dialysis was effective, she complained about everything. She said she had pain in her back, could not see well, and wasn't feeling good. She had lost her independence and all control in her life.

Guided by her faith, Mrs. A. approached the social worker about stopping dialysis. She knew this meant she would die in a relatively short period of time. For Mrs. A., life was not worth living in her condition. Her daughters did not agree with her decision. They did not want her to stop dialysis.

Ethical Questions:

What should the social worker say to Mrs. A.?
What does *beneficence* require in this case?

What does *autonomy* require in this situation?

If you were one of the two daughters, how would you respond to your mother?

There are a number of factors that make autonomy a complex issue (Childress, 1990). First, it is difficult to determine the exact preference of patients. Callahan (1995) suggests that "no one fully understands what most patients really want, including the patients themselves . . ." (p. 33). Second, patients may be ambivalent at times and express contradictory preferences. Third, patients' choices may change over time, making it difficult to know if a person's choice today will be the same choice tomorrow. Fourth, there are many types of consent (e.g., direct, implicit, or presumed), with some types indicating more acknowledgment and certainty on the part of the patient than others. Even though respecting a person's autonomy can be a complex issue, this principle will play a critical role in biomedical ethics in the future (Childress, 1990).

Justice

A final dimension of biomedical ethics involves issues of social justice. This ethical position has received much emphasis recently because people are living longer and there are more people in need of health care services. But the available resources are not plentiful enough to be equally available to all. In addition, illnesses such as acquired immunodeficiency syndrome (AIDS) have placed an increased burden on health care resources. New and expensive technologies have also brought justice issues into focus.

The justice principle refers to issues of fairness in health care. Justice demands that each individual and group receives what it rightfully deserves (Beauchamp & Childress, 1983). This principle comes into play when, for example, the government sets priorities for funding different types of national research projects. It comes into play when determining which patients, out of many waiting patients, should receive organ transplants. The justice principle also comes to the forefront when decisions are being made about which patients should be afforded the opportunity to receive certain expensive treatments.

Society is replete with examples that force health care providers to address ethical issues of justice. For example, is it fair if an 8-year-old boy dies because his parents cannot pay for a bone marrow transplant while at the same time the state in which he lives insists on spending tens of thousands of dollars to maintain an individual in a persistent vegetative state against the wishes of that individual's family? Is it fair when one family can pay for a lifesaving treatment while another family cannot? Is it just to provide extensive costly treatments to individuals in a coma when many people do not even have basic health care coverage? In a situation of limited resources, the needs of both the individual and the public cannot always be met simultaneously (Danis & Churchill, 1991).

Justice is a principle that is often interwoven with other important ethical principles such as beneficence and autonomy. In the following case study, justice issues become another factor in the decision-making process. As health care resources continue to diminish, justice issues will become even more prominent.

Mrs. C., an 87-year-old woman, lived with her husband of 50 years in a low-income apartment complex for senior citizens. They had six children and many grandchildren.

Mrs. C. had a massive stroke and was placed on a ventilator in the intensive care unit. After several weeks in intensive care, Mrs. C. showed no sign of improvement. The medical staff said that Mrs. C. would never regain consciousness and that it was futile to try to keep her alive on machines any longer. The physician, primary care nurse, and social worker all encouraged the family to allow Mrs. C. to be taken off the life support equipment.

Mrs. C.'s family, especially her husband, insisted that she be kept alive on the ventilator. They were a religious family who believed that it was not their decision nor anyone's decision to let her die. Mr. C. said, "She will die when the Good Lord wants her to and not a minute sooner."

Mrs. C.'s health care was being paid for by a health maintenance organization (HMO) for senior citizens. Over time, the cost of her care, which amounted to thousands of dollars a week, was a major concern for her financially troubled HMO. At about this time, to offset their increased expenditures, the HMO had to increase their monthly rates to subscribers, which created significant hardships for many of the subscribers who were on fixed incomes.

Ethical Questions:

How does *justice* come into play in this case?
What other ethical principles are operating in this case?
How would *benefits and burdens* be assessed in this situation?

Dealing with ethical questions in clinical settings is no easy task. It is particularly difficult because there is often not a clear answer for every question. In many situations, two or more ethical principles may conflict with one another, leaving a practitioner puzzled about which ethical principle should take precedence. The difficulty that professionals face in these cases is not a matter of ignorance about an obviously correct choice, but rather a struggle to make a responsible decision in the face of a variety of possible and plausible choices.

In summary, biomedical ethics involves the basic principles of beneficence, paternalism, autonomy, and justice. For any given case, one principle may dominate over another, or two or more of the principles may overlap. The order and relative weight that professionals give to these principles provides a picture of their ethical stance, and their ethical position dramatically affects the way in which they carry out their health care responsibilities.

▶ INFORMED CONSENT: A COMMUNICATION ISSUE

Informed consent is a legal doctrine that requires health professionals to provide information to patients so that patients themselves can determine what, if anything, will be done to them. Informed consent stresses the ethical principle of autonomy and self-determination for patients. Effective health communication is the key factor in the process of implementing informed consent. In this section, we describe the legal roots of informed consent and some of the difficulties that arise in attempting to implement informed consent procedures.

Legal Requirements

Informed consent can be traced back to a major opinion delivered by Judge Cardozo in 1914, in a case in which a physician failed to obtain a consent for surgery (*Schloendorff v. Society of New York Hospitals,* 1914). Cardozo wrote that:

....

Every human being of adult years and sound mind has a right to determine what shall be done with his (her) own body; and a surgeon who performs an operation without his (her) patient's consent, commits an assault for which he or (she) is liable in damages.

....

This case emphasized the legal obligations of providers to obtain consent from patients before administering any type of treatment to them.

In 1960, two landmark cases (*Natanson v. Kline* and *Mitchell v. Robinson*) established that patients, in addition to having the right to consent to treatment, also had the right to know exactly what they were consenting to—hence, *informed* consent. These cases established that providers need to tell patients the nature of an ailment, the nature of the proposed treatment including its risks and benefits, the probability of success of the proposed treatment, and possible alternatives to the treatment (O'Connor, 1981).

Even though the guidelines (elements) for informed consent are relatively clear, it is still difficult for providers to know exactly what is to be disclosed in any given case. A series of judgments in the 1970s (*Canterbury v. Spence*, 1972; *Cobbs v. Grant*, 1972; *Wilkinson v. Vesey*, 1972) supported the contention that informed consent means that professionals need to disclose to patients that which a "reasonable person" would need to know. These cases suggested that informed consent does not require that providers disclose information based on a professional practice standard of what would be necessary for another physician or nurse to know but rather according to an objective standard of what a reasonable person would need to know in a given circumstance (O'Connor, 1981).

Beauchamp and Childress (1983) point out that patients' autonomy is enhanced when this "reasonable person" standard for disclosure is supplemented by a standard that takes the unique information needs of individual patients into account as well. They argue that patients are well served by professionals who, in addition to providing standard information about treatments, ask patients what they want to know and answer any questions they may have (pp. 76–79).

The legal underpinnings of informed consent underscore the critical role of effective communication. In essence, the laws demand that providers communicate with patients. In addition, the laws require that they communicate certain kinds and sufficient amounts of information to patients. In Chapter 1 of this book, we defined communication as sharing information according to a common set of rules. In the case of informed consent, the laws lay out selected rules that must govern how providers are to talk to patients about receiving certain treatments for their illness.

Implementation and Improvement

The primary purpose of informed consent laws is to guarantee patients' right to self-determination in decisions about their own health. Implementing these laws to achieve that self-determination is not an easy task. For example, what constitutes being truly informed? How much information does a patient need in order to make a decision about his or her treatment? Can patients fully understand complex medical issues regarding potential risks and benefits of treatments (e.g., see the following case study)? How do professionals assess whether informed consent has been achieved? These questions highlight the difficulties that professionals face in trying to implement informed consent.

Mark, a 17-year-old boy, injured his knee while running in a high school cross-country race. Before the injury, he was an outstanding athlete who excelled in three high school sports.

Mark was scheduled for arthroscopic surgery to determine the nature and extent of his knee injury. Since the procedure was considered minor, Mark's father continued with his plans to leave on a business trip and only Mark's mother accompanied him to surgery.

During the arthroscopic procedure, the surgeon found more extensive damage than he had anticipated. The surgeon went to the waiting room and told Mark's mother that he thought that he should immediately "open the knee" to repair the torn ligaments and to remove the damaged tissue and bone chips. The surgeon assured her that this more extensive procedure was necessary and that the chances of complications were minimal.

Mark's mother felt that she was being rushed into making a decision, wondered if she should get a second opinion, and wished that her husband were there to help her think through the decision. Reluctantly, she agreed to the additional surgery and signed the consent form.

Unanticipated complications occurred as a result of the additional surgery, leaving Mark with an unstable knee joint that required a brace. The complications also caused severe curtailment of his involvement in sports. Mark was unable to run cross country, play on the hockey team, or run track.

His final year of high school fell far short of his dream of being a varsity letter-winner in three sports. He sorely missed being a part of the school's athletic programs.

Ethical Questions:

What factors influenced the informed consent process in this situation?

Should the physician have discussed with the mother the possibility that surgery would severely limit Mark's athletic activities?

Was the consent given by Mark's mother truly informed consent?

The process of informed consent has raised a number of controversies. Some clinicians believe that the requirement for full disclosure can lead to informational overkill and can add unnecessary stress to an already anxious patient (Penman et al., 1984). Clinicians have also questioned whether informed consent documents are written more to protect the investigators and institutions than to provide useful information to the patient (Penman et al., 1984). Whatever the concern, the process of implementing informed consent remains a challenge.

Comprehension

One aspect of informed consent that deserves special attention is the issue of comprehension. For patients' consent to be truly informed, it is important that patients understand the information they receive from health professionals.

Several studies point to the fact that even though informed consent is obtained from patients, they may not fully comprehend the issues and information. Cassileth and associates (1980) interviewed 200 cancer patients who were receiving chemotherapy, radiation, or surgery, and found that only half of the patients could correctly recall the purpose of their treatment 1 day after they had given informed consent. Similarly, Kennedy and Lillehaugen (1979) found that nearly half of a sample of 40 cancer patients could not adequately recall informed consent information, including whether or not they had given permission for certain drugs to be used in their treatment. In a more recent study, Lawson and Adamson (1995) found that consent form language is often not understood by patients. A sizable number of patients in their study were unfamiliar with terms such as "protocol" and "lesion." Collectively, these studies show that even though informed consent may have been obtained by professionals, many times patients do not completely comprehend the meaning of the treatment and the procedures to which they have given their consent, or the language used in the informed consent documents.

There are many factors that negatively affect or reduce the level of comprehension of informed consent. Some of the more influential factors include the patient's state of anxiety about his or her illness; the patient's level of education; the nature, amount, and clarity of the information to be disclosed; the patient–professional relationship; and the readability of consent forms. If professionals intend to provide patients with full self-determination in making health care decisions, health professionals must be aware of these factors.

Based on a review of informed consent studies to determine the factors that influence comprehension of information, Silva and Sorrell (1984) have suggested several approaches that may increase comprehension for patients.

1. A consent document should be written in a clear, brief, and direct fashion.
2. The amount of information should be neither too little nor too much.
3. Subjects should be given sufficient time (perhaps a day or longer) to digest consent information.
4. Special assistance in understanding the information should be provided to individuals who have lower educational or vocabulary levels.
5. Additional help in understanding information may need to be given to individuals who are coping with disruptive situations.

Consistent with the suggestions of Silva and Sorrell, O'Connor (1981) has recommended that comprehension is improved if the readability of the consent forms is no higher than an eighth-grade level and the form is supplemented with individualized explanation. Furthermore, O'Connor contends that informed consent is also better achieved if it is supplemented with audiovisual or written materials.

Interpersonal Relationships

Although the previous section stresses the importance of comprehension, the nature of the relationship between the professional and the patient also plays a critical role in the informed consent process. Penman and associates (1984) studied the process of informed consent and the factors that influenced 144 cancer patients' decisions to accept treatment. Patients in their study cited "trust in the physician" as the most important factor that influenced their decision to accept treatment. Other factors that were also ranked as important after the trust factor were "information given by the physician," "belief that the treatment would fight the illness," and "belief that the treatment would cure the illness." The high ranking given to physician trust was probably related to the fact that the majority of patients said that the physician had been understanding of their feelings, that they had felt comfortable with the physician, that the physician had asked if they had further questions, and that they had had sufficient time to ask all of their questions. The investigators concluded that one of the best ways to obtain patient consent was through an unhurried interview with a professional when the discussion is characterized by trust and rapport.

The nature of the relationship between providers and patients is influenced strongly by the core values of the participants (Veatch, 1995). Decisions regarding which treatment options will best serve the patient's interests are impossible to make without addressing the unique perspectives of patients. Veatch suggests that it may be valuable to pair providers and patients on the basis of their deep values (e.g., religious affiliation, philosophical orientation, and worldview). For example, a terminally ill patient with certain values about dying might utilize the services of a particular hospice whose staff subscribe to the same values. In this context, it is more likely that the patient's interests will be served. Veatch contends that obtaining informed consent is often problematic because of the wide gulf between providers' and patients' values and worldviews. However, by attending to the similarities and differences between patients' and clinicians' values, clinicians can more closely provide care that is in the best interest of patients.

Other interpersonal relationships also play a role in the consent process. Family members are often present at the time that patients receive information and consent forms, and these family members play a role in the decision of patients to accept treatment or to participate in a research protocol (Penman et al., 1984). In some instances, family members act as gatekeepers, preventing health professionals from even approaching their ill family member about a new treatment or research study or discouraging the family member from participating once they have been approached. This is especially evident with frail elderly patients for whom family members serve as guardians (Ratzan, 1981).

Kuczewski (1996) argues that the family plays an important role in the informed consent process. Rather than viewing the family's and patient's interests as conflicting, Kuczewski suggests the family be viewed as a natural partner in the development of patient autonomy. From this perspective, informed consent is a process involving shared decision making in which the values and preferences of patients and family members mutually affect each other. Through dialogue, family members assist patients in making satisfactory decisions about their health care.

To summarize, informed consent is a legal doctrine designed to guarantee patients the right of self-determination. Our legal system lays out the rules for informed consent by establishing the parameters for how professionals are to talk to patients about treatment. However, many obstacles get in the way of full implementation of these rules. The challenge for health professionals is to avoid these obstacles if they intend to make informed consent truly comprehensible and a vehicle for patients' self-determination.

▶ HONESTY AND TRUTH TELLING: A COMMUNICATION RESPONSIBILITY

Honesty and truth telling are other aspects of biomedical ethics that directly relate to communication (Jaksa & Pritchard, 1988). They play an instrumental role in achieving ethical outcomes in health care. The responsibility to tell the truth can be derived from the principle of autonomy, for to fully respect others requires being truthful with them (Beauchamp & Childress, 1994). Truth telling, also called veracity, refers to the honest disclosure of information to patients. Effective interpersonal relationships depend on honesty and trustworthiness. This is especially the case in health care relationships where patients and family members rely on health care professionals for advice in life and death situations.

Overview

Before the 1960s, it was a common practice to withhold information from patients, especially from cancer patients who were considered too frail to deal with the ramifications of a cancer diagnosis (Oken, 1961). Although today patients are generally told their diagnoses as well as their prognoses, truth telling still remains a thorny issue.

One of the ethical dilemmas related to truth telling in the 1990s involves the issue of AIDs. Who should be tested for human immunodeficiency virus (HIV) antibodies and who should know the results? What if a person agrees to be tested for HIV antibodies as a part of a research study, but also insists that he or she not be told of the results of the test? Is it ethical for the professional to tell the truth or is it ethical for this person to avoid the truth? Honoring an individual's refusal to learn information may exhibit respect for autonomy but, at the same time, it may jeopardize the health of others who are unaware that they are at risk for getting the infection (Avins & Lo, 1989).

Other ethical dilemmas related to truth telling often confront health professionals. Aroskar (1989) studied the ethical dilemmas that 319 community health nurses faced in their clinical practice with clients and discovered a number of dilemmas related to truth telling. Among the examples reported by the nurses were (1) concealing a cancer diagnosis from an elderly patient, (2) "stretching the truth" about a client's qualifications to enable the client to qualify for a certain kind of program or reimbursement, (3) concealing from one physician that a patient is seeing another physician for unorthodox cancer treatments, and (4) ignoring questionable practices of certain nurses and physicians because exposing them may lead to reprisals for the patient or the nurse. These examples illustrate that truth telling evolves around the professional's relationship with the patient as well as the professional's relationship with other health professionals and agencies.

Four Approaches to Truth Telling

In the area of patient–professional relationships, truth telling can be categorized into four different ways of conveying information to patients: (1) strict paternalism, (2) benevolent deception, (3) contractual honesty, and (4) unmitigated honesty (Goodwin, 1984). *Strict paternalism* occurs when the professional blatantly lies to the patient for the presumed well-being of the patient. For example, a physician decides not to tell a 94-year-old woman that she has cancer because he thinks that she is more likely to die from old age than cancer, and he does not want to cause her undue worry. *Benevolent deception* occurs when the professional withholds some truth, but not all of the truth, from a patient. For example, a physician may tell a patient that she has kidney cancer that can be treated, but at the same time withhold information that her prognosis is poor even with the treatment.

Contractual honesty occurs when the professional tells the patient as much information as the patient wants to know. For example, a cancer patient may say to a physician, "Give me only hopeful information; I don't want dismal percentages or statistics about my chances of surviving." *Unmitigated honesty* occurs when the professional tells the truth, whether or not the patient wants to hear it. For example, a radiation oncologist called aside the mother of a 14-year-old girl with Hodgkin's disease and said, "Your daughter has a huge tumor in her lung; there's not much I can do, and her chances of surviving are nil." Although the young girl survived the disease, her mother still angrily recalls the brutal manner in which she was given information about her daughter's condition. In recent years, unmitigated honesty is more common among some health professionals who are concerned about malpractice suits and "tell it all" as a self-protective mechanism. Speaking truthfully means giving the facts; and even though the truth can be brutal, the telling of it should not be (Jonsen, Siegler, & Winslade, 1986).

Of these four types of honesty, contractual honesty may be preferable because it respects patients' desires and patients' autonomy. Strict paternalism violates patients' rights for information, while benevolent deception deceives the patient. Unmitigated honesty, on the other hand, overrides the patients' preferences for information (Goodwin, 1984).

Some authors caution against relying too much on patient preferences for information for fear that a person may end up with insufficient information to make informed decisions (Garrett, Baillie, & Garrett, 1989). Rather, they argue for a dialogue between professional and patient that assumes that the patient has a sufficient amount of information to make a decision from the patient's point of view. Dialogue such as this is similar to contractural honesty but is more informing. In other words, the patient receives the kind of information that any prudent person would need to know but within the context of what is important to the particular patient. According to Jonsen, Siegler, and Winslade (1986), the ideal ethical relationship is one in which patients provide certain information to professionals who, in turn, analyze the information and inform patients about their conditions, creating a reciprocal relationship between two autonomous people.

Before leaving the discussion of truth telling, it is important to consider the ethical dilemma that occurs when a patient asks another health professional for information that was withheld from them by their primary health care provider. For many years, nurses often found themselves in this intermediary position with patients. Terminally ill patients would often ask the nurse if they were dying, and the nurse would either refer the patient's questions to the physician, counter the patient's questions with further questions to determine what the patient already knew, or distract the patient to avoid answering the question (High, 1989).

The influence of the hospice movement in recent years has resulted in terminally ill patients being more fully informed about their situation, and nurses are less apt to be caught in the middle of these difficult dilemmas. In addition, physicians are realizing that they do not work alone but rather interdependently with other team members. If physicians choose to withhold information from patients, it may be met with the disapproval of the rest of the team. Furthermore, with the availability of ethics committees and consultants, nurses and other professionals now have resource people to help them explore ways of dealing with these dilemmas.

Truth telling continues to pose a series of ethical dilemmas for patients, family members, and professionals (e.g., see the following case study). Sharing information in a manner that respects the autonomy of patients and their preferences for information remains a challenge.

M̲r. B., a 67-year-old man, was diagnosed with kidney cancer. He lived with his second wife who was partially disabled due to multiple sclerosis. For many years, Mr. B. operated a small manufacturing business but he retired early to help care for his wife. Mr. B. had two stepchildren from his second marriage.

By the time of diagnosis, the cancer had already spread to Mr. B.'s lungs and was causing him considerable respiratory difficulty. Mr. B. was started on radiation therapy to control further spread of the cancer. Even though Mr. B.'s health was deteriorating, he wanted to maintain hope for a cure at all costs. He was very guarded about any kind of information about his situation and refused to let his stepdaughters meet with the physician. He said adamantly, "I'll tell you what the doctor tells me."

The stepdaughers became increasingly anxious about Mr. B.'s illness and also about their mother's living situation should he not recover. In desperation, they called the physician and asked about their stepfather's prognosis. The physician told them that Mr. B.'s prognosis was poor and that he would probably not live for more than 4 to 6 months. The physician said that he did not want to give this information to Mr. B. because he thought Mr. B. had a very strong need to maintain hope and he knew Mr. B. did not want the information.

Ethical Questions:

Was the physician right in not sharing this information with Mr. B.?

Was the physician engaged in *benevolent deception* or *contractual honesty*?

Was it ethical for the physician to tell the stepchildren Mr. B.'s prognosis?

How will the physician's communication with the family affect the family's communication with Mr. B.?

► ETHICS COMMITTEES: THE PROCESS OF ETHICAL DECISION MAKING

Throughout this chapter, we have been discussing the principles of bioethics—the underlying assumptions of ethical decisions. Although ethical choices and decisions are made every day at patients' bedsides and throughout the health care system, the formal process of ethical decision making is often carried out through the use of formal committees on medical ethics. These committees provide the structure for discussing and making decisions about bioethical issues. In the following sections, we will discuss the background of institutional ethics committees, the functions of these committees, and some of the common issues they are frequently asked to confront.

Background

An ethics committee is an interdisciplinary group of individuals that addresses some of the most difficult ethical problems that are confronted in clinical care by health professionals, patients, and those close to them. The membership of ethics committees is usually comprised of physicians, nurses, social workers, and chaplains experienced in ethics; but members may also include patient advocates, administrators, attorneys, and lay persons. The basic assumption on which ethics committees are founded is that cooperative, reasoned reflection by a group is likely to benefit decision makers and help them in reaching better conclusions (Cohen, 1988).

Although the history of the use of ethics committees in hospitals and other health care organizations is short, it reveals a rapidly growing phenomenon. As recently as the early 1980s, only a small percentage of the country's hospitals had ethics committees (Cranford & Doudera, 1984); however, it is commonplace today for nearly every hospital to have an ethics committee.

The rapid growth of ethics committees can be traced to several key events (Cranford & Doudera, 1984; Ross, Bayley, Michel, & Pugh, 1986). One of the first events that gave impetus to the emergence of ethics committees was the Karen Ann Quinlan (1976) case. In this case, which was concerned with whether or not to remove life-support measures, the court quoted an article by Teel (1975), which emphasized the importance of the use of hospital ethics committees to enhance medical decision making. Further interest in ethics committees was spurred by the cases of Infant Doe, Indiana (1982); and Baby Jane Doe, New York (*Weber v. Stony Brook Hospital*, 1983), both of which concerned the legal issues surrounding parents' and health professionals' choices to treat or not to treat handicapped infants. These cases highlighted the need to provide physicians and parents with as much help as possible in making decisions.

At about the same time, the President's Commission for the Study of Ethical Problems in Medicine and Biomedical and Behavioral Research (1983) issued a report which declared that, in order to protect patients who did not have the capacity to make their own decisions, medical staff and administrators of health care institutions should explore the use of ethics committees for decisions that have life and death consequences. The Commission's Report, along with the court cases on the treatment of infants, were the primary forces behind establishing a growing number of ethics committees. Today, the mood in health care continues to support the need for established ethics committees in health care institutions.

Functions

The work of ethics committees falls primarily in three areas: education, policy, and case consultation. The educational role involves providing information on ethical questions to health professionals and staff, as well as to individuals in surrounding communities. It would include, for example, an in-service hospital workshop on "withdrawing life support" or a community program on "living wills." In the area of policy, ethics committees propose, analyze, and review institutional policies on ethically difficult issues. An example of policy work might be the development of a policy statement for an institution on DNR orders. The third function of ethics committees, case consultation, involves the discussion of patient care situations that have ethical dimensions. In this role, the committee reviews difficult patient cases and makes recommendations about possible alternative courses of action (see the following case study), or in the case of retrospective reviews, evaluates the already chosen course(s) of action. Because the case review role is closer to the action and is probably more rewarding than the education or policy roles, case review is often the role that ethics committees want to take on (Ross, Bagley, Michel, & Pugh, 1986).

The following case about Ms. B. illustrates the case consultation function of ethics committees. It highlights the important role committees play for providers.

Ms. B., a 75-year-old woman, was transferred from a nursing home to the hospital when she developed a urinary tract infection from an indwelling catheter placed to control incontinence. She was extremely weak in all four limbs due to multiple strokes that related to uncontrolled hypertension, poorly controlled diabetes, and cigarette addiction. She was unable to speak because of her brainstem infarctions and a permanent tracheostomy. Although she opened her eyes, she gave no consistent nonverbal responses to simple verbal or visual questions. A neurological consultant indicated that there was no chance that Ms. B.'s neurological function would improve.

There had been no prior contact between Ms. B. and her current caregivers, and they had no indication of her wishes concerning the use of life-sustaining treatment. The attending physician attempted to meet with her adult children, but they failed to keep several appointments. When they finally met, Ms. B.'s family was unable to supply information about her values and preferences concerning the use of life-sustaining treatment. Her children did consent to the insertion of a feeding gastrostomy to replace her nasogastric feeding tube, but they steadfastly refused to make their mother a DNR candidate. They stated that she was worth saving at all costs.

The attending physician and the primary care nurse told Ms. B.'s children that the former planned to consult with the hospital ethics committee to gain its support in writing a DNR order to override their wishes. To their surprise, the family did not resist, but agreed to an ethics committee consult. (*Hastings Center Report*, 1989, *19* (5), p. 24. Used with permission.)

Ethical Questions:

What is the role of the ethics committee in this situation?

What kind of communication should take place between the physician, family, and members of the ethics committee?

Principle-based Versus Case-based Approaches

Bioethics committees employ two major approaches to ethical decision making: the principle-based approach and the case-based approach. The *principle-based approach,* by far the most common in health care, is a deductive method of reaching a decision by applying ethical principles and rules (e.g., autonomy and beneficence) to a particular case. It attempts to find answers by confronting the dilemmas that emerge from opposing ethical positions. In the principle-based approach, universal principles act as a guide to the ethical duties of health professionals. Although widely employed, principle-based ethics has been challenged by some scholars for not being helpful in dealing with real human problems (Smith, 1991; Veatch, 1989).

The *case-based approach,* sometimes referred to as the casuistic method, has received increased attention in recent years although its history dates back to before Aristotle. Unlike the principle-based approach, which applies universal principles, the case-based approach begins with the case and moves outward toward principles. It places great emphasis on the details and particularities of each case (Murray, 1988), including, for example, questions such as: What is the nature of the illness? What are the patient's values? What are the concerns of family members? What are the preferences of the health providers? From these particulars, decisions are reached based on the degree to which a case compares or fails to compare in an analogous way to previous cases.

The case-based approach has several unique features (Jonsen, 1986). First, it draws from a series of established cases, moving from the clear and obvious to the more problematic. Second, it draws on both the consensus and divergent opinions of colleagues on model cases. Third, it expresses decisions on ethical issues with a degree of probability. A major strength of the case-based approach is that it is sensitive to the many complex facets of clinical cases (Fowler, 1989; Murray, 1987; Smith, 1991). However, there are some weaknesses to this approach. It has the potential to be used in self-serving ways (Murray, 1987) and it fails to use a theoretical basis for decision making (Arras, 1991).

Communication Within Ethics Committees

There is ample evidence that communication plays a central role in the work of ethics committees. In a review of the mission statements of nine ethics committees, Van Allen, Moldow, and Cranford (1989) found that committees saw their role as that of being a "forum" for the discussion of ethical dilemmas and concerns. Similarly, the California Medical Association (1983) has stated that the purpose of ethics committees is to "facilitate communication between concerned parties regarding treatment decisions, to assist in the decision-making process when ethical conflicts occur, and to retrospectively review decisions for the purpose of establishing guidelines." Likewise, in Minnesota, the ethics committee at one large hospital lists as its primary purpose to promote and facilitate communication and sharing of information so mutual understanding between health care providers and receivers is achieved. In a Hastings Center Report, Murray (1988) argues that 80 to 90 percent of the work of ethics committees revolves around clarifying facts and fostering communication. In essence, effective communication is an inseparable part of the workings of ethics committees.

How ethics committees function is influenced by the goals they are trying to achieve. As discussed in the chapter on group communication (Chap. 6), the goals of the group as well as the task versus process orientation of the group have a major influence on the inner workings of the group. Bayley and Cranford (1984, 1986) pointed out that ethics committees are unlike most typical hospital committees that have a strong task orientation. Ethics committees are required to deal with problems that are bound up in emotions and other issues that are not subject to scientific analysis. Their function to serve as a forum for communication on difficult issues emphasizes the process dimensions of communication.

Throughout this book we have seen that the way or the process that professionals use to talk about issues has an effect on the outcome of those issues. For example, if a committee member is discussing the necessity of a certain treatment for a patient with a family member, the way the professional talks about the treatment implies a great deal about the professional's ethics. If a professional takes a strong position for patient autonomy but does so in a paternalistic way, one has to question whether the professional strongly believes in patient autonomy. Similarly, if a professional argues strongly for patient participation in treatment decisions but insists on setting the agenda for patient–professional discussions about treatment, the strength of the professional's insistence on autonomy should be questioned.

In considering ethical questions in health care contexts, it is important for committees to be attuned to the complex nature of the communication process (see the following case study). Ethics committees deal with highly charged issues that have serious implications for the well-being of patients and family members. As a result, it is not uncommon for individual committee members to become very emotionally involved in the case being reviewed. Emotions run high, and this can sometimes make communication difficult. Furthermore, members often have different beliefs or values that can conflict with one another. To be effective members of the committee, individuals need to be willing to listen closely to others, to set aside their own positions and agendas, and to be open to others' viewpoints on difficult issues. Members also have to pay attention to "how" they communicate (the process), as well as to "what" (the content) they are communicating.

P̃aul, a 25-year-old single man, was admitted to the hospital after being seriously injured in a motorcycle accident. He was living with two roommates and working at an automotive plant just prior to the accident. Paul was an only child who had been rebellious as a teenager. Over the past several years, he had grown quite distant from his parents, who lived in a rural area about an hour away.

Paul had been riding his motorcycle without a helmet and had suffered multiple fractures as well as a severe head injury that left him in a deep coma. Paul's prognosis was poor and even if he did survive he would live in a persistent vegetative state for the rest of his life. Paul's parents were extremely distraught and maintained a constant vigil at their son's bedside.

The neurologist covering Paul's case requested a consult from members of the ethics team because the parents were having difficulty understanding medical information and accepting the patient's prognosis. In the conference with the family, issues of quality of life and benefit versus burden were raised in light of the grim prognosis. A follow-up conference was held 1 week later and again the parents were told of the grim prognosis. At this point, the parents appeared to understand the situation and they expressed their feelings that Paul would not want to live "this way," but they were unable to make the decision to remove the ventilator. The following day, an attending physician who was not at the family conference, met with the parents and encouraged them to permit their son to have a tracheostomy and gastrostomy. Although the parents agreed to these procedures, they were confused by the inconsistent recommendations that they were receiving from various health professionals. Paul's situation was again brought to the attention of the ethics committee for further discussion and recommendations.

....

Ethical Questions:

How does the communication of various health professionals affect the family in this case?

How could an ethics committee remedy this situation?

How would *case-based ethics* be used in dealing with this case?

Overall, ethics committees have had a positive impact on health care institutions. Although their specific role is still emerging, their legitimate position in health care is firmly established. Ethics committees have altered the moral climate of institutions by breaking down barriers to effective sharing of values among patients, physicians, nurses, other professionals, and society at large (Bayley & Cranford, 1986).

► SUMMARY

Biomedical ethics is one of the fastest growing areas of health care and an area in which communication plays a pivotal role. Ethics is concerned with applying principles of "right" and "wrong" to the complex problems that occur in a highly sophisticated health care system in which resources are sometimes scarce or limited.

The major dimensions of biomedical ethics include beneficence, autonomy, and justice. Beneficence refers to professionals' making health care choices that benefit patients and family members. When actions are taken on behalf of patients without determining whether patients indeed want help, those actions are described as paternalistic. Autonomy emphasizes self-determination for patients and underscores that individuals should be in charge of matters related to their own health. The principle of justice refers to fairness in health care, to giving each individual what he or she rightfully deserves, and to distributing society's resources equitably.

A cornerstone of bioethics is the legal doctrine of informed consent. It requires that health professionals communicate certain kinds and amounts of information to patients so that patients themselves can determine what, if anything, will be done to them. For consent to be truly informed, it is essential that patients comprehend the information they receive from health professionals. Effective interpersonal relationships will also facilitate patients' understanding and willingness to give consent. The opportunity to obtain full informed consent is enhanced when health professionals pay attention to who provides information to the patient, to the readability of consent forms, to the opportunity to allow patients to ask questions, and to the supplemental audiovisual and written materials that accompany consent information.

Honesty and truth telling refer to the honest disclosure of information to patients. Respect for autonomy requires that providers attend closely to patients' needs regarding the amount of information they want and how they want it expressed.

Bioethics committees provide the structure for discussing and making decisions about complex ethical dilemmas in health care. The primary functions of these committees are education, policy, and consultation. Bioethics committees do their work by applying principles to cases, the principle-based approach, or by starting with the case and comparing it to previous cases, the case-based approach. Overall, bioethics committees provide an effective forum for the discussion of difficult and often highly charged ethical dilemmas.

One thing is clear. In the future, humanistic health care will depend on patients, family members, and professionals who are able to communicate effectively with one another to promote the ethical distribution and delivery of health care resources.

▶ REFERENCES

Aroskar, M. A. (1989). Community health nurses: Their most significant ethical decision-making problems. *Nursing Clinics of North America, 24*(4), 967–975.

Aroskar, M. A. (1994). Ethical decision-making in patient care. *The American Nurse, 26,* March, 10.

Arras, J. D. (1991). Getting down to cases: The revival of casuistry in bioethics. *Journal of Medicine and Philosophy, 16*(1), 25–91.

Avins, A. L., & Lo, B. (1989). To tell or not to tell: The ethical dilemmas of HIV test notification in epidemiologic research. *American Journal of Public Health, 79*(121), 1544–1548.

Bayley, C., & Cranford, R. E. (1984). Techniques for committee self-education and institution-wide education. In R. E. Cranford, & A. E. Doudera (Eds.), *Institutional ethics committees and health care decision making* (pp. 149–156). Ann Arbor, MI: Health Administration Press.

Bayley, C., & Cranford, R. E. (1986). Ethics committees: What we have learned. In *Making choices: Ethics issues for health care professionals.* Chicago: American Hospital Publishing.

Beauchamp, T. L., & Childress, J. F. (1983). *Principles of biomedical ethics* (2nd ed.). New York: Oxford University Press.

Beauchamp, T. L., & Childress, J. F. (1994). *Principles of biomedical ethics* (4th ed.). New York: Oxford University Press.

California Medical Association. (1983). *Guidelines on hospital ethics committees.* San Francisco, CA: California Medical Association.

Callahan, D. (1995). Once again, reality: The lessons of the SUPPORT study. *Hastings Center Report, 25*(6), S33–S36.

Canterbury v. Spence, 464 F.2d 772 (1972).

Caplan, A. L. (1983). Can applied ethics be effective in health care and should it strive to be? *Ethics, 93,* 311–319.

Cassileth, B. R., Zupkis, R. V., Sutton-Smith, K., & March, V. (1980). Informed consent—Why are its goals imperfectly realized? *The New England Journal of Medicine, 302,* 896–900.

Childress, J. F. (1979). Paternalism and health care. In W. L. Robison & M. S. Pritchard (Eds.), *Medical responsibility* (pp. 15–27). Totowa, NJ: Humana.

Childress, J. F. (1990). The place of autonomy in bioethics. *Hastings Center Report, 20*(1), 12–47.

Cobbs v. Grant, 8 Cal.3d 229 (1972).

Cohen, C. B. (1988). Birth of a network. *Hastings Center Report, 18*(1), 11.

Cranford, R. E., & Doudera, A. E. (1984). *Institutional ethics committees and health care decision making.* Ann Arbor, MI: Health Administration Press.

Danis, M., & Churchill, L. R. (1991). Autonomy and the common weal. *Hastings Center Report, 21*(1), 25–31.

Fowler, M. D. M. (1989). Ethical decision making in clinical practice. *Nursing Clinics of North America, 24*(4), 955–965.

Garrett, T., Baillie, H., & Garrett, R. (1989). *Health care ethics.* Englewood Cliffs, NJ: Prentice-Hall.

Goodwin, G. L. (1984). *Ethics in medicine.* Unpublished manuscript, College of St. Scholastica, Duluth, MN.

Hastings Center. (1989). Committee consultation to override family wishes. *Hastings Center Report, 19*(5), p. 24.

High, D. M. (1989). Truth telling, confidentiality, and the dying patient: New dilemmas for the nurse. *Nursing Forum, 24*(1), 5–10.

Infant Doe, No. GU 8204–00 (Cir. Ct. Monroe County, Ind., April 12, 1982).

Jaksa, J. A., & Pritchard, M. S. (1988). *Communication ethics: Methods of analysis.* Belmont, CA: Wadsworth.

Jonsen, A. R. (1986). Casuistry and clinical ethics. *Theoretical Medicine, 7,* 65–74.

Jonsen, A. R., Siegler, M., & Winslade, W. (1986). *Clinical ethics* (2nd ed.). New York: Macmillan.

Katz, J. (1984). *The silent world of doctor and patient.* New York: Macmillan.

Kennedy, B. J., & Lillehaugen, A. (1979). Patient recall of informed consent. *Medical and Pediatric Oncology, 7,* 173–178.

Kuczewski, M. G. (1996). Reconceiving the family: The process of consent in medical decision making. *Hastings Center Report, 26*(2), 30–37.

Lawson, D. L., & Adamson, H. M. (1995). Informed consent readability: Subject understanding of 15 common consent form phrases. *IRB, 17*(5–6), 16–19.

Mitchell v. Robinson, 334 S.W.2d 11 (Mo., 1960).

Murray, T. H. (1987). Medical ethics, moral philosophy and moral tradition. *Social Science and Medicine, 25*(6), 637–644.

Murray, T. H. (1988). Where are the ethics in ethics committees? *Hastings Center Report, 18*(1), 12–13.

Natanson v. Kline, 187 Kan. 186 (1960).

O'Connor, R. J. (1981). Informed consent: Legal, behavioral, and educational issues. *Patient Counselling and Health Education, 3*(2), 49–56.

O'Connor, K. F. (1996). Ethical/moral experiences of oncology nurses. *Oncology Nursing Forum, 23*(5), 787–794.

Oken, D. (1961). What to tell cancer patients. *Journal of the American Medical Association, 175,* 1120–1128.

Orem, D. E. (1995). *Nursing: Concepts of practice* (5th ed.). St. Louis: Mosby.

Penman, D. R., Holland, J. C., Bahna, G. F., Morrow, G., Schmale, A. H., Derogatis, L. R., Carnrike, C. L., Jr., & Cherry, R. (1984). Informed consent for investigational chemotherapy: Patients' and physicians' perceptions. *Journal of Clinical Oncology, 2*(7), 849–855.

President's Commission for the Study of Ethical Problems in Medicine and Biomedical and Behavioral Research. (1983). *Deciding to forego life-sustaining treatment: Ethical, medical and legal issues in treatment decisions.* Washington, DC: U.S. Government Printing Office.

Quinlan, 355 A.2d 647 (N.J. 1976).

Ratzan, R. M. (1981). The experiment that wasn't: A case report in clinical geriatric research. *The Gerontologist, 21*(3), 297–302.

Ross, J. W., Bayley, C., Michel, V., & Pugh, D. (1986). *Handbook for hospital ethics committees.* Chicago: American Hospital Publishing.

Schloendorff v. Society of New York Hospitals, 211 N.Y. 125 (1914).

Shatz, D. (1986). Autonomy, beneficence, and informed consent: Rethinking the connections. I. *Cancer Investigation, 4*(3), 257–269.

Sherry, D. (1990). Autonomy versus beneficence: The dilemma and its implications in home care. *Home Healthcare Nurse, 8*(6), 13–15.

Silva, M. C., & Sorrell, J. M. (1984). Factors influencing comprehension of information for informed consent: Ethical implications for nursing research. *International Journal of Nursing Studies, 21*(4), 233–240.

Smith, D. H. (1991). Stories, values, and patient care decisions. In C. Conrad (Ed.), *The ethical nexus: Values in organizational decision making.* Norwood, NJ: Ablex.

Teel, K. (1975). The physician's dilemma—A doctor's view: What the law should be. *Baylor Law Review, 27,* 6, 9.

Thomasma, D. C. (1983). Beyond medical paternalism and patient autonomy: A model of physician conscience for the physician–patient relationship. *Annals of Internal Medicine, 98,* 243–248.

Van Allen, E., Moldow, D. G., & Cranford, R. (1989). Evaluating ethics committees. *Hastings Center Report, 19*(5), 12–13.

Veatch, R. M. (1989). *Medical ethics.* Boston: Jones and Bartlett.

Veatch, R. M. (1995). Abandoning informed consent. *Hastings Center Report, 25*(2), 5–12.

Weber v. Stony Brook Hospital, 52 U.S.L.W. 2267 (N.Y., October 28, 1983).

Wilkinson v. Vesey, 295 A.2d 676 (1972).

Winters, G., Glass, E., & Sakurai, C. (1993). Ethical issues in oncology nursing practice: An overview of topics and strategies. *Oncology Nursing Forum, 20*(10), 21–34.

Intercultural Communication 9
and Health Care

In the last two decades, cultural sensitivity has been a growing concern for organizations. According to Porter and Samovar (1997), intercultural communication demands attention for several reasons. For example, advanced transportation systems have given us easy access to all parts of the globe. New communication technologies, such as the World Wide Web, allow us to communicate instantaneously with other people throughout the world. The U.S. economy is rapidly becoming a global economy, and we are becoming interdependent with other countries. Immigration patterns are changing and bringing more people with diverse backgrounds into the United States. For these reasons, people today, more than ever, are coming into contact with people from cultures different than their own. These changes have led organizations to place more emphasis on cultural sensitivity and cultural awareness for their employees.

Culture plays a significant role in the communication that occurs in health care settings (Geist, 1997; Kavanagh & Kennedy, 1992; Kreps & Kunimoto, 1994; Leininger, 1990). It has a major impact on the communication in provider–patient, provider–provider, and provider–family member relationships. As a result, it is a factor that affects everyone in health care.

We are devoting an entire chapter to intercultural communication because cultural diversity has become one of the most salient and urgent concerns of today's health organizations. Cultural diversity plays an integral role in the three major components—relationships, transactions, and contexts—of the health communication model we discussed in Chapter 1. For these reasons, health professionals need to make intercultural communication more effective.

Keeping in mind the models of communication discussed in Chapter 1, this chapter will discuss various ways in which culture influences health communication. We begin by providing a definition of intercultural communication and then discuss two closely related concepts: ethnocentrism and prejudice. Next, we describe how cultures vary in regard to whether they are individualistic versus collectivist, and in how they use contexts to interpret messages. We also briefly review some of the research in three broad areas of intercultural communication: perception, verbal communication, and nonverbal communication. In the final section of the chapter, we discuss strategies that can be used by health professionals to improve intercultural communication.

► INTERCULTURAL COMMUNICATION DEFINED

Anthropologists, sociologists, and many others have debated about the meaning of the word *culture*. Because it is an abstract term, it is hard to define and it is often defined in different ways by different people. For our purposes, we will define culture as the learned beliefs, attitudes, values, rules, norms, and behaviors that are common to a group of people. Culture is dynamic and transmitted to others. In short, culture is the way of life, customs, and script of a group of people (Gudykunst & Ting-Toomey, 1988).

Related to culture are the terms *multicultural* and *diversity*. Multicultural refers to the existence of multiple cultures such as African-American, Arab, Asian, European-American, Native American, and others. Multicultural can also refer to a set of subcultures defined by race, gender, ethnicity, sexual orientation, and age. Diversity refers to the existence of different cultures or ethnicities within a group or organization. Health organizations have a wide range of diversity among the physicians, nurses, administrators, and staff within each organization, but each also serves patient populations that are also highly diverse. Throughout this chapter we will be addressing issues related to multiculturalism and its effect on health communication.

We have chosen to frame our discussions in this chapter around the process of intercultural communication—in other words, communication between people of different cultures. In Chapter 1, we defined communication as "the process of sharing information using a set of common rules." In this chapter we are concerned with how individuals from different cultures share information with one another. It becomes readily apparent that "using a set of common rules" is a major challenge for individuals of diverse cultures. This chapter deals with how people who come from different cultures with different rules can still share information, find meaning, and obtain high-quality health care.

► RELATED CONCEPTS

Before beginning our discussion of the various facets of intercultural communication, this section describes two human tendencies that are closely related to intercultural communication: ethnocentrism and prejudice.

Ethnocentrism

As the word suggests, *ethnocentrism* is the tendency for individuals to place their own group (ethnic, racial, or cultural) at the center of their observations of others and the world. People tend to give priority and value to their own beliefs, attitudes, and values, over and above those of other groups. Ethnocentrism is a universal tendency and each one of us is ethnocentric to some degree.

Ethnocentrism is like a perceptual window through which individuals from one culture make subjective or critical evaluations of people from another culture (Porter & Samovar, 1997). For example, an Asian man recalled the embarrassment he was made to feel when he wanted to eat with chopsticks in the hospital (Chrisman, 1991). Although this was a normal eating utensil for him, it was not the standard utensil used in the white middle class hospital where he was a patient. Ethnocentrism accounts for why we tend to think our own cultural values and ways of doing things are "right" and "natural" (Gudykunst & Kim, 1997).

On the other hand, ethnocentrism is a major obstacle to effective intercultural communication because it prevents people from fully understanding the world of others. For example, if one person's culture values individual autonomy, it may be difficult for that person to understand another individual whose culture emphasizes community values over individualism. Similarly, if one person believes strongly in the biomedical model, he or she may find it difficult to understand an individual who places his or her faith in folk-healing methods. The more ethnocentric we are, the less open or tolerant we are of other people's cultural traditions or practices. An example of ethnocentrism is illustrated in the case below.

F atma, a 65-year-old Arab woman, developed chest pain while visiting her relatives in the United States. When she arrived at the hospital, she was wearing a traditional Arab dress and had her head covered with a scarf. She was accompanied by several family members.

After being seen in the emergency room, she was admitted to the cardiac unit and scheduled for immediate cardiac surgery.

While on the unit, a young male electrocardiogram (ECG) technician entered her room to do a preoperative ECG. After introducing himself, he explained what he needed to do and why the physician wanted it done immediately. Then, the technician asked Fatma to open her gown so he could attach the leads for the ECG. At this point, one of the family members in the room, strongly objected to her disrobing in front of the technician and demanded a female technician. Aware of the urgency of the test, the technician left the room feeling very frustrated without conducting the test.

As he walked down the hall, he felt angry that he had let a third party get in the way of his work. He also wondered why this older woman would not want a procedure that was so important in this situation.

As this example illustrates, the technician had his own ethnocentric viewpoint and was unable to understand why Fatma's family requested a female technician or why Fatma placed so much importance on her privacy. Ethnocentrism hits at the core of the nature of communication—the more ethnocentric we are, the less we are able to empathize, share information, and understand others from different cultures.

Prejudice

Closely related to ethnocentrism is prejudice. *Prejudice* refers to making a judgment about others based on previous decisions or experiences. It is a relatively fixed attitude, belief, or emotion held by an individual about another individual or group which is based on faulty or unsubstantiated data. Prejudice involves inflexible generalizations that are resistant to contrary evidence or change (Ponterotto & Pedersen, 1993). Prejudice is often thought of in the context of race (e.g., European-American versus African-American) but it also applies in areas such as sexism, ageism, homophobia, and other independent prejudices. Although prejudice can be positive (e.g., thinking positively about another culture without sufficient evidence), it is usually negative.

As with ethnocentrism, we all hold prejudices, to some degree. Sometimes, our prejudices allow us to keep our partially fixed attitudes undisturbed and constant. In addition, prejudice can reduce our anxiety because it gives us a familiar way to structure our observations of others. One of the main problems with prejudice is that it is self-oriented rather than other-oriented. It helps us achieve balance for our selves at the expense of others. Moreover, attitudes of prejudice inhibit understanding by creating a screen that filters and limits our ability to see multiple aspects and qualities of other individuals, as indicated in the following case study.

A social worker was entering information on a patient's chart on one of the nursing units when she overheard the staff discussing a patient who was recently admitted to the unit.

The nursing staff was not certain if the patient was Chinese, Taiwanese, or Vietnamese. The nurse manager called the supervisor of International Services, who helped clarify that the patient was Taiwanese, and needed a Taiwanese interpreter.

As the staff continued to discuss the patient, one staff member said, "So she doesn't speak any English at all? How does she get along in this country if she can't speak English?" Another staff member responded, "She doesn't need to get along here. They are all on welfare" (Walker, 1996).

As this example illustrates, prejudice often shows itself in crude or demeaning comments that people make about others. Both ethnocentrism and prejudice interfere with our ability to understand and appreciate the human experience of others.

▶ TWO MAJOR CHARACTERISTICS OF CULTURES

Of the many factors that have been set forth to explain intercultural communication, *individual* versus *collective* values and *context* are two of the most common. Researchers have found that each of these can be used to explain how cultures differ from one another, and how communication is changed by these differences. In this section we will discuss how each of these variables plays a role in intercultural communication.

Individualism versus Collectivism

One of the primary characteristics of cultures is the degree to which they are focused on the individual or on the group. Individualistic cultures, as the name implies, are centered on the individual and the individual's interests, needs, and values (Figure 9–1). They place the individual's good above the collective good or the good of the community, and value individual goals over group goals. For example, in the U.S. health care system, the ability of

Individualistic Cultures	Collectivistic Cultures
• Focus on the individual • Emphasize individual needs • Stress autonomy in health care decision making • Examples: United States, Canada, and Western European countries	• Focus on the group • Emphasize group harmony • Stress consensus in health care decision making • Examples: Japan, Pakistan, Thailand, and South American countries

Figure 9–1. Comparison between individualistic and collectivistic cultures.

individuals to make autonomous decisions about their treatment is highly supported and promoted. Individualism stresses that people are supposed to take care of themselves and their immediate families, paying less attention to the larger community or society as a whole (Gudykunst & Kim, 1997). North American countries, such as the United States and Canada, and Western European countries such as the Netherlands, Italy, and Belgium are examples of cultures that are considered highly individualistic.

On a continuum, collectivistic cultures are on the opposite end of the continuum from individualistic cultures. In collectivistic cultures the interests of community are paramount. Individuals attend to their own needs and aspirations only after first attending to the concerns of the group (Gudykunst & Ting-Toomey, 1988). In collectivistic cultures, the social norms of the group supersede individual pleasure; group cooperation is more important than individual initiative (Triandis, 1986). For example, in the area of health care, Japanese value the welfare of the *group* and emphasize consensus decision making, which takes into account the impact of treatment decisions on those close to the ill person (Kagawa-Singer, 1996). Collectivistic cultures value harmony and cooperation before individual self-realization. Examples of collectivistic cultures include Asian countries, such as Japan, Pakistan, and Thailand, and South American countries such as Colombia and Chile.

Several implications can be drawn about intercultural communication based on the culture's individualism–collectivism characteristics. Collectivistic cultures promote communication that is consistent with the norms of the group. The communication rules within the group (both implicit and explicit) are followed more closely by people from collectivistic cultures. More attention is given to appropriate ways to talk to one another as well as ways to address authority.

On a nonverbal level, intercultural differences are also apparent. Andersen (1997) lists several differences drawn from the research literature. For example, people in collectivistic cultures tend to carefully regulate their nonverbal displays. They tend to show emotions that facilitate group cohesiveness and harmony more than people do in individualistic cultures. They also try to make sure their nonverbal communication is appropriate to status hierarchies. In response to conflict, people from collectivistic cultures frequently use avoidance strategies and face-saving displays. Overall, nonverbal communication is directed more toward group solidarity in collectivistic cultures but toward spontaneity and independence in individualistic cultures.

The following case illustrates in a vivid way how collectivistic characteristics of a culture can affect health outcomes. In the example, the woman receiving care is Hmong. The Hmong, originally from Southern China, have lived primarily in the high country of northern Laos for several generations. The two largest groupings of Hmong in the United States are found in St. Paul, Minnesota, and Sacramento, California.

A 35-year-old Hmong woman is admitted to the hospital with severe lower abdominal pain. Her evaluation reveals that she has an ectopic pregnancy. She rapidly becomes unstable with intra-abdominal bleeding, and the recommendation is made for her to undergo emergency surgery.

Before surgery, she will need a central line and possibly intubation. The entire extended family, 25 individuals, gathers in the waiting room of the intensive care unit. The senior male member of her family states that he will not give permission for surgery unless the surgeon can guarantee two results: (1) that she live through the surgery, and (2) that she remain fertile after the surgery.

In the meantime, the patient becomes more unstable. The surgeon, growing frustrated, proceeds with intubating the patient, placing a central line and taking her to emergency surgery. The patient recovers well medically.

Subsequently it is determined that the patient is infertile. Her husband, angry over her infertility, seeks a divorce and takes custody of the children. She is left alone in the United States with no relatives and no financial support. Without an extended family support system, she feels depressed and of little value (Walker, 1996).

This case points out the importance of collectivism in certain cultures. It also underscores how certain "correct" medical decisions can result in far-reaching negative outcomes for patients and their families. Health professionals need to be sensitive to the issue of individualism or collectivism and its impact health care outcomes.

Context

A second major characteristic of cultures is found in the way they use contexts in interpreting messages. Cultures can be placed on a continuum from high to low, based on the extent to which they use contexts in communication (Hall, 1976). High-context cultures interpret messages based on a broad set of culturally based rules, which reside within the individual and the environment (Fig. 9–2). Low-context cultures, on the other hand, do the reverse; they rely primarily on the specific content of messages and pay far less attention to the culturally based contextual rules. On a continuum from high to low context, cultures such as Japanese, Arab, Greek, and Spanish are considered high-context cultures, and Swiss, German, Scandinavian, and American cultures are considered low-context cultures.

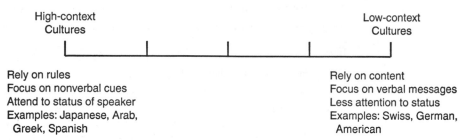

Figure 9–2. Comparison between low-context and high-context cultures.

Hall (1976) has suggested that people use contexts to help them manage the demands associated with complex information and information overload. To give structure to incoming information, people engage in "contexting," the process of responding to information based on a set of preprogrammed rules. For example, in Asian cultures there are often norms that suggest that passive acceptance or acquiesence is an appropriate response to conflict. Thus, in an interpersonal dispute it is likely that an Asian participant would respond with accommodation. In other words, the norms of the culture give the individual a way to structure his or her response to the conflict.

Another way of thinking about context is in regard to rules. In high-context cultures, there are many rules for communication and in low-context cultures there are few rules. For example, in high-context cultures respect for the status of the speaker is clearly established, whereas in low-context cultures this may not be the case. Furthermore, a high-context culture may have many established nonverbal rules whereas a low-context culture may have fewer nonverbal rules. The point is that high-context cultures have a "map" that resides either within the individual or the environment; this map gives the person some direction on how to interpret the meaning of messages. Low-context cultures, on the other hand, are less dependent on a map. For people in low-context cultures, meaning emerges solely from the content of the message.

An example of differences between high- and low-context cultures is illustrated in the following example from Gervais (1996). She advocates that providers from Western cultures show respect and be sensitive to the viewpoint of patients from non-Western cultures. For example, Gervais points out that some Asian ethnic groups believe that bad news given by an authority figure can have the impact of a curse. She suggests, "rather than saying, 'your son is dying,' physicians should use less direct phrases like, 'Your family will have a difficult time in the next week or so'" (p. 50). This example, in addition to recognizing the role of authority and family in high-context cultures, highlights an approach to framing messages in less direct ways for patients from certain non-Western cultures. Although this recommendation may be in conflict with our Western cultural values (e.g., autonomy and truth-telling), it underscores the critical role of context in provider–patient communication.

Context has several implications for intercultural communication (Porter & Samovar, 1997), particularly in health care situations. First, people in high-context cultures are better at reading nonverbal and environmental cues than people in low-context cultures. They may attend more closely to the nonverbal behavior exhibited by professionals. Second, people in high-context cultures do not speak as much as those in low-context cultures because they expect others to be able to understand the unstated rules, just as they do. In health care situations, professionals may need to spend more time clarifying or validating such clients' beliefs to avoid misunderstandings. Third, in low-context cultures verbal messages are very important because people in these cultures do not receive as much information from the environment. Obviously, patient teaching modules, written pamphlets, and other sources of information may be perceived as very valuable by patients from low-context cultures. Lastly, people from low-context cultures are seen by people from high-context cultures as less attractive, perhaps because people from low-context cultures more frequently violate the rules of people from high-context cultures. There are no "hard and fast" rules of how to incorporate context into health care practice; rather, it is another characteristic of cultures which, if understood, can inform health professionals and enhance their understanding of intercultural communication.

▶ ELEMENTS IN INTERCULTURAL COMMUNICATION

Three elements of intercultural communication are discussed in this section: perception, verbal communication, and nonverbal communication. Culture influences each of these elements and ultimately the quality of the interpersonal communication that occurs in health care relationships. In cross-cultural settings, patients and providers often hold different ideas about the meaning of illness and how an illness may affect a person's life (Huttlinger et al., 1992).

Perception

There is a growing body of research that suggests that our sociocultural background can have a profound influence on how we perceive symptoms, explain the cause of illnesses, and determine what type of treatment is needed. For example, Hubbell and colleagues (1996) found that the beliefs about breast cancer held by Latinas and Anglo women were very different. Latinas were more likely than Anglo women to believe that breast cancer was caused by trauma to the breast or breast fondling than by the "medically accepted" risk factors, such as a family history of breast cancer. The particular beliefs held by Latina women about breast cancer seemed to correspond more closely to a moral interpretation of the illness (punishment for improper behavior) than to a biomedical interpretation of illness.

Another example of how culture is a factor during illness can be seen in some of the research findings on how African-American women view breast cancer. In a study of African-American women's perceptions of mammography and breast cancer, Price and colleagues (1992) found that the majority of women did not perceive breast cancer to be a severe disease, in part because of their strong religious beliefs that God would take care of them. Long (1993) contends that African-Americans have a great tolerance for symptoms and are more likely to assume responsibility for their illness and recovery than to seek out medical "experts" for help. In addition, Long contends that African-Americans from lower socioeconomic backgrounds tend not to legitimize illness because they perceive a greater necessity to provide for their families first.

In a qualitative study of Native Americans with diabetes, Huttlinger and colleagues (1992) found that the traditional biomedical view of diabetes had little meaning for Native Americans. They believe that mind, body, and soul are in harmony or balance, and that when this balance is disrupted, illness occurs. The researchers found that Native Americans viewed diabetes as a "white man's" disease that came upon them in recent years as they became more assimilated into mainstream American culture and lifestyles. For Native Americans, the proper treatment for diabetes depended on using both their traditional medicines as well as "Anglo" medicines. However, for some Native Americans who viewed diabetes as an "Anglo" disease, the proper treatment was only "Anglo" medicines (Huttlinger et al., 1992).

These studies illustrate how perceptions of illness can vary across cultures. It is important to understand patients' perceptions of the origins of their illnesses because they can influence how receptive patients are to various treatments. Patients from one culture may be labeled "noncompliant" by a health professional from another culture, when in fact the patient and professional have different views about the cause of an illness and the treatment needed for it. The following case study illustrates how differing beliefs about illness between a patient and a health care professional can have a pronounced impact on treatment and recovery.

J im Eagle was a 22-year-old Native American man who lived in a rural area on the outskirts of a large urban city in the Southwest. He was employed as a construction worker but his behavior started to become increasingly erratic and he said that he was hearing voices. Jim's family thought that an evil spirit was affecting Jim and wanted to take him to a shaman or spiritual healer in New Mexico for treatment. Jim's boss told the family to get him psychiatric help or he would be fired from his job.

With much hesitancy, Jim's family had him admitted to a psychiatric unit at a university hospital where he was placed on a locked unit. Jim was diagnosed as schizophrenic and placed on Thorazine to manage his psychotic symptoms. He also received one-to-one therapy from a psychiatrist, but was not able to develop rapport with him. Jim frequently appeared dazed during their sessions, would not talk, often walked out before the time was up, and was considered "uncooperative."

Jim's family became more and more worried about him. He was not getting any better, looked "drugged" from the medication, and frequently tried to get off the unit. Although the family members tried to talk with the psychiatrist about their concerns about the medication and their beliefs about an evil spirit, the psychiatrist minimized their concerns and stated that Jim was schizophrenic and the treatment of choice was Thorazine. After another week with no change in Jim's condition, his family signed him out against medical advice (AMA) and took him to a shaman out of state. A social worker who followed up on Jim's case a few weeks later found out that Jim was still in New Mexico but doing much better and no longer hearing voices.

As illustrated in this case study, the family and psychiatrist were operating from different beliefs or perceptions about Jim's illness. They were unable to understand one another's differing views about the cause or the treatment; as a result the family stopped treatment and removed Jim from the setting. This example underscores the importance of acknowledging different frames of reference, and the importance of attempting to form an alliance to achieve a common goal of helping the client recover.

Verbal Communication

A second element of intercultural communication that is affected substantially by culture is the words, language, and verbal processes that we use to share information. As the cultural distance between the patient and provider increases, there is a greater likelihood of communication problems (Pachter, 1994).

One of the more obvious communication problems occurs when two people do not share a common language (Fig. 9–3). Even when an interpreter is used, words from one language often cannot be translated into another language with the exact same meaning. Language barriers are espe-

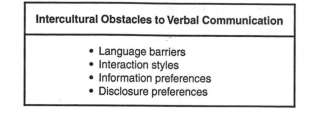

Figure 9–3. Obstacles that inhibit effective intercultural communication.

cially problematic in health care situations for a number of reasons (Trill & Holland, 1993). First, being ill is often a frightening experience under any circumstance. However, being ill and unable to communicate fears and needs or to understand the language of the provider is especially traumatic. Second, a language barrier makes it difficult for patients to communicate their symptoms and for health professionals to make accurate assessments. Third, without a common language, a free exchange of questions and answers between patient and provider is blocked, and this can ultimately impair the effectiveness of a therapeutic relationship.

The communication problems associated with language barriers were evident in an ethographic study conducted by Herselman (1996) with white physicians and black patients in South Africa. The physicians spoke primarily English and Afrikaans, the dominant language of the whites in that particular region. The patients spoke primarily isiXhosa, the traditional language of the blacks located in that region. Although some of the patients spoke English and Afrikaans, only one physician spoke isiXhosa. Even with the help of an interpreter, physicians and patients did not have a common language to use to communicate freely. For example, patients tried to communicate symptoms that were not understood by physicians. Subtle differences in the meanings of symptoms lead to misunderstandings and misdiagnoses. In a number of instances, patients were given diagnoses they did not understand, which were explained in unfamilar medical terminology. Furthermore, because physicans did not understand the language, they did not understand the beliefs of the people, or would only acknowledge beliefs as "interesting" ideas, but would not incorporate the patients' beliefs into clinical care. The research by Herselman points out how important a common language is in order to share information and provide high-quality care.

Even when two cultural groups can communicate in the same language, such as English, their cultural background can influence the *manner* in which they communicate. For example, Native Americans often begin discussions with others by giving a lengthy discussion of family lineage and clan or by telling lengthy stories. They consider it rude to rush into discussions of their business or health problems (Huttlinger et al., 1992). Anglo practitioners, on the other hand, often neglect this formality and hustle the communication process, which is frustrating to the Native Americans.

In addition to stories, Native Americans often use metaphors as a means of communicating. Huttlinger and associates found that metaphorical images about battles (e.g., "battling the disease") and wars (e.g., "winning the war against the disease") were often used by Native Americans to describe how they managed their illnesses. According to Huttlinger and others, health professionals need to understand the communication patterns used by patients and, where possible, incorporate these communication patterns into treatment. For example, they suggest that patients' metaphors be incorporated into teaching plans (e.g., take the medication as a "weapon" to fight the disease), in order to make the information more relevant to the patients. It is also important to allow time for patients to "tell their stories" whenever possible as a way to establish rapport and understanding between patients and providers.

Another area of verbal communication, affected by culture, is comfort with asking questions. Although people from some cultural backgrounds, such as European-Americans, often feel comfortable asking questions and actively seeking out information, people from other cultures may be more hesitant and not directly question health professionals—even when they do not understand the information they have been given. Among Mexican-Americans, for example, *respecto* (respect) is a very important component of communication. Mexican-American culture encourages the use of diplomacy and discourages confrontation in conversations with others (Burk, Wieser, & Keegan, 1995). As a result, Mexican-American clients may be hesitant to question health care providers or disagree with treatment plans.

A hesitance to ask questions has also been reported in other research studies. Among Native Americans, Huttlinger and co-workers (1992) found that it was rude to question professionals because they were considered the "experts." Among South African patients, Herselman (1996) noted that some patients, who initially appeared disinterested in wanting information, were actually hesitant to ask questions. As a result, communication between physicians and patients became one-sided, with the physician dominating the interaction and receiving little verbal feedback from the patients. Given that some patients may hesitate to ask questions or seek clarification, the provider needs to assess more closely patients' understanding of information and treatment plans.

Within the area of verbal communication, different subcultures may use different dialects or verbal expressions. According to Giger and Davidhizar (1990), the dialect spoken by some African-Americans, with its unique pronounciation, grammar, and syntax, is significant enough to be considered "Black English." Although the extent to which Black English is used depends on many factors such as geographical location, education, and socioeconomic status, it plays a role in ethnic identity. Black English is characterized by a tendency to change the pronounciation of certain words such as *th*'s in "these" and "them" to a *d* sound such as "des" or "dem" or to drop the *g* sound from such words as laughing so they sound like "laughin." According to Giger and Davidhizar, it is important for health professionals not to regard Black English as substandard or ungrammatical. In addition, they caution health professionals not to mimic the person using Black English because it can be seen as ridiculing their mode of expression. Rather, health professionals need to develop a sensitivity to the dialect variations that exist among people from different cultural backgrounds. It is essential that health professionals and patients understand each other for the sake of good health outcomes.

A final area in which verbal communication can be affected by culture is in the preferences for disclosure of information. Researchers studied the information preferences of 800 American senior citizens in California who were of Korean, Mexican, European, and African descent and found differences in the extent to which they wanted information about a fatal illness or the likelihood they would die (Blackhall et al., 1995). Only 35 percent of the Korean-Americans and 48 percent of the Mexican-Americans believed that patients should be told they were going to die, in contrast to 63 percent of the African-Americans and 69 percent of the European-Americans. Also, in contrast to the latter two groups, Korean-Americans and Mexican-Americans (who are generally more collectivistic) were more likely to believe that family members, in addition to the patient, should be very involved in making medical decisions. This study underscores how culture influences preferences for information and the extent to which family members are viewed as key participants in health care decisions.

Nonverbal Communication

Nonverbal communication is the third element of intercultural communication. Our interpretation of nonverbal cues is greatly affected by how we interpret or decode nonverbal messages. There is a greater likelihood that we will misinterpret nonverbal cues in cross-cultural interactions because of the different encoding and decoding rules each person uses (Lee et al., 1992). Furthermore, for some nonverbal behaviors, such as facial expression, culturally based "display rules" may be operating that influence how or what emotions are expressed in social situations. For example, in one study both American and Japanese participants showed nonverbal disgust when viewing a negative situation (which was set up as a part of the study). However, when a higher-status individual was present in the experimental situation, the Japanese participants altered their expressions to smiles whereas the Americans continued to display disgust (Ekman, 1972; Friesen, 1972). Apparently, the Japanese participants changed their expression in the latter situation because of a culturally based display rule that says, in the presence of higher-status individuals, negative emotions should be masked (Lee et al., 1992).

One particularly important area of nonverbal behavior associated with culture is in the area of expressing pain. Culture influences the experience and *expression* of pain. Some ethnic groups have been described as more likely to show their pain by grimacing and crying, whereas other cultural groups are more likely to hide their pain (Trill & Holland, 1993). The cultural diversity apparent in the expression of pain has been associated with role modeling in early pain experiences, which influences and shapes response to pain in later years (Trill & Holland, 1993).

Villarruel (1995) conducted a qualitative study to gain a better understanding of the meaning and expression of pain among Mexican-Americans. Among the participants there was a strong expectation that pain be hidden and stoically endured, as one of the respondents indicated:

....

. . . when my family used to come to the hospital . . . I would be thinking, I hurt, but I wouldn't ask the nurse for anything. . . . I would say everything was all right . . . because I didn't want them to worry. (p. 432)

....

Accepted expressions of pain among the Mexican-Americans included withdrawing from others, going to bed, and changing one's activity or demeanor. A person was considered to be in pain, not by what he or she said, but by what was *not* said, or by the attempts the person used to hide the pain. Crying, complaining, or not carrying out one's usual responsibilities were considered signs of weakness and were likely to be ridiculed and scorned by others. The ability to endure pain was viewed as a strength among the Mexican-Americans, in part, because bearing pain was a cultural expectation and in part, because it would protect family members from additional worry and burden.

One of the challenges facing health professionals is how to help people from different cultures obtain adequate pain relief when they often hide their pain from others. This is especially relevant for Hispanic patients in light of reports that they are much less likely to receive pain medications than non-Hispanic patients with the same medical problem (Todd, Samavod, & Hoffman, 1993). Villarruel (1995) cautions health professionals not to equate the absence of pain behaviors with the absence of pain. Rather, she encourages professionals to find ways to administer pain relief measures, while at the same time helping the patient maintain personal integrity. For example, emphasizing the value of analgesics in "quicker recovery, the performance of responsibilities, and as a means to keep strong" (p. 433) may be more acceptable to Mexican-American patients than focusing solely on pain relief. The overriding issue is to attempt to provide care in a way that is sensitive to the beliefs and values of the particular cultural group.

Perceptions, verbal communication, and nonverbal communication all are influenced by culture and are key elements in intercultural communication. We have presented research that has attempted to look at cultural influences in each of these areas. In the next section, we will discuss general guidelines for communicating in multicultural situations.

▶ WAYS TO PROMOTE EFFECTIVE INTERCULTURAL COMMUNICATION

Although there are many ways to promote effective intercultural communication, we have identified three general approaches that we believe are essential: (1) recognizing the transactional influence of culture on interpersonal relations, (2) fostering culturally sensitive care, and (3) enlisting culturally based resources to supplement existing resources. Each of these approaches will be addressed in this section.

Transactional Influence of Culture on Interpersonal Relations

Separate clinical realities and individual cultural beliefs influence the interactions that occur between providers and patients in health care settings. According to DeSantis (1994), there are three cultural influences that operate in each interaction: the beliefs, values, and worldview of the health professional; the beliefs, values, and worldview of the patient; and the context in which the provider–patient interaction takes place (e.g., hospital, clinic, or community setting). From a transactional perspective, health professionals respond to patients on the basis of their own perceptions of clinical reality and their expectations of patients, while at the same time, patients respond to professionals on the basis of their beliefs and their expectations of health professionals. Furthermore, their interactions are influenced by the cultural norms (e.g., active patient participation or passive compliance) that operate within the various health care settings.

Transactions between individuals in health care are influenced strongly by the participants' cultural or ethnocentric viewpoints. The term "dual ethnocentrism" has been used to describe the different cultural orientations that may exist between providers and patients (DeSantis, 1994). It recognizes that each person brings his or her unique perspective to the clinical encounter and that no one operates from a blank slate. As health professionals acknowledge their own values and beliefs and become more consciously aware of them, they are in a better position of determining where cultural conflicts may occur with clients. They are also more likely to see their views of health and health practices as only *one* perspective (not necessarily the "right" perspective) among a number of possible perspectives on a particular health issue.

Given the different perspectives that are likely to occur in health encounters, health professionals need to develop skills that will enable them to negotiate and work through differing points of view. This skill has been labelled "cultural brokerage" (Tripp-Reimer & Brink, 1985) and refers to the ability to link, bridge, and negotiate between the typically more standard biomedical perspective of the health care provider and the cultural orientation of patients.

Cultural brokerage is essentially a process whereby professionals continually attempt to clarify their own as well as patients' perspectives. In this process, the professional tries initially to understand the patient's view of the health problem, compares the patient's view with his or her own view, and then tries to establish a working alliance with the patient, bridging the differences that may exist. Obviously, the closer the professional's and patient's perspective on the health problem, the more likely and the more rapidly they will be able to establish a common understanding about the health problem and a plan of treatment. Likewise, the greater the disparity in their views, the more negotiating and reclarification will be needed (Tripp-Reimer & Brink, 1985). The process of understanding, clarifying, and negotiating is essentially a communication process. It requires an awareness of the ongoing, transactional nature of communication and recognizes that each person in an interaction affects the other.

Culturally Sensitive Care

According to Chrisman, culturally sensitive care is based on three interrelated principles: knowledge, respect, and negotiation (1991). Health professionals need to have knowledge about patients' cultural beliefs, and practices in order to provide care that is congruent with patients' expectations and sensitive to their beliefs. One way to obtain this knowledge is to view the patient as a cultural informant, who can share his or her particular beliefs with the health professional (DeSantis, 1994). The patient is the most knowledgeable source about the cultural beliefs that are important to him or her. This approach moves beyond a more stereotypical, cookbook approach to culture (e.g., Asians always want this information, Hispanics never want this information) to an approach that recognizes the individual's unique point of view that is shaped by his or her culture and personal experiences (DeSantis, 1994). In providing culturally sensitive care, health professionals need to be aware that certain beliefs may be held by various cultural groups, but then determine the extent to which these beliefs are held by *a specific patient* during *a specific illness* (Pachter, 1994).

One way to become more knowledgeable about patients' beliefs is to elicit from them explanations about their own illness. Table 9–1 lists some questions that can be used to learn more about patients' views of their illness and their expectations about treatment. Answers to questions such as these provide health professionals with knowledge about patients' particular beliefs, the extent to which patients believe in a biomedical model, and the particular language and terminology that patients use to describe their illness (Chrisman, 1991). Based on the information obtained from these assessment questions, health professionals will be more knowledgeable about

TABLE 9–1. LEARNING THE PATIENT'S PERSPECTIVE

1. What do you think caused your illness?
2. When did it start?
3. How severe is your illness?
4. How have you been treating your illness?
5. What kind of treatment do you think you need now?
6. What do you fear most about your illness?

Adapted with permission from Kleinman, A. (1980). Patients and healers in the context of culture: An exploration of the borderland between anthropology, medicine, and psychiatry. *Copyright © 1980 The Regents of the University of California. Berkeley, CA: University of California Press.*

the patient and the particular approach to pursue in providing culturally sensitive care.

In addition to knowledge, culturally sensitive care is also based on respect. According to Chrisman (1991), respect is mutual between provider and patient in a culturally sensitive relationship. Professionals are much more likely to show respect to clients when they understand why clients hold particular beliefs or behave in certain ways. Likewise, patients are more likely to show respect for professionals when they believe that the professional is sensitive to their beliefs and is trying to learn more about their cultural practices.

Respect moves beyond just giving lip-service to cultural orientations or being tolerant of cultural differences. Rather, it implies actually trying to incorporate cultural beliefs into health care practices. The following case study of *empacho*, a folk illness decribed in various Latino cultures, (associated with symptoms of nausea, loss of appetite, and stomach cramps), illustrates how cultural beliefs were incorporated into standard health care treatment.

A 20-month-old Puerto Rican boy was admitted to the inpatient unit for failure to thrive after a weight loss of 1.6 kilograms (kg), associated with a decrease in appetite. The child was admitted to the inpatient unit for dietary and behavioral observation. On questioning, the mother expressed the opinion that a possible cause of her child's weight loss and poor appetite was his eating some pork a few weeks earlier. She believed that the pork was spoiled and caused *empacho* in her son. She was so certain about this that she and her husband were planning to send for her husband's mother—a *santiguadora* (healer)—to visit from Puerto Rico to see the child and perform the treatment that cures *empacho*.

As the husband's mother could not come immediately, the mother was asked if she would like a local *santiguadora* to come to the hospital to treat the child. She readily agreed to this, and with the help of the owner of a local *botanica* (a shop in the Puerto Rican community that sells herbs, remedies, and various religious objects, and is an informal source of information about many folk beliefs and practices) a local *santiguadora* was contacted, who came to the hospital and performed the ritual healing massage on this child.

Two days later the child was discharged from the hospital after showing a moderate weight gain during hospitalization, and follow-up medical, behavioral, and dietary management was arranged in a private physician's office. (Adapted with permission from Pachter, LM. Culture & Clinical Care: Folk Illness Beliefs and Behaviors and Their Implications for Health Care Delivery. JAMA 1994; 271:690-694.)

Culturally sensitive care does not mean that the health professionals need to agree with the logic or efficacy of cultural beliefs or practices, but it does imply that the professional respects the importance of the practices to the patient or family and, where possible, incorporates nonharmful practices into the care (Pachter, 1994). Folk practices can be utilized along with the standard biomedical approaches to provide culturally congruent health care (Leininger, 1988) (Fig. 9–4). The ability to bridge these two systems of health care delivery will help to ensure that patients receive high-quality care that is compatible with their cultural beliefs.

Culturally sensitive care also involves negotiation. As discussed in the previous section, negotiation refers to the ability to develop an effective working alliance even though the cultural beliefs and practices of the provider and patient may differ. Health professionals who make an effort to become knowledgeable about clients' cultural beliefs, and treat their beliefs

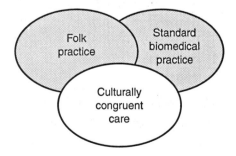

Figure 9–4. Blending practices to promote culturally congruent care.

with respect, will be in a better position to negotiate different approaches to treating health problems.

Culturally Based Resources

A third approach that is essential to providing effective intercultural communication is to enlist culturally based resources to supplement existing services. One resource that is frequently used in health care settings is an interpreter/translator. The term *translator* is used when referring to written communication and the term *interpreter* is used when referring to oral communication. This bilingual person is very valuable in facilating communication and understanding between patients and providers. Patients feel less isolated when they know someone is available to help them understand the complex and oftentimes confusing health-related information.

Although interpretation and translation are extremely important, there are a few issues that Kagawa-Singer (1996) believes need to be taken into consideration in this area. For example, a number of languages have male and female syntax and the interpreter needs to be fluent enough to use the vocabulary correctly. Where possible, the interpreter should be of the same gender and social class as the patient. According to Kagawa-Singer, social class differences can be a major barrier to communication, especially when the interpreter is from a higher class than the patient. In some cultures this would be perceived as placing the interpreter in a position of authority and would be considered inappropriate by the patient and awkward for the interpreter. Although family members often are used as interpreters, family members may be biased in their interpretation. Furthermore, family members may not understand medical terminology. Even though there are potential problems to using an interpreter, the benefits far outweigh the potential problems that may occur.

In addition to interpreters, another valuable resource is people in the community who have the same cultural background as the patient. For example, in our community, a group of volunteers has joined together to provide a range of services to hospitalized people who are from different cultures. The organization these volunteers have founded, called International Neighbors, is coordinated by a nurse. This organization is contacted by hospital staff when a person or a family from one culture has difficulty communicating or understanding medical procedures, as illustrated in the following case study.

An 18-year-old woman from France was an exchange student at a local university. She lived with a family whose home was located 1 hour from campus. She was commuting to class with a friend when their car was involved in an automobile accident. The young woman was seriously injured and hospitalized in critical condition. She sustained multiple fractures, internal head injuries, and was in a coma.

The young woman's mother was contacted by the host family and told about the accident. The mother was a nurse, originally from Hungary, who had moved to France recently to find a more stable life. She was a single parent to her 18-year-old daughter and a 13-year-old son; her husband had died three years previously. She had an extremely close relationship with her daughter and had shared her daughter's dream of wanting to be a physician.

The mother and her son flew to the United States to see her daughter. The son accompanied his mother because there was no one for him to stay with in France. Although the mother was a nurse, she was panic-stricken by her daughter's condition. Because she spoke no English (she was fluent in Hungarian and spoke some French), she had difficulty understanding what was happening to her daughter. A social worker contacted the International Neighbors group who arranged for two Hungarian-speaking people to assist the mother. They not only helped her with the language but they became what she described as her "lifeline."

Group members helped the mother and her son find a place to stay for an extended period of time, invited them to their homes for meals, and assisted them with the transition when the daughter was moved from the acute care setting to a rehabilitation facility.

The young woman remained in a coma and eventually the mother and her son needed to return to France for the mother to retain her job. Members of International Neighbors helped her find resources to set up a legal guardianship for her daughter, who remained in the United States while the mother and her son returned to France.

As illustrated in this example, a network of community volunteers provided a strong, temporary system of support for this family. Their support went beyond the translation of language to a broader safety net of services that provided social, emotional, and legal resources to the family. This example points out the kind of creative resources that exist within communities and that can be utilized to provide culturally sensitive care to patients and their family members.

In recent years, there has also been an attempt to supplement existing health care services by bringing community-based services to various cultural groups, such as the Hispanic community, the Native American community, and the African-American community. These agencies are often administered and staffed by people who share the same culture as the recipients. For example, Burk, Wieser, and Keegan (1995) describe a comprehensive community and migrant health center in Southern Texas that serves 30,000 clients annually, 94 percent of whom are Mexican-American and 50 percent of whom are uninsured. In addition to their regular primary care services, the agency has a highly respected birthing center that provides culturally sensitive care to the women and families in the community. The success of this program has been attributed to the fact that the birthing center is located in the predominantly Mexican-American community, 85 percent of the staff are Mexican-American, and most of the staff are native to the region, thus they share a common cultural and regional background with the clients. Burk and co-workers describe a number of positive health outcomes that have occurred as a result of this community-based program, such as a higher use of early prenatal care.

Community-based programs not only provide direct services for members of their community, but they also serve as advocates in the broader health care arena. For example, in a recent program to increase the use of screening mammograms in the community as a whole, representatives of a Mexican-American health center and the Native American health center were invited to attend a community-wide planning session. These representatives discussed specific approaches that would be sensitive to members of their community and would increase their participation in screening programs.

Providing effective intercultural communication involves understanding the transactional influence of culture on both provider and patient as well as the environment in which the care is provided. By increasing our knowledge and awareness of the cultural beliefs and practices of various cultural groups, we will be more sensitive to their needs and more respectful of their health care practices. We need to know our own limits for providing culturally sensitive care and actively seek out additional resources within our agencies or the community to ensure that a range of resources and services is available to patients and their families.

► SUMMARY

This chapter is about multiculturalism and the implications of cultural diversity for health care. Discussion in the chapter is structured around the nature of intercultural communication, which is defined as the process whereby people from different cultures share information using a set of common rules.

Intercultural communication is influenced by ethnocentrism and prejudice. Ethnocentrism is the universal tendency for people to place their own group at the center of their observations of others and, in so doing, to give priority and greater value to their own perspective. It is an obstacle to effective health communication because ethnocentrism distorts one's view of others and limits one's ability to be fully empathic with others' circumstances. Prejudice is the individual's tendency to make judgments of other individuals or groups which are faulty or not fully substantiated. Prejudice is an obstacle that gets in the way of our ability to be other-oriented and to fully understand others and communicate effectively.

Individualism versus collectivism and high versus low context are two major characteristics of cultures. Individualistic cultures place the individual's interests, needs, and values above those of the group. In collectivistic cultures, social norms and group concerns supersede the interests of the individual.

Cultures can also be distinguished by the way they incorporate contexts in communication. High-context cultures interpret messages based on a broad set of culturally based rules, which reside in the individual and the environment. Conversely, low-context cultures rely primarily on the specific content of messages, paying far less attention to culturally based rules. When compared to people from low-context cultures, people from high-context cultures are more effective at reading nonverbal cues, talk less, and place less emphasis on verbal messages.

Culture is inextricably related to three aspects of communication: perception, verbal communication, and nonverbal communication. Perception has a profound influence on how health professionals and patients view symptoms, causes of illness, and types of treatment. For health professionals the challenge is to develop an alliance with patients, while acknowledging and giving respect to the patient's different frame of reference.

Perhaps the greatest barrier to effective intercultural communication is language differences. Language barriers make being ill even more traumatic for patients; language problems make it difficult for health professionals to make accurate assessments and treament decisions; and they make it difficult to develop a helping relationship with the patient. Language and how it is used affects the quality of health care in many ways. For example, patients need to be able to "tell their stories" whenever possible. In addition, patients need to be able to ask questions freely, and they need the freedom to use their own dialect. Lastly, patients need to be able to disclose information and involve themselves in decision making to the extent that is appropriate for them within their own culture.

Cultural differences are also demonstrated in nonverbal communication. Facial displays are different across cultures and provide a real challenge for health professionals. Providers need to be sensitive to how patients use facial expressions to smile and to express pain.

We have identified three general ways of promoting more effective intercultural communication. First, it is essential to recognize the transactional influence of culture. This requires that health professionals seek to find ways to understand, clarify, and negotiate the disparities between their own perspective and the perspective of the patient. Each party affects and is affected by the other. Second, it is essential to foster culturally sensitive care, which occurs when health professionals seek information, show deep respect, and negotiate their differences with patients. Lastly, it is essential to enlist culturally based resources whenever possible. Health professionals need to actively seek out additional resources within their organizations or within the community to promote the health and well-being of patients and their families.

► REFERENCES

Andersen, P. (1997). Cues of culture: The basis of intercultural differences in nonverbal communication. In L. A. Samovar & R. E. Porter (Eds.), *Intercultural communication: A reader* (8th ed., pp. 244–255). Belmont, CA: Wadsworth.

Blackhall, L. J., Murphy, S. T., Frank, F., Michel, V., Azen, S. (1995). Ethnicity and attitudes toward patient autonomy. *Journal of American Medical Association, 274*(10), 820–825.

Burk, M. E., Wieser, P. C., & Keegan, L. (1995). Cultural beliefs and health behaviors of pregnant Mexican-American women: Implications for primary care. *Advances in Nursing Science, 17*(4), 37–52.

Chrisman, N. J. (1991). Cultural systems. In R. McCorkle, M. Grant, M. Frank-Stromborg, & S. B. Baird (Eds.), *Cancer nursing: A comprehensive textbook,* (pp. 45–54). Philadelphia: Saunders.

DeSantis, L. (1994). Making anthropology clinically relevant to nursing care. *Journal of Advanced Nursing, 20,* 707–715.

Ekman, P. L. (1972). Universals and cultural differences in facial expression of emotion. In J. Cole (Ed.), *Nebraska symposium on motivation* (Vol. 19, pp. 207–283). Lincoln, NE: University of Nebraska Press.

Friesen, W. V. (1972). Cultural differences in facial expressions in a social situation: An experimental test of the concept of display rules. Unpublished doctoral dissertation, University of California, San Francisco.

Geist, P. (1997). Negotiating cultural understanding in health care communication. In L. A. Samovar & R. E. Porter (Eds.), *Intercultural communication: A reader* (8th ed., pp. 340–349). Belmont, CA: Wadsworth.

Gervais, K. G. (1996). Providing culturally competent health care to Hmong patients. *Minnesota Medicine, 79,* 49–51.

Giger, J. N., & Davidhizar, R. (1990). Developing communication skills. *The ABNF Journal, 1*(2), 33–35.

Gudykunst, W. B., & Kim, Y. Y. (1997). *Communicating with strangers: An approach to intercultural communication* (3rd ed.). New York: McGraw-Hill.

Gudykunst, W. B., & Ting-Toomey, S. (1988). *Culture and interpersonal communication.* Thousand Oaks, CA: Sage.

Hall, E. T. (1976). *Beyond culture.* New York: Doubleday.

Herselman, S. (1996). Some problems in health communication in a multicultural clinical setting: A South African experience. *Health Communication, 8*(2), 153–170.

Hubbell, F. A., Chavez, L. R., Mishra, S. I., & Valdez, R. B. (1996). Differing beliefs about breast cancer among Latinas and Anglo women. *Western Journal of Medicine, 164,* 405–409.

Huttlinger, K., Krefting, L., Drevdahl, D., Tree, P., Baca, E., & Benally, A. (1992). "Doing battle": A metaphorical analysis of diabetes mellitus among Navajo people. *The American Journal of Occupational Therapy, 46*(8), 706–712.

Kagawa-Singer, M. (1996). Cultural systems. In R. McCorkle, M. Grant, M. Frank-Stromborg, & S. B. Baird (Eds.), *Cancer nursing: A comprehensive textbook* (2nd ed., pp. 38–52). Philadelphia: Saunders.

Kavanagh, K. H., & Kennedy, P. H. (1992). *Promoting cultural diversity: Strategies for health care professionals.* Thousand Oaks, CA: Sage.

Kleinman, A. (1980). Patients and healers in the context of culture: An exploration of the borderland between anthropology, medicine, and psychiatry. Berkely, CA: University of California Press.

Kreps, G. L., & Kunimoto, E. N. (1994). *Effective communication in multicultural health care settings.* Thousand Oaks, CA: Sage.

Lee, M. E., Matsumoto, D., Kobayashi, M., Krupp, D., Maniatis, E. F., & Roberts, W. (1992). Cultural influences on nonverbal behavior in applied settings. In R. S. Feldman (Ed.), *Applications of nonverbal behavioral theories and research* (pp. 239–261). Hillsdale, NJ: Erlbaum.

Leininger, M. M. (1990). The significance of cultural concepts in nursing. *Journal of Transcultural Nursing, 2*(1), 52–59.

Leininger, M. M. (1988). Leininger's theory of nursing: Cultural care diversity and universality. *Nursing Science Quarterly, 1*(4), 152–160.

Long, E. (1993). Breast cancer in African-American women: Review of the literature. *Cancer Nursing, 16*(1), 1–24.

Pachter, L. M. (1994). Culture and clinical care: Folk illness beliefs and behaviors and their implications for health care delivery. *Journal of the American Medical Association, 271*(9), 690–694.

Ponterotto, J. G., & Pedersen, P. B. (1993). *Preventing prejudice: A guide for counselors and educators.* Thousand Oaks, CA: Sage.

Porter, R. E., & Samovar, L. A. (1997). An introduction to intercultural communication. In L. A. Samovar & R. E. Porter (Eds.), *Intercultural communication: A reader* (8th ed., pp. 5–26). Belmont, CA: Wadsworth.

Price, J. H., Desmond, S. M., Slenker, S., Smith, D., & Steward, P. W. (1992). Urban black women's perceptions of breast cancer and mammography. *Journal of Community Health, 17*(4), 191–204.

Todd, K. H., Samavod, N., & Hoffman, J. R. (1993). Ethnicity as a risk factor for inadequate emergency department analgesia. *Journal of American Medical Association, 269,* 1537–1539.

Triandis, H. (1986). Collectivism vs. individualism: A reconceptualization of a basic concept in cross-cultural psychology. In C. Bagley & G. Verma (Eds.), *Personality, cognition, and values: Cross-cultural perspectives of childhood and adolescence.* London: Macmillan.

Trill, M. D., & Holland, J. (1993). Cross-cultural differences in the care of patients with cancer: A review. *General Hospital Psychiatry, 15,* 21–30.

Tripp-Reimer, T., & Brink, P. J. (1985). Culture brokerage. In B. M. Bulechek & J. C. McCloskey (Eds.), *Nursing interventions* (pp. 352–364). Philadelphia: Saunders.

Villarruel, A. M. (1995). Mexican-American cultural meanings, expressions, self-care and dependent-care actions associated with experiences of pain. *Research in Nursing & Health, 18,* 427–436.

Walker, P. F. (1996). *Clinical case studies.* Unpublished work. (St. Paul-Ramsey Medical Center, 640 Jackson Street, St. Paul, Minnesota, 55101).

Author Index

A

Aaronson, L., 104
Abbey, A., 54
Ackerman, N., 112
Adamson, H. M., 269
Adesman, P., 51
Aiken, L. H., 249
Alagna, F., 148
Alexander, J. F., 34
Allekian, C. I., 142, 143
Allen, D. C., 39
Ancoli, S., 148
Andersen, P., 290
Anderson, G., 23, 29
Anderson, M. A., 103
Antonovsky, A., 37
Archer, D., 138, 141
Argyle, M., 140, 141
Arnston, P., 38, 181
Aroskar, M. A., 259
Arras, J. D., 278
Attwell, J. R., 39
Avins, A. L., 272
Azen, S., 298

B

Baca, E., 293, 294, 296
Backus, D. K., 169
Bahna, G. F., 268, 270
Baird, S. B., 113
Baker, C. F., 156
Baker, S. J., 183
Bales, R. F., 215
Ballard, K., 154
Barnlund, D. C., 173, 201
Barrett-Lennard, G. T., 25, 26
Bartol, G. M., 92

Baun, M. M., 38
Bayley, C., 275, 276, 278, 280
Beauchamp, T. L., 259, 260, 264, 267
Beavin, J., 6, 7, 34
Beck, L., 53
Becker, M. H., 13, 15
Bedell, S. E., 88
Beisecker, A. E., 39, 87, 89, 107
Benally, A., 293, 294, 296
Benjamin, A., 164, 173, 175, 181, 182, 186
Benne, K. D., 204, 207
Bennett, R. L., 39
Bennis, W. G., 215, 218
Bensing, J. M., 140
Berelson, B., 183
Berger, P., 90, 92
Berlo, D. K., 5, 9
Bernstein, L., 191
Bernstein, R., 191
Billings, J. A., 165
Billiu, G. A., 168
Bishop, C., 4
Blackhall, L. J., 298
Blake, R. R., 244
Blanchard, C. G., 106–107
Blanchard, E. B., 106–107
Blanchard, K., 203
Bloom, J. R., 53, 103, 195
Bolzani, R., 139
Bond, S., 106
Bottorff, J. L., 23, 29, 147
Bourgeault, I. L., 87, 89
Bowen, M., 106, 117
Bowen, S., 246, 247
Bowker, J., 38
Bradac, J. J., 56
Braithwaite, D. O., 54
Brammer, L. M., 190
Brehm, J. W., 32, 33

Breu, C., 104
Brickman, P., 84, 85, 86
Brink, P. J., 300, 301
Broome, M. E., 32
Brown, C. T., 227
Brown, S. J., 182
Buber, M., 61
Buller, D. B., 127, 132, 145
Burgoon, J. K., 145
Burk, M. E., 297, 306
Burnside, I., 204
Bzdek, V. M., 148

C

Calhoun, J. G., 168
Callahan, D., 264
Cancini, M., 139
Canedy, B. H., 213
Cannell, C. F., 164
Cantor, R. C., 36, 44
Caplan, A. L., 259
Carew, D., 203
Carlson, R. R., 217, 221
Carnrike, C. K., Jr., 268, 270
Carpentier, W. S., 80
Carr, V., 174
Carrocci, N. M., 229, 235
Cartwright, D., 196, 201
Cassem, N., 114
Cassileth, B. R., 53, 269
Cella, D. F., 214
Chaikin, A. L., 50, 51, 54
Chalmers, K., 173, 178
Charron-Moore, C., 111
Chavez, L. R., 293
Cherry, R., 268, 270
Childress, J. F., 259, 260, 262, 264, 267
Chrisman, N. J., 301, 302
Churchill, L. R., 264

Cipolli, C., 139
Cissna, K. N., 60
Clark, B., 230
Clark, S., 101
Clift, E., 4
Cline, R. J. W., 196
Coates, D., 54, 84, 85
Cohen, C. B., 275
Cohen, S. A., 172, 174, 177, 178
Cohn, E., 84, 85
Compton, K., 106
Cook, M., 140, 141
Coser, L. A., 226
Courts, N. F., 92
Cozby, P. C., 49–51
Craig, K. D., 136, 138
Cranford, R. E., 259, 275, 278, 280
Creaser, J., 172
Cronenwett, L., 85
Cruzen, D., 39

D

Dabbs, J. M., 33
Danis, M., 264
Danziger, S., 90
Davidhizar, R., 297, 298
Davis, M. H., 25
Dawson, C., 53
Degner, L. F., 37
Delbanco, T. L., 88
Dennison, P. D., 180
Derlega, V. J., 50, 51, 54, 127
Derogatis, L. R., 268, 270
DeSantis, L., 300, 301
Desmond, S. M., 294
Deutsch, M., 42, 226, 235, 236
DeVellis, R., 33
DeWever, M., 149
Dewey, J., 242
DiMatteo, M. R., 40, 86, 127–129, 138, 141
DiSalvo, V. S., 169
Dorris, G., 111
Dosovitz, I., 211
Doudera, A. E., 259, 275
Downs, C. W., 167, 168
Dracup, K., 35, 104
Draper, E., 93, 102
Drew, N., 64, 67
Droge, H. E., 181
Dunkel-Schetter, C., 54
Dyck, S., 107

E

Eagin, C., 93
Ekman, P., 136, 137, 140
Ellsworth, P., 136

Engel, N. S., 60
Epstein, N., 24
Estabrooks, C. A., 151
Evans, J. W., 33

F

Fagin, C., 97
Fahlberg, N., 24
Fairbairn, S., 174
Farran, C., 174
Filley, A. C., 236, 240, 243, 251
Finnegan, J. L., 4
Fisher, B. A., 215, 219, 220
Fisher, J., 148, 149, 153
Flanigan, R. C., 39
Fletcher, C., 174
Folger, J. P., 226, 250, 253
Forchuk, C., 171, 172, 180
Formo, A., 115
Forsyth, G. L., 23, 26
Fowler, M. D. M., 278
Frank, F., 298
Frankel, R., 147
Frankl, V., 61
Fraser, K., 67
Freedman, K., 115
Freeman, S., 115
Freimuth, V., 4
French, R. P., 87
Friedman, H. S., 40, 127, 128
Friesen, W. V., 136, 137, 140

G

Galbraith, M. E., 39
Gallop, R., 67
Garfinkle, K., 104
Garvin, B. J., 60, 68, 71, 156
Geist, P., 285
Gernstein, F., 104
Gervais, K. G., 292
Gibb, J. R., 46
Giffin, K., 42
Giger, J. N., 297, 298
Gilliam, N. R., 178
Gladstein, G. A., 25
Glass, E., 260
Glicksman, A. S., 53
Goffman, E., 131, 253
Goldberg, A. A., 196
Gonzalez, S., 211
Goodwin, G. L., 272, 273
Gordon, V. C., 213
Gotcher, J. M., 54, 111, 118
Gottheil, E., 53, 195
Gould, H., 108
Graen, G. B., 203
Green, C. P., 115
Greenfield, S., 39

Grennberg, R., 51
Grotz, J., 43
Gudykunst, W. B., 286, 287, 290

H

Hackett, T., 114
Hadlow, J., 90
Haiman, F. S., 173, 201
Halaris, A., 139
Hall, E. T., 142, 144, 145, 291, 292
Hall, J. A., 127, 138, 141, 182
Halstead, L. K., 32
Hammond, D. C., 187, 188
Hammond, M. A., 113
Hampe, S. O., 104
Hanna, K. M., 80
Hansson, R., 24
Hardin, S., 139
Harlow, H., 147
Harrigan, A. K., 217, 221
Harrison, R. P., 137, 140
Hawks, I. K., 203
Hays, R. D., 127
Heemer, A., 231
Heidt, P., 148
Heineken, J., 60, 64, 233
Hejl, J., 80
Helms, L., 103
Henley, N., 151
Hepworth, D. H., 187, 188
Herman, F., 51
Herselman, S., 296, 297
Hersey, P., 203
Herzog, J., 80
Heslin, R., 149, 153
High, D. M., 273
Hilton, B. A., 119
Hobart, C. W., 24
Hocker, J. L., 226–228, 251
Hoffman, J. R., 299
Hogan, R., 24
Holland, J., 268, 270, 296, 299
Hosman, L. A., 56
House, R. J., 199
Howard, L., 172
Howell, T., 102
Hubbell, F. A., 293
Huttlinger, K., 293, 294, 296
Hwang, T., 138

I

Ingham, R., 140, 141

J

Jackson, D. D., 6, 7, 34, 116
Jackson, I., 34
Jacob, M. C., 181

Jacobsen, P. B., 104
Jaksa, J. A., 271
James, S. A., 181
Jandt, F. E., 236
Jay, S. S., 148
Jezewski, M. A., 65
Johnson, E. T., 113
Johnson, F. L. P., 143
Johnson, J. E., 33
Johnson, J. L., 35
Johnson, M., 56, 155
Jones, S., 112
Jones, S. B., 145
Jones, S. E., 201
Jonsen, A. R., 273, 277
Jourard, S. M., 50, 52, 56

K

Kagawa-Singer, M., 290, 304
Kahn, R. L., 164
Kalisch, B. J., 23, 26, 29, 101
Kalisch, P., 101
Kaplan, G. D., 33
Kaplan, S. H., 39
Karus, D., 115
Karuza, J., Jr., 84, 85
Katon, W., 39
Katz, J., 260
Katzman, E. M., 98, 101, 249
Kavanagh, K. H., 285
Keefe, M., 156
Keegan, L., 297, 306
Keeling, A. W., 180
Keller, E., 148
Keller, P. W., 227
Kelner, M. J., 87, 89
Kendon, A., 139
Kennedy, B. J., 269
Kennedy, C. W., 60, 68, 71, 156
Kennedy, P. H., 285
Kerssens, J. J., 140
Kidder, L., 84, 85
Kilmann, R. H., 244, 245, 248
Kim, Y. Y., 287, 290
King, B. W., 245
King, I. M., 15
Kirscht, J. P., 33
Klein, R. H., 199
Kleinman, A., 39
Klotkowski, D., 56
Knapp, M. L., 137, 149, 154, 155
Knauss, W. A., 93, 102
Kneisl, C. R., 170, 172
Knutson, T., 231
Kobayashi, M., 298
Kraemer, H. C., 53
Kramer, H. D., 195
Kramer, M., 94

Kraus, D., 117
Krefting, L., 293, 294, 296
Kreps, G. L., 285
Krevdahl, D., 293, 294, 296
Krieger, D., 148
Krisjanson, L., 173, 178
Kritek, P. B., 87
Krupp, D., 298
Kuczewski, M. G., 271
Kulik, J. A., 86
Kunimoto, E. N., 285

L

Labreque, M.S., 106–107
LaFasto, F. M. J., 198
Laing, G. P., 148
Laing, R. D., 61
Lamb, G. S., 41, 98, 249
Lamb, S. A., 212
LaMonica, E. L., 23
Lane, P. L., 149
Langer, E. J., 31, 32, 39
Larsen, J. K., 169
Larson, C. E., 60, 62, 196, 198
Lasakow, P., 52
Laschinger, H. K. S., 97
Lashbrook, V., 231
Latanich, T., 101
Latham, C. P., 80
Lauer, P., 92
Lawson, D. L., 269
Lazure, L. L., 38
Leary, T., 88
Leavitt, M. B., 212
Lee, M. E., 298
Lego, S., 177
Leininger, M. M., 285, 303
Lepper, H. S., 86, 128, 129
Leutgert, M. J., 172
Levanthal, H., 33
Lewis, F., 33, 113
Lieberman, M. A., 203
Lillehaugen, B. J., 269
Limandri, B. J., 54
Lipps, T., 23
Lister, L., 99
Litman, T., 113
Lo, B., 272
Long, E., 294
Loomis, M. E., 174, 197, 200, 202
Loveridge, C. E., 60
Lowery, B. J., 33
Lucas, B. A., 39
Luce, R. D., 42
Luckman, T., 90, 92
Lulofs, R. S., 226, 253
Lyall, W., 115
Lynch, A., 37–38

M

MacDonald, M., 168
Maguire, P., 174
Mahler, H. I. M., 86
Mahoney, D. F., 102
Maides, S. A., 33
Maiman, L. A., 13, 15
Maisto, S. A., 33
Makoul, G., 38
Malone, D., 113
Maniatis, E. F., 298
Mannes, S. L., 104
March, V., 53, 269
Martin, E., 167, 168
Martin, L. R., 86, 128, 129
Maslow, A., 232
Matsumoto, D., 298
Matthews, K. E., Jr., 24
Matwychuk, A. K., 213
Mauksch, H., 44, 53, 82
Mauksch, I., 101
Maxson, E., 174
May, C., 87
McCorkle, R., 113
McDonald, A. P., 33
McDonald, J. C., 106
McIlveen, K. H., 23, 29
McLellan, L., 80
McRoberts, J. W., 39
Mechanic, D., 90, 249
Mehrabian, A., 24, 127, 146
Mercer, S. R., 138
Meyerowitz, B. E., 33
Michel, V., 275, 276, 298
Miles, M. B., 203
Millar, F. E., 6
Minckley, B., 143, 156
Minuchin, S., 106, 111, 157
Mishra, S. I., 293
Mitchell, G. W., 53
Mlott, S. R., 33
Mlott, Y. D., 33
Moldow, D. G., 278
Montagu, A., 149
Montbriand, M. J., 37
Moore, W. P., 107
Moos, R. H., 95, 100, 102
Moreland, J. R., 115
Morganstern, O., 236
Morrow, G., 268, 270
Morse, J. M., 23, 29, 35
Morton, T. L., 34
Moser, D. K., 35
Mouton, L. S., 244
Murphy, S., 92, 298
Murray, T. H., 277, 278
Musser, D. B., 100
Mutinelli, P., 139

N

Naber, S. J., 32
Nanni, C., 89
Napodano, R. J., 41, 98, 249
Nehren, J., 178
Northouse, L. L., 53, 84, 85, 104, 111, 113
Northouse, P. G., 43, 53

O

Oberst, M. T., 148
O'Brien, B., 23, 29
O'Connor, R. J., 260, 266, 267, 270
Okun, D., 108, 271
Olson, J. K., 26, 27
Orem, D., 86, 262

P

Pachter, L. M., 295, 301, 303
Parisi-Carew, E., 203
Pascale, L., 115, 117
Pattison, J., 148
Payne, J. G., 4
Pearce, W. B., 41
Pedersen, P. B., 288
Penman, D. R., 268, 270
Penny, K., 149
Peper, E., 148
Peplau, H., 189, 191
Pepler, C. J., 37–38
Peters-Golden, H., 54
Pettegrew, L. S., 3
Phillips, C. Y., 98
Pitts, M., 90
Piziak, V. K., 80
Polivka, B. J., 156
Ponterotto, J. G., 288
Poole, M. S., 226, 250, 253
Porter, R. E., 285, 287, 293
Powers, M., 92
Pratt, L., 119
Prescott, P. A., 98, 246, 247
Price, J. H., 294
Prince, L. M., 127
Pritchard, M. S., 271
Prkachin, K. M., 136, 138
Pugh, D., 275, 276
Putnam, S. M., 181

Q

Quinlan, Karen A., 275

R

Rabinowitz, V., 84, 85
Raiffa, H., 42
Rand, C. S., 127
Rankin, E. D., 172, 174, 177, 178
Rankin, G. W., 174
Rapoport, A., 236
Ratliffe, S. A., 199
Ratzan, R. M., 271
Ratzan, S. C., 4
Raudonis, B. M., 27
Raveis, V. H., 115, 117
Raven, R., 87
Ray, E., 146
Ray, G., 146
Raymond, G., 101
Redd, W. H., 104
Reed, P. G., 214
Rehwaldt, M., 32
Reiss, D., 211
Richardson, B. Z., 24
Roberts, J. I., 98, 101, 249
Roberts, W., 298
Robinson, C. A., 107
Rock, D. L., 33
Rogers, C., 12, 23, 24–26, 29, 169
Rogers, E. M., 3, 4
Rogers, J., 115
Rogers, L. E., 6
Rogers, P. L., 138, 141
Rosenstock, I. M., 13
Rosenthal, R., 138, 141
Ross, H., 156, 157
Ross, J. W., 275, 276
Roter, D. L., 127, 182
Roth, C. H., 172
Rotter, J. B., 32, 33, 43
Ruben, B. D., 79
Ruckdeschel, J. C., 106–107
Russell, C. A., 37
Ryan, J. W., 98
Ryan, P. Y., 105
Rytting, M., 153

S

Sachs, E. G., 213
Sakurai, C., 260
Saltzman, C., 172
Samavod, N., 299
Samovar, L. A., 285, 287, 293
Satir, V., 116
Sayre, J., 175, 176, 178
Schaefer, J. A., 95, 100, 102
Schirner, M., 53
Schmale, A. H., 268, 270
Schofield, T., 38
Schultheiss, P., 101
Schutz, W. C., 215–217, 219, 221, 234
Schutzenhofer, K. K., 100
Schwankovsky, L., 39, 89
Schwebel, A. I., 115
Seeman, M., 33
Seeman, T. E., 33
Seibold, D. R., 56
Seligman, M. E. P., 32
Sharf, B. F., 90, 154, 182
Shatz, D., 263
Shaw, M. E., 201, 215
Sheats, P., 204, 207
Shepard, H. A., 215, 218
Sherman, S. E., 24
Sherry, D., 260
Sieburg, E., 60, 62, 63
Siegel, K., 115, 117
Siegler, M., 273
Silva, D., 101
Silva, M. C., 269, 270
Simington, J. A., 148
Skinner, G., 80
Slenker, S., 294
Smeyak, G. P., 167, 168
Smith, D., 277, 278, 294
Smith, V. G., 187, 188
Sobolew-Shubin, A., 39
Solberg, S. M., 23, 29
Solomon, P. S., 138
Sommer, R., 156, 157
Sorrell, J. M., 269, 270
Spiegel, D., 53, 195
Spitz, R., 147
Staver, S., 99, 100
Stech, E., 199
Steckel, S. B., 174
Stein, L. I., 102
Steiner, G. A., 183
Steinglass, P., 211
Stern, M., 115, 117
Stetz, K., 106
Steward, P. W., 294
Stiles, W. B., 181
Stillman, J. J., 142, 143
Stoeckle, J. D., 165
Stotland, E., 24
Street, R. L., 80, 106, 127, 132, 145
Strickland, B. R., 33
Strodtbeck, F. L., 215
Stross, J. K., 168
Stuart, G. W., 171, 172, 175, 177, 178
Stutman, R. K., 226, 250, 253
Sundeen, S. J., 171, 172, 174, 175, 177, 178
Sundell, W., 68
Sutton-Smith, K., 53, 269

T

Tagliacozzo, D., 44, 53, 81
Tardy, C. H., 56
Tate, J. W., 143

Taylor, D. A., 50
Taylor, S., 36, 81
Teel, K., 275, 276
Templeton, B., 168
Templin, E., 81
Thomas, K. W., 244, 245, 248
Thomasma, D. C., 262
Thompson, K. O., 98
Thompson, S. C., 39, 89
Thompson, T. L., 31, 32, 56, 60, 79
Thorne, S., 107
Ting-Toomey, S., 286, 290
Todd, K. H., 299
Toghill, P., 108
Tree, P., 293, 294, 296
Triandis, H., 290
Trill, M. D., 296, 299
Tripp-Reimer, T., 300, 301
Tuckman, B. W., 215, 216, 218–220
Tuozzi, G., 139

U

Uhl-Bien, M., 203

V

Vachon, M., 115
Valdez, R. B., 293

Van Allen, E., 278
van der Pasch, M., 140
Veatch, R. M., 260, 270
Vess, J. D., 115
Villarruel, A. M., 299
Vinacke, W. E., 42
Viswanath, K., 4
Von Neumann, J., 236
Voss, B. S., 212

W

Wagner, D., 93, 102
Walker, P. F., 289, 291
Wallston, B. S., 33
Wallston, K. A., 33
Ware, J. E., Jr., 39
Watts, D. T., 102
Watzlawick, P., 6, 7, 34
Weiss, S., 99, 147, 149
Welch, D., 110
Wenburg, J. R., 51
Werner-Beland, J. A., 64
West, C., 181
Weston, W., 97
Wheeless, L. R., 42, 43, 52
Whitcher, S. J., 149
White, A. B., 82
Wicas, E., 148
Wieser, P. C., 297, 306
Williams, C., 25, 26

Williams, M. A., 153, 156, 157
Wilmot, W. W., 35, 51, 226–229, 251
Wilson, H. S., 170, 172
Winslade, W., 273
Winters, G., 260
Wishnie, H., 114
Wispe, L., 24
Witcher, S., 148
Woods, N. F., 113
Wooliscroft, J. O., 168
Wortman, C. B., 32, 33, 51, 54, 84, 85
Wozniak, D. A., 233
Wright, K., 107

Y

Yalom, I. D., 195, 198, 201, 203, 211–220
Yellen S. B., 214
Yonge, O., 23, 29
Young, C. A., 214

Z

Zander, A., 196, 199
Zimmerman, J. E., 93, 102
Zimmermann, R., 147
Zupkis, R. V., 53, 269

Subject Index

A

Access to information, 107–111
Accommodation as a conflict style, 247–248
Admissions interviews, 166
Affectional ties and small group communication, 221
Affiliation issues and relational conflict, 234–235
African-Americans and intercultural communication, 294, 297–298
Agreement about content as a confirming response, 62, 70
Alcoholics Anonymous, 85
Alienation, feelings of, 26
Altruism in small group communication, 212
Amount aspect of self-disclosure, 52
Animal communication, 2
Aristotle and trust, 42
Assertiveness as a conflict style, 244
Authority, hierarchical lines of, 39
Autonomy
ethics and patient, 262–264
professional-professional relationships, 101–103
Avoidance as a conflict style, 245–246

B

Baby Jane Doe case, 275
Baker model of silence, 183, 184
Barrett-Lennard Relationship Inventory, 26

Behavioral control, 31–32
Behavioral cues, nonverbal, 130–131
Beliefs and values, conflict regarding, 229–231
Beneficence, principle of, 260–262
Benevolent deception, 272
Bioethics. *See* Ethics
Black English, 297–298
Borderline personality disorder (BPD) and confirmation, 67
Breast cancer victims and self-disclosure, 54
Buber, Martin, 61

C

California Medical Association, 278
Cancer patients
access to information, 110
African-American women and breast, 294
closed communication patterns, 115–118
control issues, 37
enlightenment model of helping and coping, 85
perceptions of, 92
role flexibility, 114–115
role uncertainty in professional-client relationships, 82
self-disclosure from, 53, 54
Canterbury vs. Spence in 1972 (informed consent), 267
Cardiac patients and control issues, 35
Cardozo, Judge, 266

Caring and leadership role, 203
Case-based approach to ethical decision making, 277–278
Certainty *vs.* provisionalism, 49
Change
conflict related to, 225
small group communication, 211–215
Clarification
as a confirming response, 62, 67
of group goals, 199
interview process, 189
Client centered therapy, 12–13, 169
Clients in health care settings. *See also* Family-client relationships; Family-professional relationships; Professional-client relationships
as active participants in health care, 38–39, 86–87
confirmation, 64–67
control issues, 35–39
defining, 18
empathy influencing, 26–29
nonverbal communication, attentiveness to, 128
self-disclose, 53–56
significant others to, 18
trust issues, 44
Closed questions in interview process, 181–182
Cobbs vs. Grant in 1972 (informed consent), 267
Cognitive control, 32, 38
Cognitive perceptual process, 25
Cohesiveness, small group, 201–202, 213–214, 219–220

Collaboration as a conflict style, 248–249
Collectivistic and individualistic cultures, comparing, 289–291
Commitment and small group communication, 221
Communication, defining, 1–2. *See also* Health communication; Human communication; *various subject headings*
Communication and Interpersonal Relations (Haney), 93
Community-based programs, 304–306
Compensatory model of helping and coping, 84, 85
Competition as a conflict style, 246–247
Complementary relationships, 34, 40–41
Comprehension and informed consent, 269–270
Compromise as a conflict style, 248
Confirmation, 72
    applications in health care, 63
    client's perspective, 64–67
    conceptual frameworks of, 61–63
    defining, 60
    professional's perspective, 68–71
Conflict
    change related to, 225
    content areas, 228
        beliefs and values, 229–231
        goals, 231–232
        defining, 226–228
        game theory, 236
        relational level
            affiliation issues, 234–235
            control issues, 233–234
            esteem issues, 232–233
        resolving
            differentiation, 249–251
            face-saving, 253–255
            Filley's model of conflict resolution, 236–243
            fractionation, 251–253
        small group communication, 217–219
        styles of approaching, 243–245
            accommodation, 247–248
            avoidance, 245–246
            collaboration, 248–249
            competition, 246–247
            compromise, 248
            summary, 255–256

Conflict Resolution Through Communication (Jandt), 236
Congruence, 12–13
Connectedness, confirmation and a sense of, 65–66
Consent, informed, 266–271
Content dimension of messages, 7–8, 33–34, 197
Contexts, health communication, 19–20, 291–293
Contexts, human communication, 3–4
Contracts with clients, 174
Contractual honesty, 272, 273
Control, 71
    applications in health care, 35
    client's perspective, 35–39
    conflicts over, 233–234
    defensive climates created, 47
    personal, 30–33
    power differences in professional-client relationships, 87–89
    professional's perspective, 39–41
    relational, 33–35, 41
    small group communication, 217–219, 221
Coping skills, 84–86, 176
Covert norms, 199
Creative problem-solving, 242–243
Cues, nonverbal, 130–131
Cues stimulating preventive health activity, 13–15
Cultural brokerage, 300–301
Cultural differences. See Intercultural communication

D

Decision making and ethics committees, 274–280
Defensive climates, 46–47
Depersonalization in patients, 36
Depth dimension of self-disclosure, 52
Descriptive communication, 47
Deviants, group, 202
Differentiation process in conflict resolution, 249–251
Direct acknowledgment as a confirming response, 62, 67, 70
Directive interviewing, 167–169
Disclosure of information and intercultural communication, 298

Disconfirming responses. See Confirmation
Distance zones and nonverbal communication, 143–145
Diversity. See Intercultural communication
Dominant communicative behaviors, 10–11, 88
Dying, control over, 88–89
Dynamics of Interviewing: Theory, Technique and Cases (Kahn & Cannell), 164

E

Education and service, gap between, 94
Emotional stimulation and leadership role, 203. *See also* Feelings
Empathy, 71
    applications in health care, 26
    client's perspective, 26–29
    conceptual frameworks of, 24–26
    neutrality *vs.*, 48
    professional's perspective, 29–30
    Rogerian theory, 12, 23–24
Enabling norms, 200
Enlightenment model of helping and coping, 85
Environment's impact on patient care, 153–157, 173
Esteem and recognition, need for, 232–233
Ethics, 259
    autonomy, patient, 262–264
    committees and decision making process, 274–280
    defining, 260
    Hippocratic tradition and beneficence, 260–262
    honesty and truth telling, 271–274
    informed consent, 266–271
    paternalism, 262
    social justice, 264–266
    summary, 280–281
Ethnocentrism, 286–288
European-Americans and intercultural communication, 297
Evaluative communication, 46–47
Executive functioning and leadership role, 203

Existential factors in small group communication, 214
Exploration phase in interview process, 175–177
Expression of the Emotions in Man and Animals, The (Darwin), 136
Extent in paralinguistics, 146
External locus of control, 32, 33
Eye contact, 139–141

F

Face-saving process in conflict resolution, 253–255
Facial expressions, 136–139
Family-client relationships, 111
   closed communication patterns, 115–120
   disruption of family member roles, 112–115
   informed consent, 270–271
Family-professional relationships, 103
   access to information, 107–111
   change process in small group communication, 212
   limited contact with professionals, 104–107
Family systems theory, 106
Feelings. *See also* Conflict; Empathy
   alienation, 26
   confirming response and positive, 62, 70
   exploration phase in interview process, 176
   nonverbal communication and expressing, 130
   vocabulary of, 188
Felt conflict, 238–239
Filley's model of conflict resolution
   antecedent conditions, 236–238
   lose-lose strategies, 241
   manifest behavior, 239
   perceived and felt conflict, 238–239
   resolution aftermath, 243
   win-lose strategies, 239–241
   win-win strategies, 241–243
Filtered communication, 107, 109
Folk illness, 302–303
Formal settings, 154
Forming phase and small group communication, 215–217

Fractionation process in conflict resolution, 251–253
Frankl, Viktor, 61
Furniture arrangement, 156–157

G

Game theory, 42, 236
Gaze, 139–141
Gender
   nonverbal communication, 141
   touch, receptivity to, 149
Gestures, 135–136
Goals
   conflict regarding, 231–232
   establishing mutual, 174
   small group communication, 198–199
Goblet issues and small group communication, 216–217
Grief Responses to Long-Term Illness and Disability (Werner-Beland), 64
Group goals, 198–199. *See also* Small group communication

H

Handicapped infants, treating, 275
Hateful behavior, 10–11, 88
Health belief model of health communication, 13–15
Health communication
   defining, 3–4
   health belief model, 13–15
   King's interaction model, 15–17
   a model of, 17–21
      contexts, 19–21
      relationships, 17–18
      transactions, 19
      summary, 20–21
   therapeutic model, 12–13
   transactions, 19
Health Locus of Control (HLC) scale, 33
Health professional, defining a, 18. *See also* Professional-client relationships; Professional-professional relationships
Helping and coping, models of, 84–86
Hierarchical lines of authority, 39, 102
Hippocratic tradition and beneficence, 260–262

History-taking interviews, 166
Honesty and truth telling, 271–274
Honesty dimension of self-disclosure, 52
Hospice settings, 27, 273
Human communication
   closed communication patterns, 115–120
   defining, 2–3
   Leary's model, 10–11
   is multidimensional, 6–8
   Shannon-Weaver model, 8–9
   SMCR model, 9–10
   summary, 20–21
   transactional nature of, 5–6

I

Imitative behavior in small group communication, 213
Impersonal disconfirming responses, 63, 66, 70
Impervious disconfirming responses, 63, 66, 70
Incoherent disconfirming responses, 63
Incongruous disconfirming responses, 63
Individual goals, 198
Individualistic and collectivistic cultures, comparing, 289–291
Individual roles, 206
Infant Doe, Indiana case, 275
Information
   access to, 107–111
   control of, 32
   exchange process between providers/patients, 38
   intercultural communication and disclosure of, 298
   interviews and sharing, 165–167
   small group communication and imparting, 212
Informed consent, 266–271
Initiation phase in interview process, 172–175
Instillation of hope in small group communication, 211
Intensity in paralinguistics, 146
Intentional nonverbal communication, 130
Intention aspect of self-disclosure, 52

Intercultural communication, 285
 contexts in interpreting messages, 291–293
 defining, 286
 ethnocentrism, 286–288
 individualism vs. collectivism, 289–291
 nonverbal communication, 298–300
 perceptions and sociocultural backgrounds, 293–295
 prejudice, 288–289
 resources, culturally based, 304–306
 sensitive care, culturally, 301–304
 summary, 306–308
 transactional influence of culture on interpersonal relations, 300–301
 verbal processes, 295–298
Internal-External (I-E) scale, 32
Internal locus of control, 32, 33
Interpersonal communication, 4
Interpersonal learning in small group communication, 213
Interpersonal Reactivity Index, 25
Interpersonal trust, 43
Interpreters, 304
Interpreting messages
 content and relationship dimensions of messages, 7–8
 context and intercultural communication, 291–293
 interview process, 189–191
 nonverbal cues, 141
 words, differing meanings to common, 91–92
Interprofessional understanding, lack of, 97–100
Interruptive disconfirming responses, 63
Interview process
 blocking effective interviewing, 191
 defining the, 163–165
 exploration phase, 175–177
 information-sharing interviews, 165–167
 initiation phase, 172–175
 preparation phase, 170–172
 summary, 192–193
 techniques used to conduct interviews, 181
 clarification, 189

interpretation, 189–191
 questions, 181–183
 reflection, 186–188
 restatement, 185–186
 silence, 183–185
 termination phase, 177–179
 therapeutic interviews, 167–169
Intimate distance, 144
Intrapersonal communication, 4
Irrelevant disconfirming responses, 63, 66, 70
Isolation myth about nonverbal communication, 133

J
Japanese people and intercultural communication, 298
Jargon used by professionals, 90
Jourard's Self-Disclosure Questionnaire, 52
Justice, social, 264–266

K
Key to success myth about nonverbal communication, 133
Kinesic dimensions of nonverbal communication
 facial expressions, 136–139
 gaze, 139–141
 gestures, 135–136
King's interaction model of health communication, 15–17, 20–21
Korean-Americans and intercultural communication, 298

L
Laing, R. D., 61
Language barriers, 295–296
Latino cultures and empacho (folk illness), 302–303
Leadership and small group communication
 cohesion phase, 220
 conflict phase, 219
 defining, 202–203
 differing behaviors for different groups, 203–204
 orientation phase, 217
 termination phase, 220–221
 working phase, 220
Leary's model of human communication, 10–11, 20, 88

Life-support controversies, 275
Linear communication, 5, 8
Locus of control perspective, 32–33
Lose-lose approach to conflict, 241
Loving behavior, 10–11, 88

M
Maintenance roles, 205–206
Manifest behavior and Filley's model of conflict resolution, 239
Mass communication, 3–4
Meaning-attribution and leadership role, 203
Medical model of helping and coping, 84–85
Message perspective on self-disclosure, 50, 52
Metaphorical images and intercultural communication, 297
Mexican-Americans and intercultural communication, 297–299, 306
Midrange groups, 197
Mitchell vs. Robinson in 1960 (informed consent), 266
Modifying factors in health belief model of health communication, 15
Moral model of helping and coping, 84, 85
Multiculturalism. See Intercultural communication
Multidimensional communication, 6–8, 20
Multidimensional view of empathy, 25

N
Natanson vs. Kline in 1960 (informed consent), 266
Native Americans and intercultural communication, 294, 296–297
Neutrality vs. empathy, 48
Noise, negative impact of, 155–156
Noise in Shanon-Weaver model of human communication, 8, 9
Nondirective interviews, 169
Nonverbal communication, 127
 defining, 129–130
 environmental and physical factors, 153–157

Nonverbal communication
    (cont.)
    intercultural communication,
        298–300
    kinesic dimensions, 135–141
    myths about, 133–135
    paralinguistic dimensions, 146
    patients' attentiveness to, 128
    professionals' attentiveness
        to, 128–129
    proxemic dimensions,
        142–146
    purposes of, 130–133
    summary, 157–158
    touch, 146–153
Norms in group communica-
    tion, 199–201, 219–220
Nurse practitioners, 101
Nurses. *See also* Professional-
    client relationships;
    Professional-profes-
    sional relationships
    families working with, 107
    King's model of health com-
        munication, 16–17
    nonverbal communication,
        128
    preconceptions in therapeutic
        relationship, 171

O

Older adults and small group
    communication, 204
Open questions in interview
    process, 182–183
Organizational communication,
    4
Orientation phase and small
    group communication,
    215–217
Overt norms, 199

P

Pain and intercultural commu-
    nication, 299
Pain communicated through fa-
    cial cues, 138–139
Paralinguistic dimensions of
    nonverbal communica-
    tion, 146
Parallel relationships, 41
Paternalism, 262, 272
Patient care assistants (PCAs),
    252–253
Patient-controlled analgesia
    (PCA), 39

Patients. *See* Clients in health
    care settings; Family
    listings; Professional
    listings
Patient's Bill of Rights, 83
Perceptions
    of the environment, 154–155
    Filley's model of conflict reso-
        lution, 238
    health belief model of health
        communication,
        13–15
    King's model of health com-
        munication, 16
    sociocultural backgrounds
        and intercultural
        communication,
        293–295
    unshared meanings in profes-
        sional-client relation-
        ships, 89–92, 93
Performance appraisals, 166
Personal control, 30–33
Personal distance, 144
Personality theorists view of
    empathy, 24–25
Personal space and territoriality,
    142–143
Phatic communication, 173
Pitch height in paralinguistics,
    146
Positive feelings expressed as a
    confirming response,
    62, 70
Positive regard, 12
Power differences in profes-
    sional-client relation-
    ships, 87–89, 151–152,
    154
Preconceptions in professional-
    client relationships, 171
Prejudice, 288–289
Preparation phase in interview
    process, 170–172
President's Commission for the
    Study of Ethical Prob-
    lems in Medicine and
    Biomedical and Behav-
    ioral Research (1983),
    275
Preventive health activity, cues
    stimulating, 13–15
Principle-based approach to ethi-
    cal decision making, 277
Prisoner's Dilemma game, 42
Privacy fostering communica-
    tion, 55–56, 154
Privileged communication,
    107–109

Problem-oriented communica-
    tion, 47
Problem-solving, creative,
    242–243
Procedural conflict, 231–232
Process, communication as a dy-
    namic, 5–6, 20, 197
Process of Communication, The
    (Berlo), 9
Professional-client relationships,
    79. *See also* Clients in
    health care settings;
    Family-client relation-
    ships; Family-profes-
    sional relationships
    disconfirming communica-
        tion, cyclical process
        of, 69–70
    empathic communication,
        25–26
    information exchange process,
        38
    informed consent, 270
    interpersonal communication
        influencing, 4
    interpreting messages, 7–8
    nonverbal communication,
        128–129
    power differences, 87–89
    preconceptions, 171
    process, communication as a
        dynamic, 5
    responsibility conflicts, 83–87
    role uncertainty, 80–83
    self-disclosure, patients',
        56–57
    self-disclosure, reciprocal,
        58–59
    touching, 151
    trust issues, 44–48
    unshared meanings, 89–92, 93
Professional-professional rela-
    tionships
    autonomy struggles, 101–103
    confirmation, 68–71
    control issues, 39–41
    empathic communication,
        29–30
    interpersonal communication
        influencing, 4
    interpreting messages, 7–8
    interprofessional understand-
        ing, lack of, 97–100
    process, communication as a
        dynamic, 5
    role stress, 93–97
    self-disclosure, 60
    strategic *vs.* spontaneous com-
        munication, 47–49

symmetrical relationships, 34–35
touching, 151–152
Profile of Nonverbal Sensitivity (PONS), 141
Protectiveness of family members toward one another, 117
Provisionalism vs. certainty, 49
Proxemic dimensions of nonverbal communication, 142–146
Psychological distance, 155
Public communication, 4
Public distance, 145

Q

Questions in interview process, 181–183

R

Reality Shock (Kramer), 94
Reciprocal self-disclosure, 58–59
Reflection in interview process, 186–188
Reflexive model of human interaction, 10–11
Regulation of interaction and nonverbal communication, 130–131
Relational control, 31, 33–35, 41
Relational perspective on self-disclosure, 50–52
Relationship dimension of messages, 7–8, 33–34, 60
Relationships, health care. See also Professional-client relationships; Professional-professional relationships
  behavior of individuals in, 6
  conflict in, 232–235
  effectiveness of interpersonal communication influenced by, 7–8
  family-client relationships, 111–120
  family-professional relationships, 103–111
  health communication, a model of, 17–18
  nonverbal communications and maintaining, 132–133
  summary, 120–121
  touch enhancing/violating, 147–148, 151–152

Resolution of Conflict, The (Deutsch), 236
Resources, culturally based, 304–306
Responses to illness, confirmation and client, 65
Responsibility conflicts in professional-client relationships, 83–87
Restatement in interview process, 185–186
Restrictive norms, 200
Retrospective control, 32, 38–39
Rogerian therapeutic model, 12–13, 20, 23–24
Role(s)
  disruption of family member
    role ambiguity, 112–113
    role flexibility, 114–115
    role rigidity, 113–114
    underfunctioning/overfunctioning roles, 114
  interprofessional understanding, lack of, 97–100
  small group communication, 204
    assessment checklist, 207–208
    individual roles, 206
    maintenance roles, 205–206
    task roles, 205
  stress, 93
    role conflict, 94–95, 97
    role overload, 95–97
  uncertainty in professional-client relationships, 80–83
Rotter Interpersonal Trust Scale, 43

S

Scheduling and workload stressors, 95–97
Schloendorff vs. Society of New York Hospitals in 1914 (informed consent), 266
Seating arrangements, 157
Selection interviews, 166
Self-care, 86–87
Self-disclosure, 72
  applications in health care, 53
  client's perspective, 53–56
  conceptual frameworks of, 50–53
  defining, 49
  professional's perspective, 56–60
Self-help groups, 211

Self-image and nonverbal communication, 131–132
Sensitive care, culturally, 301–304
Shannon-Weaver model of human communication, 8–9, 20
Significant others, clients', 18. See also Family-patient relationships; Family-professional relationships
Silence in interview process, 183–185
Single meaning myth about nonverbal communication, 134–135
Small group communication
  change process, therapeutic factors crucial to, 211–215
  cohesiveness, 201–202, 219–220
  conflict phase, 217–219
  defining, 196
  goals, 198–199
  leader behavior, 202–204
  member behavior, 204–208
  networks existing among group members, 208–210
  norms, 199–201
  orientation phase, 215–217
  summary, 222
  termination phase, 220–221
  types of groups, 196–197
  working phase, 220
Small talk, 173
SMCR model of human communication, 9–10, 20
Social Construction of Reality, The (Berger & Luckman), 90
Social distance, 144–145
Socializing techniques in small group communication, 212–213
Social justice, 264–266
Social workers and role stress, 95
Sociocultural backgrounds. See also Intercultural communication
  perceptions, 293–295
  touch, reactions to, 149–150
Sociograms and small group communication, 209–210
Sounds in health care settings, 155–156
Source credibility, 42–43

South Africans and intercultural communication, 296, 297
Spontaneous communication, 47–48
Storming and small group communication, 217–219
Strategic communication, 47–48
Stress, role, 93–97
Strict paternalism, 272
Structural design of health care settings, 156–157
Subgrouping, 202
Submissive communicative behaviors, 10–11, 88
Substantive conflict, 232
Summarizing issues and accomplishments, 178
Superiority, communicating, 48
Supportive climates, 46–47, 173
Supportive response as a confirming response, 62, 67, 70
Survey interviews, 166
Symbolic language, 2–3
Symmetrical relationships, 34–35, 40
Sympathy contrasted with empathy, 24

T

Tangential disconfirming responses, 63, 70
Task groups, 197
Task roles, 205
Telephone interviews, 180
Termination phase and small group communication, 220–221
Termination phase in interview process, 177–179
Territoriality and personal space, 98–99, 142–143
Theory and Measurement Methodology of Interpersonal Communication (Leary), 10
◄ Theory For Nursing, A (King), 17
Therapeutic interviews directive, 167–169
nondirective interviews, 169

Therapeutic model of health communication, 12–13
Thompson's typology of control, 31–32
Touch
gender and receptivity to, 149
healing based on, 148–149
human development influenced by, 147
messages conveyed by types of, 150–151
relationships enhanced through, 147–148
sociocultural factors and reactions to, 149–150
variety of forms, 146–147
Transactional communication
conflict, 225–226
defining, 5–6, 19, 20
intercultural communication, 300–301
variables, communication, 23
Transparency myth about nonverbal communication, 133–134
Transparent Self, The (Jourard), 49
Trust, 71–72
applications in health care, 43–44
client's perspective, 44
conceptual frameworks of, 42–43
defining, 41
initiation phase in interview process, 173
professional's perspective, 44–49
Truth telling, four approaches to, 272–273
Two-person process, communication as a, 6

U

Uncertainty about roles and expectations, 83
Understanding and empathic process, 24
Unintentional nonverbal communication, 130

Unique persons, confirmation recognizing clients as, 64
Universality in small group communication, 211–212
Unmasking the Face (Ekman & Friesen), 137
Unmitigated honesty, 272
Unshared meanings, 89–92, 93

V

Valence aspect of self-disclosure, 52
Validation of verbal messages using nonverbal communication, 131
Variables in health care communication process
confirmation, 60–71
control, 30–41
empathy, 23–30
self-disclosure, 49–60
summary, 71–72
trust, 41–49
Verbal processes and intercultural communication, 295–298
Victims, people's reactions to, 54

W

Warm environments, 154
Weber vs. Stoney Brook Hospital in 1983 (treating handicapped infants), 275
Whose Life Is It Anyway? (Clark), 230, 234, 262
Wilkinson vs. Versey in 1972 (informed consent), 267
Win-lose strategy of conflict resolution, 239–241
Win-win strategies in conflict resolution, 241–243
Words, differing meanings to common, 91–92
Workload and scheduling stressors, 95–97